"The authors have succeeded in writing another masterpiece on Metacognitive Interpersonal Therapy (MIT). The book is a natural and well-written extension of its predecessors focusing on the therapeutic mechanisms of MIT with particular attention to the therapeutic relationship when treating individuals manifesting personality pathology and related symptoms. The authors master the balance between offering up-to-date theory and research while at the same time providing several, helpful case examples and concrete clinical techniques. This way, the book is of great interest to a wide audience of researchers and clinicians interested in MIT and experiential practices more broadly. I thoroughly recommend this!"

Majse Lind, *Ph.D., Department of Communication and Psychology, Aalborg University, Denmark*

"This book is a much needed addition to the literature on psychotherapy. This is an innovative, insightful, and sophisticated approach to the interpersonal issues involved in therapy that often can be used or misused in the therapeutic relationship. Both scholarly and practical, this book should be required reading for any therapist who wants to deepen the quality of the work that they do. There was much wisdom to be gained here. Bravo!"

Robert L. Leahy, *Ph.D., Director, American Institute for Cognitive Therapy, Past-President, Association for Behavioral and Cognitive Therapies*

"Wow. When I read this book, I could not help but wish I had written it myself. Integrative, pragmatic, and authentic, DiMaggio manages to strike a balance between the flexible humanity of classical psychodynamic therapeutic approaches with the precision and incisiveness of modern technically driven manualized therapies. Both imaginative and directive simultaneously, metacognitive interpersonal therapy (MIT) preserves the humanistic spirit of a psychotherapeutic intervention which aims to heal the burden of early and current adversities that all people face when their personality problems cause them to trip and fall, from time to time throughout their life trajectory."

Lois W. Choi-Kain, *M.D. M.Ed.*

Experiential Techniques in Metacognitive Interpersonal Therapy with Personality Disorders

This book provides a guide to using experiential techniques, such as imagery rescripting, chairwork, body work, and mindfulness in metacognitive interpersonal therapy to treat personality disorders and PTSD, along with their many comorbid conditions.

Psychotherapy for patients with personality disorders and their associated symptom disorders needs (1) a tailored case formulation, continuously updated and shared with the patient; (2) the use of experiential techniques to challenge embodied, automatic, hard-to-change interpersonal patterns; and (3) active attention to the therapeutic relationship. This book will help readers work along these dimensions, acting as a guide to constructing a client-first model of their own psychological functioning that can be used as a roadmap to change. It includes specific procedures for addressing problems in the therapeutic contract, devising and enacting imagery rescripting and other techniques, interrupting repetitive thinking, and so on. It also includes real case examples, with rich and detailed clinical exchanges for the procedures described.

This comprehensive text will help practicing clinicians of any orientation in working with patients suffering from personality disorders and their associated symptoms.

Giancarlo Dimaggio is editor-in-chief of the *Journal of Clinical Psychology: In Session*; senior associate editor for the *Journal of Psychotherapy Integration*; and associate editor for *Psychology and Psychotherapy: Theory, Research and Practice*. He is a co-founding member of the Center for Metacognitive Interpersonal Therapy.

Antonella Centonze is a clinical psychologist at the Center for Metacognitive Interpersonal Therapy.

Paolo Ottavi, psychologist and psychotherapist, is the main developer of two published treatments with empirical support: Metacognition Oriented Social Skills Training and Metacognitive-Interpersonal Based Mindfulness Training.

Raffaele Popolo is a co-founding member of the Center for Metacognitive Interpersonal Therapy, a trainer at the Società Italiana di Terapia Comportamentale e Cognitiva (SITCC), and a trainer of the psychotherapy school 'Studi Cognitivi'.

Experiential Techniques in Metacognitive Interpersonal Therapy with Personality Disorders

The Therapeutic Relationship

Giancarlo Dimaggio, Antonella Centonze, Paolo Ottavi and Raffaele Popolo

Routledge
Taylor & Francis Group

LONDON AND NEW YORK

Designed cover image: Getty Images

First published 2026
by Routledge
4 Park Square, Milton Park, Abingdon, Oxon OX14 4RN

and by Routledge
605 Third Avenue, New York, NY 10158

Routledge is an imprint of the Taylor & Francis Group, an informa business

© 2026 Giancarlo Dimaggio, Antonella Centonze, Paolo Ottavi and Raffaele Popolo

The right of Giancarlo Dimaggio, Antonella Centonze, Paolo Ottavi and Raffaele Popolo to be identified as authors of this work has been asserted in accordance with sections 77 and 78 of the Copyright, Designs and Patents Act 1988.

British Library Cataloguing-in-Publication Data
A catalogue record for this book is available from the British Library

ISBN: 978-1-032-94481-4 (hbk)
ISBN: 978-1-032-94480-7 (pbk)
ISBN: 978-1-003-57096-7 (ebk)

DOI: 10.4324/9781003570967

Typeset in Times New Roman
by Apex CoVantage, LLC

Contents

Preface

There are cautious, very cautious therapists. They use the concepts of connection, empathy, and validation with sensitivity. They listen to patients, welcome them, and gently accompany them along the painful path of the world. Only with much caution and care will they help them, they say, to change. These very cautious therapists usually claim that all therapies are equally effective. So they push little toward active change because, in the end, they believe they will still get optimal results. They have a protective attitude, which is, behind the mask, paternalistic and concerned. Parents who see their children as more fragile than they are imagine them in a dangerous, painful world. And so they keep them in a cocoon where the lashing wave of reality will not be able to hurt them.

There are active, very active therapists. Healthy and enthusiastic executors of techniques, they look forward to applying the short, intensive protocols they have studied. These very active therapists press their foot on the accelerator. They visualize the path to entering a world of less pain and push the patient in that direction. To hear them tell it, they take that path with the patient in a collaborative way, but it is clear that the real motivation is their need to be effective: "Cure fast, as the manual dictates." Often, however, patients have not made up their minds to follow them and dig in their heels. And so these very active therapists experience frustration, helplessness, guilt, shame, and anxiety. They push a little harder on the accelerator, and they hit the wall more painfully.

Cautious therapists draw on common factor theory and insist on the equivalence of psychotherapies: all manualized therapies work the same; the real driver of change is the quality of the therapeutic relationship and its ability to provide corrective emotional experiences in a validating, empathic climate. Easily guiding them is attachment theory; they want to be the secure base that the patient lacks. Another concept dear to *cautious* therapists is the *window of tolerance*. Stephen Porges' term says that if emotionality is too high or too low, patients are unable to attach meaning to what is happening in therapy and remember it. So, therapists pay extreme attention to the fact that the patient does not step outside that window, preventing or nipping states of dysregulation and dissociation in the bud. The concept of the window of tolerance is a fairly emblematic case of reinventing the wheel. That emotion plays tricks at the opposite poles of hypoarousal and hyperarousal has long been known to cognitive science and psychotherapists. The *cautious* therapist type is reticent to apply experiential techniques, which are too dangerous. And after all, if the main driver of change is the therapeutic alliance, why risk it?

Active therapists focus on techniques. They follow manualized, short, time-limited approaches and rely on empirically supported protocols, using the specific tools the manual demands, as these tools are the therapy. These are approaches aimed at reducing symptoms: obsessions and compulsions, rumination, anxiety, post-traumatic symptoms, eating disorders, and so on. For these therapists, the main drivers of change are adherence to the protocol and patient engagement in tasks, mainly exposure: exposure with response avoidance for compulsions, imagery exposure for anxiety disorders, use of eye movements or prolonged exposure for post-traumatic stress disorder, and attentional techniques and mindfulness for anxiety disorders. For many *active* therapists, the therapeutic relationship has marginal value. All it takes is a little attention to cooperative work, which actually consists of explaining the rationale to patients, inviting them to engage in the task without exerting undue pressure, and motivating them by explaining the cause-and-effect relationship between therapeutic work and possible positive outcomes.

Active therapists are skeptical about the importance of paying much attention to the relationship; they recognize its value, but they are unlikely to spend time discussing what is happening between themselves and patients. They recognize relational ruptures with difficulty and are not very skilled at repairing them. If therapy does not work, especially on the target symptom for which patients asked for help, they oscillate between blaming themselves for incompetence or patients for lack of commitment. Both reactions are most useful in further deteriorating the relationship and holding back progress that was already stalling.

Yet, there is ferment in the field. There seems to be a third type of therapist who dislikes the polarization: "It's almost all in the relationship" versus "It's almost all in the techniques." They are found mainly in the third wave of cognitive-behavioral therapies, in Gestalt, sensorimotor therapy, and EMDR. These therapists use active techniques aimed at change and exposure-based approaches extensively: guided imagery with rescripting, role-play, chairwork, behavioral experiments, and so on. They do this while paying attention to the therapeutic relationship, detecting alliance ruptures early and trying to repair them.

Metacognitive Interpersonal Therapy (MIT), as we formalized it in *Metacognitive Interpersonal Therapy: Body, Imagery and Change* (Dimaggio et al., 2020), fits squarely in the zeitgeist of the *experiential revolution* (Dimaggio, 2022). What was missing, however, was an accurate description of how MIT works immersed in reflection on the therapeutic relationship and its regulation. We needed to fill this gap.

Therapists ask themselves questions such as "What schemas are guiding that patient to construct me in a certain way?"; "Is a relational rupture taking place?"; "In what way am I reacting? Am I constructing the patient through the lens of my own schemas?"; "What can I do to repair that rupture?"; "Will I proceed with the technique or set aside the experiential work to focus on the relationship until it is repaired?"; "Am I hesitating too much to use a technique just because of my fears?"; "What impact has this imagery exercise had on the relationship? Can it be that the patient feels closer to me now that we passed together through so much?"

But what do we know about the role of experiential work? Is it safe and effective? Does it add effectiveness to talk-only psychotherapy? The answer is positive about safety and effectiveness, while it is too early to say with certainty that such approaches offer anything more. Our volume, in a sense, is an attempt to push the psychotherapeutic field in this direction: these approaches are safe, and it is possible that they will contribute to therapies that are more effective and faster, provided that they operate in a context of ongoing attention to the relationship.

The entire volume revolves around the following principles:

1. Every therapeutic action should be performed from an accurate, detailed case formulation shared with the patient and updated continuously.
2. Every therapeutic action should be carried out by monitoring the alliance. Therapists must make sure that patients have understood the treatment goals and explicitly share them. They must also make sure that patients have decided to commit themselves to working to achieve goals.
3. The experiential technique should be proposed after assessing the state of the alliance and its consistency with the case formulation. Therapists first assess whether patients have fully agreed to engage in that experiment, then make predictions about the potential impact of the technique: Will it push patients toward health? Or does it risk confirming their dysfunctional ideas about relationships?
4. From the moment therapists propose the use of a technique, they monitor the therapeutic relationship.

In summary, therapists have an eye on the relationship before, during, and after the experiential work. Sometimes, the technique has no impact on the relationship, and patients implement it in a cooperative atmosphere. In general, we hypothesize five patterns of relationship-technique interaction:

1. The very proposal to use a technique or the initiation of its execution generates a deep and prolonged rupture in the relationship, which therapists must attend to until it is repaired. Patients read the proposal in the light of their own schemas, or, more simply, the technique is not compatible with their preferences.
2. Patients initially accept the technique and practice it. However, during its execution, they experience negative effects that create a rupture in the relationship because they are inclined to fear that the therapist's intervention is only painful.
3. The proposal of the technique or its execution generates transient negative emotions and thoughts. At some moments, patients construct the therapist as, for example, harmful, critical, or dominant. However, patients can tolerate these negative reactions and thus agree to begin the experiential practice or to continue it until they discover its beneficial effects, at which point the rupture is followed by consolidation.

4. The experiential technique immediately reinforces the therapeutic relationship, either from the proposal itself or later during its execution. Patients are curious about experiential work, find it stimulating, understand that therapists are guided by a sincere interest in helping them overcome suffering and relational problems, and are grateful to have done active work to this end. Patients also sense the therapists' ability to remain present and well-regulated in the face of the emergence of painful emotions during experiential work.

5. The technique has a positive impact on the relationship because of the beneficial effects patients experience after having practiced it. Returning home after in-session exposure, they notice that symptoms are less disturbing and relationship problems are easier for them to deal with. Trust in the therapists increases.

To maximize the positive impact of the techniques on the relationship and, looked at from the other end, to reduce the risk of ruptures or to repair them more quickly, it is necessary that everything be executed from a solid and clear shared case formulation. In this volume, we will describe how to arrive at such a formulation and how to use it as a guide for experiential techniques. We will discuss in detail the therapeutic contract and how it should be continually updated based on the formulation and how patients respond to proposals to engage in experiential work. We will show a variety of techniques and how to use them in combination with each other. For example, during *imagery rescripting*, we can invite patients to work through their body to bring out the healthy parts and encourage schema rewriting.

We move in the context of the experiential revolution in psychotherapy, and we hope that our volume will give impetus to this way of practicing psychotherapy: a combination of activity, relational attunement, and a never-ending attention to building every step on a truly shared and continuously updated case formulation.

Chapter 1

Interactions between experiential techniques and the therapeutic relationship

A classification

Can we say that experiential work is effective and safe? Are approaches that adopt experiential techniques at least as safe as conversational ones? And are they more effective? Beyond the *conversation-only vs. experiential work* poles, there are now psychotherapies that pay attention to both poles.

To be clear, what do we mean by *experiential*? We refer to the part of the work on interpersonal patterns that does not just invite patients to narrate them and reason about them or observe them as they unfold in the therapy relationships. Rather, it is active work, which includes patients revisiting past episodes in the therapy room to the point that arousal mounts and then rewrites them. Some of the practices we use for this purpose are (a) guided imagery alone or with rescripting, (b) role-play, (c) chairwork, (d) working with the body, (e) mindfulness and attentional regulation techniques, and (f) behavioral experiments. We do not use experiential interventions focused solely on symptom reduction, such as exposure with response prevention, behavioral activation, or mindfulness. Our approach emphasizes modifying interpersonal schemas to promote lasting change.

Why use experiential techniques? Can't the same results be achieved through purely cognitive or relational work, that is, getting the patient to think differently until he or she changes patterns? Our answer is no. Treating patients with personality disorders (PD) or complex post-traumatic disorders involves rewriting dysfunctional interpersonal patterns; essentially, updating their system of predictions: "I suffer because I fear that when I show my vulnerability, the other will ignore me, humiliate me, neglect me"; "I suffer because when I seek resources and support to explore the world, the other will hinder me, paralyze me, not support me."

These are predictions based on memories and learned experiences. We know that memories are not just for remembering the past. They are maps of the world that we use to predict, as far as possible, the future (Solms, 2021). Therapeutic work is a rewriting of these world maps. The structure of the maps that guide patients' needs to change for memories to lose the power to drive action.

Studies on memory reconsolidation (Nader & Einarsson, 2010) explain a key part of therapeutic change. When a memory is reactivated and arousal increases, the memory is in a phase of instability. When altering its content in this phase, the actual rewriting and adjusting of the associated emotions allow the memory

DOI: 10.4324/9781003570967-1

to be re-embedded in a new format. However, it is necessary to first reactivate the memory before rewriting it. Techniques such as imagery rescripting, EMDR, role-play, and chairwork all share this characteristic. They evoke a scene from the past until negative arousal increases and the patient experiences the memory as if it were happening now. The instability phase begins. Writing alternative endings or adjusting emotions that were going out of control up to that point will cause that memory to return to "stock" modified! We open the *World Map* app and update it; the prediction system changes, and so does the attitude toward the future.

Is this way of promoting change safe and effective? Is it safer and more effective than other approaches? Does it have side effects? Is it suitable for everyone? Let the data speak.

The experiential techniques/reporting interface: empirical evidence

The therapeutic alliance is the most studied predictor of outcome, but its quality explains a very small part of the outcome, about 7% (Flückiger et al., 2018). It is clear that effective therapy requires many other components. A meta-analysis (Pascual-Leone & Yeryomenko, 2017) found that the depth of emotional experience in therapy, one of the key aspects of experiential work, predicts therapy outcomes. Deepening emotional experience is, therefore, part of successful therapy.

But let's get to the heart of the matter: are experiential techniques safe and effective? The answer is largely positive. The next question is do experiential techniques bring additional effectiveness over relationship work alone? We predict that in the future, the answer will be a definite yes, especially if clinicians work at the techniques-relationship interface. Our volume is an attempt to tip the needle in this direction.

Effectiveness and safety

The background here is often the division between *very cautious* and *very active* clinicians. To move the former, it is necessary to provide evidence for why using the techniques not only helps patients but also avoids causing unwanted effects: dysregulation, dissociation, and, ultimately, dropout. The most frequent phrase is, "If I offer her an exposure-based technique (e.g., guided imagery), she might drop out of the window of tolerance." To quell the latter's ardor, data on side effects and dropouts are necessary: what if their enthusiasm is counterproductive? In light of the available data, we will see that it is more necessary to encourage *cautious* therapists to move out of their safety zone and dare more.

In a meta-analysis, Morina and colleagues (2017) evaluated the effectiveness of imagery rescripting in a variety of disorders, mostly post-traumatic stress disorder (PTSD) and social anxiety disorder. In general, rescripting was effective compared with passive control groups but not when compared to other treatments. These were very short interventions, four to five sessions on average, making it difficult for the superiority of a therapy to emerge within such a short time frame. Romano and colleagues (Romano et al., 2020) considered patients with social anxiety disorder who had randomly received a single session of imagery rescripting, imaginal exposure without imagery rescripting, and supportive counseling. Well, only the two imagery interventions changed the nuclear self-representations related to social anxiety. Moreover, only the imagery interventions, and not the supportive counseling, facilitated the retrieval of positive memories. Overall, data from Morina and colleagues (2017) seem to indicate the potential efficacy of this technique, although the lack of data on dropout and adverse events leaves questions about its potential safety and tolerability.

Let us now examine the details of the various pathologies and see that the data about safety is really encouraging. The most significant studies are in PTSD, where experiential interventions are the most widely used, with established efficacy and safety data. In fact, current guidelines recommend exposure interventions as first-line treatment. Let's go into the specifics.

In one randomized control trial (RCT), two forms of Emotion Focused Therapy (EFT; Greenberg, 2002) were tested on patients with a history of childhood abuse trauma (Paivio et al., 2010). One was expository, involving imaginative confrontation with the abuser; the other was limited to empathic exploration of traumatic memories. Both approaches were effective, with a slight advantage for the imaginative exposure group and a slightly lower dropout rate for the arm focused on empathic exploration. This result re-iterates our point: exposure might increase efficacy while relationship might provide more stability and thus make therapy more tolerable. Another RCT (Markowitz et al., 2015) compared a *non-exposure therapy*, that is, interpersonal therapy, with prolonged exposure. We note that the alleged *non-exposure therapy* used role-play in session, and thus, we consider it an experiential therapy *de facto*. In any case, outcomes were similar for both arms, and the only minor differences were that prolonged exposure produced faster results while interpersonal therapy had slightly lower dropout rates.

Two RCTs brought significant data in favor of the efficacy and safety of exposure approaches. In the first, female patients with complex trauma received either exposure therapy, trauma-adapted dialectical-behavioral therapy (DBT), or cognitive therapy (Bohus et al., 2020). DBT showed less dropout (25% *vs* 39%) and better symptomatic response. Thus, exposing patients to memories of episodes, often characterized by sexual abuse, had no negative impact and actually increased efficacy. It's also important to note that great attention was paid to safety in the DBT arm; exposures began after about 20 sessions. The message is that once the appropriate climate is created, exposure is possible, necessary, and safe.

The second study (Boterhoven de Haan et al., 2020) compared imagery rescripting and EMDR in a population of adults with a history of childhood trauma, a sample with significant distress and relational problems, exactly the kind of patients with whom "cautious" therapists are wary of risking experiential practices. The two therapies were equally effective, and dropout rates were very low (7.7%), again indicating that they were appropriate and well tolerated.

Regarding safety, Tripp and colleagues (2020) explored whether treating patients with PTSD and alcohol abuse with exposure therapy exacerbated symptoms compared with non-exposure therapy. It did not. Symptomatic worsening during treatment was identical in the two groups. Is it better to avoid exposure in this population to avoid the risk of worsening? No, exposure is safe.

In cases of war trauma, *in vivo* re-immersion is obviously impossible, so how can we counteract avoidance tendencies? Rizzo and colleagues (2009) performed virtual reality exposure to create trauma scenes that were very similar and arousing. A meta-analysis (Deng et al., 2019) indicated that such a program was effective and generated no adverse effects. However, it was not shown whether it had superior efficacy to classic exposure interventions, and dropouts were high, as in traditional interventions. This finding brings us back to the other problem: exposure work alone may be insufficient if it is not accompanied by sustained attention to the therapeutic relationship and individualized case formulation.

Harned and colleagues (2021) compared two different forms of DBT on patients with PTSD: the classic one and one that included an exposure component. Patients were asked to express their preferences at the beginning of the study, and they preferred the one with the added exposure component. Dropout rates were the same in the two groups, around 25%: exposure did not make the treatment less tolerable. Safety was also good; no reported suicides and the rate of deterioration was equal in the two groups. Experiential DBT was more effective than the standard form for both PTSD symptoms and other variables.

In an RCT (Van Vliet et al., 2021), two groups of PTSD patients received either stabilization first and then EMDR or direct EMDR. The stabilization intervention was group-based and psychoeducational in nature, centered on the regulation of affects and interpersonal problems. Results were equivalent, both in terms of dropout (about 20%) and effectiveness. The results indicate that a well-designed intervention can be carried out directly and safely without the added caution of the stabilization phase.

The definitive word regarding the safety of expositional therapies for PTSD comes from a meta-analysis by Hoppen and colleagues (2022) on the risk of deterioration, adverse events, and serious adverse events of psychotherapies. The efficacy studies analyzed were overwhelmingly exposure-based in nature, mainly from the cognitive-behavioral family. The results left no doubt that interventions for PTSD were safe and effective, and adverse events, including serious life-threatening ones, were rare. Exposure interventions were as safe as non-exposure interventions. Until proven otherwise, this should be enough of a reminder that those who claim that experiential techniques are risky are speaking without empirical support. The real risk is in delaying the start of empirically supported treatment for the disorder! Not acting is more dangerous than acting.

Beyond PTSD, what do we know?

Let us begin with personality disorders (PD), which are the core target of MIT. Schema Therapy (Young et al., 2003) uses imagery rescripting and chairwork and is effective across the PD spectrum, both on symptoms and relational aspects, minimizing dropouts (Bamelis et al., 2014). Adverse events were not reported in published randomized trials. The study described earlier by Bohus and colleagues (2020) on DBT for PTSD in people with a history of abuse supports the use of experiential approaches for PD since an inclusion criterion was the presence of three or more criteria for borderline PD.

With regard to other pathologies, a meta-analysis (Kip et al., 2023) showed that imagery rescripting is as effective as other exposure treatments for anxiety, depression, and eating disorders. Significant data comes from a review of self-compassion interventions on pathological self-criticism (Wakelin et al., 2022). Compassion-focused therapy (CFT) belongs to the family of therapies we describe here: it pays attention to the therapeutic relationship and uses imagery, meditation, and role-play (Matos & Dimaggio, 2023). Overall, it was slightly more effective in reducing self-criticism than waiting list or *treatment as usual (TAU)*.

One experiential therapy, among the first to generate empirical data, is EFT (Greenberg, 2002), which incorporates chairwork. Patients reenact unresolved conflicts and problems and either turn to significant others, such as critical parents, or engage in dialogue among parts of themselves. In addition to the previously mentioned study on trauma, EFT was effective and tolerable in the treatment of depression (Watson et al., 2003), and initial results with eating disorders are emerging (Osoro et al., 2021).

Imagery rescripting is also finding application in eating disorders. These are preliminary studies with ultra-short interventions or where imagery is self-guided without therapist assistance, so their real clinical value is yet to be verified. One pilot study showed that a single session of cognitive restructuring or imagery rescripting was equivalent in reducing negative emotions and beliefs (Dugué et al., 2019). A second study (Zhou & Wade, 2021) illustrates, in our opinion, what happens if one uses exposure without taking into account the therapeutic relationship and the case formulation. The authors compared two groups with eating disorders in a pilot RCT: one received the usual treatment and the other the usual treatment with the addition of an imagery rescripting session at the end of the first week. The group with imagery rescripting experienced a slowdown in therapeutic progress. The finding is not surprising, and we stand by the words of a patient quoted in the article who noted how working in imagery on a past event "was like opening Pandora's box" and that she felt "unresolved" after the session. This is one of the reasons at the root of our book: it makes little sense to use experiential interventions outside the therapeutic relationship, and in a session with a therapist the patient will never see again!

In another study (Kadriu et al., 2022), women with sub-clinical eating disorders received three different types of interventions in the laboratory. They were asked to evoke either an autobiographical memory related to eating disorder themes or an intrusive image about the same problem. At that point, one group received imagery rescripting based on received autobiographical memories, one imagery rescripting based on intrusive images, and the third group focused on a generic positive memory. Overall, the imagery interventions were equally effective. The authors expected greater effectiveness in rescripting autobiographical memories, but this was not the case, and they were surprised by the 25% dropout rate. To us, the data are predictable: experiential interventions were used in the study for a short period and without attention to the therapeutic relationship. It is easy to assume that many patients experienced suffering in reenacting symptom-related scenes and, in the absence of a therapist, the task was too stressful.

Brand and colleagues (2021) used six sessions of trauma-focused imagery in patients with auditory hallucinations. The exposures began as early as session 2. Few of the patients who were offered the treatment accepted it. For those who started treatment, the effect on hallucinations was overall very good. Dropouts were in line with other treatments for the same disorder (25%). There were adverse events: 25% of patients experienced distress that they could not regulate. The feasibility of imaginal exposure in this population needed to be better investigated. Although efficacy was good, most people either refused to start treatment, dropped out, or experienced significant adverse events. It is possible that the problems in the research design were the following: a) this was a protocol in which exposures began in a predetermined manner in session 2, so there was no time to establish a solid relationship or to organize exposures based on case formulation; b) imaginal exposure was a classically behaviorally derived intervention based on the principle of stress habituation, rather than on meaning reattribution. This, on the one hand, may be too stressful for patients with auditory hallucinations and, on the other hand, does not provide them with the opportunity to understand and process personal meanings and relational fears related to hallucinations.

Overall, these preliminary studies summarize both poles of our argument well: experiential techniques are effective and safe, and the absence of relational work, at least in some pathologies, can generate stress, increased dropouts, and reduced efficacy. Yet the stabilization phase with attention to the therapeutic relationship is not necessarily helpful, as seen in the study where it was unnecessary to stabilize patients before starting with EMDR (Van Vliet et al., 2021). There is a clear need to explore the relationship between experiential techniques and the therapeutic relationship in more detail.

Experiential techniques and the therapeutic relationship: incremental effectiveness or alternative pathways?

Do techniques provide anything more than a therapy simply centered on dialogue, or even on common factors alone such as empathy and the therapeutic relationship? It clearly emerges that empathy alone serves little purpose. A meta-analysis (Elliott et al., 2023) showed that empathic mirroring interventions alone contributed almost nothing to progress. Duffy and colleagues (2023) showed that humanistic treatments, primarily based on empathic and relational aspects, were only slightly more effective than TAU for depression. At the end of therapy, outcomes were comparable to cognitive behavioral therapy (CBT) interventions. But at follow-up,

CBT was superior. In short, active treatment ingredients seem indispensable. But what do we know about the experiential elements?

Experiential elements seem to add power to treatment. The previously cited study by Harned and colleagues (2021) on DBT with an experiential component versus standard DBT showed that the experiential form was more effective. We re-iterate, neglecting the relational component is a problem: exposure interventions carried out prematurely and without attention to the relational element seem either to reduce the effectiveness of ongoing treatment or to cause adverse events. Our book seeks to address and, where appropriate, prevent these issues.

What do studies on psychotherapy processes convey about the interaction between techniques and relationships or their mutual role in making treatment effective? Research is in its nascent state. Stiegler and colleagues (2018) showed how anxiety and depression improved more after the use of the two-chair technique compared to the initial sessions that centered only on alliance building, empathic attunement, and other common factors. The most interesting work (Harrington et al., 2021) involves analyzing sessions of patients with a history of childhood abuse treated with trauma-adapted EFT, which uses the two-chair technique to encourage confrontation with internalized traumatizing figures. Which was found to be effective: relationship work or two-chair? Previous studies have shown that both experiential work and therapeutic alliance predict therapeutic change (Paivio et al., 2010; Pascual-Leone & Yeryomenko, 2017). What emerged here? Patients who already had good abilities to process emotions at the beginning of therapy, for example, described them in detail and reported pain congruently, did not need chairwork to improve. These patients did not need experiential work to do something they were already capable of. However, the study did not allow the authors to explain how it fostered change in patients who entered therapy with both good alliance and good ability to experience emotions. The authors suggested that in patients who started therapy with low alliance, the work should have aimed at repairing and consolidating it; in patients with emotional processing difficulties, the work should have aimed at increasing the ability to experience emotions. We add probably also to write different endings to painful stories after reenacting them. These are initial data; research on the psychotherapeutic process does not offer much more, but it is encouraging. The time is ripe to design treatment procedures that guide the clinician in moving between relationship and experiential techniques and lend themselves to empirical testing.

But what do we know about the empirical status of MIT?

MIT effectiveness: state of the art

Empirical evidence for MIT is growing. Early studies had been encouraging (Dimaggio et al., 2017; Gordon-King et al., 2018; Popolo et al., 2018, 2019), with good results and very low dropouts. Subsequent studies have confirmed the initial trends. In an RCT of MIT in group (MIT-G), all 20 patients in the MIT arm completed treatment, and MIT was more effective than TAU in terms of symptoms, interpersonal problems, and alexithymia (Popolo et al., 2022). MIT-G was tested in a pilot study in Spain with 10 patients (Inchausti et al., 2020). There was only one dropout, and patients improved in interpersonal problems, depression, metacognition, and impulsivity. We then adapted MIT to the treatment of eating disorders and tested the protocol through a pre-registered pilot trial (MIT-ED; Fioravanti et al., 2023), comparing it with CBT-E (Fairburn et al., 2003). Results were equivalent to CBT-E in terms of symptoms, but MIT-ED had fewer dropouts and more improvement in personality disorders (Fioravanti et al., submitted). A new single-arm pre-registered study of MIT-ED is underway, including underweight patients (Fioravanti et al., 2024).

MIT is being tested in adolescents. In a pilot study, a combination of CBT and MIT principles was compared against TAU. Patients in the MIT-informed arm had an 11% dropout rate against 23% for TAU, and they had larger symptom improvement (Marconi et al., 2023). In an RCT, Inchausti and colleagues (2024) delivered MIT in a group for adolescents with PD (MIT-GA) and tested it against a waiting list in a sample of 100 adolescents. MIT-GA included family meetings and the use of an app to facilitate homework. MIT-GA led to broad improvements in symptoms, social functioning, interpersonal problems, metacognition, and alexithymia (i.e., the ability to name one's emotions), and in most of these domains, it was more effective than the control group. The dropout rate in MIT-GA was 30%, which is considered relatively good. For example, it is comparable to the 26–27% obtained in a study on borderline PD based on individual treatment, which generally tends to have higher adherence rates (Schmeck et al., 2023). This rate is possibly better than the 39% associated with always applying individual therapy (Chanen et al., 2008), and surely better than the 57% of patients with borderline PD who dropped out prematurely from a group treatment of mentalization therapy (Beck et al., 2020). MIT has also been applied to early psychosis (Inchausti et al., 2023). In this study, 23 adolescent patients received up to 40 individual sessions accompanied by some meetings with family members. The dropout rate was very low, with 21 out of 23 patients completing treatment. The subjective sense of recovery increased, metacognition improved, and positive and negative symptoms as well as emotional distress diminished.

MIT has also been delivered in combination with other approaches. A single-arm study was conducted in Denmark on patients with avoidant PD (Simonsen et al., 2022) who received one and a half years of individual MIT plus mentalization-based therapy in group format. Of the 30 patients selected, six failed to start the group, and two dropped out again because of the group. None refused or discontinued individual MIT. Patients improved in various personality dimensions, such as the ability to feel pleasure and establish relationships and self-respect. Symptoms were largely reduced, and social functioning improved. Note that in this study, the therapists applied pre-experiential MIT (Dimaggio et al., 2015). MIT has been applied with good outcomes in two single case studies: a domestic violence perpetrator (Pasetto et al., 2021) and a schizotypal disorder (Cheli et al., 2019), both with good outcomes. In a case series for male domestic offenders, all three patients ceased acts of violence when receiving MIT and up to a 2-month follow-up (Pasetto et al., 2024).

The effectiveness of the combined in-group mentalization and individual MIT format on avoidant PD was also tested in a study in Norway (Wilberg et al., 2023). One of us (GD) supervised the MIT component even though the therapists had not received formal training. Twenty-two out of 28 patients completed therapy; this was a severe population with numerous failed treatments prior. Total symptoms of anxiety and depression were reduced, psychosocial functioning improved, and many patients returned to work or study at the end of therapy. The patients' ability to recognize emotions also improved, and various aspects of their personality pathology were reduced, although to a lesser extent than in the study by Simonsen and colleagues (2022). The authors noted that this may be because, in the Danish MIT study, it was applied more systematically and with more supervision.

A different manualization of MIT (Carcione et al., 2021) than ours was applied to BPD and tested in an RCT versus a control group receiving structured clinical management. The dropout rate in the MIT arm was 27%. MIT reduced emotional dysregulation, borderline disorder severity and symptoms, and improved metacognition; results largely overlapped with the control group (Rossi et al., 2023).

Overall, MIT as we manualized it (Dimaggio et al., 2015, 2020) is extremely well accepted by patients, and dropouts are very low. Significant changes in symptoms, social and interpersonal functioning, and, where measured, metacognition or alexithymia were observed in all studies.

A classification of patterns of interaction between techniques and relationship

The intertwining of experiential and relational work is important for various approaches (Matos & Dimaggio, 2023; Steindl et al., 2023). In EFT, a balance is sought between providing a safe relational context and helping patients experience and process intense and painful emotions (Goldman & Goldstein, 2023). In CFT, experiential work is essential, similar to MIT, and the therapist works on the relationship to remove blocks and fears of taking a self-compassionate stance that hinders it (Matos et al., 2023). In CBT therapy, focused on compassion, Leboeuf and Antoine (2023) described how applying imagery created relational ruptures that the therapist then repaired before returning to the use of imagery. Pugh and colleagues (2023) questioned the assumption that a good relationship is necessary to work experientially and proposed that sometimes it is experiential work such as chairwork that strengthens the relationship.

Systematic and formalized work was needed to describe how in MIT the active work to treat personality disorders and symptoms intertwines with the work on the therapeutic relationship. Above all, we needed to show how we use experiential work while being mindful about the therapeutic relationship. That is why we wrote this book. The literature review, summarized in this chapter, was the starting point. The mainstay of our work has been dismantling the misconception that experiential techniques are risky or deteriorate the therapeutic relationship. In light of the results, this is, in general, a false claim. At the same time, some studies have shown that the absence of relational work can contribute to dropout or treatment ineffectiveness.

Thus, the idea is that experiential techniques and therapeutic relationships interact in various ways that need to be described and categorized. In doing so, the therapist will have an easier time understanding what he or she will be up against, both in the positive and negative aspects, when proposing and implementing an experiential technique. At the same time, research on the therapeutic process aimed at understanding what happens when we propose, implement, and evaluate the consequences of a technique, both in terms of the effectiveness of the therapy and its impact on the relationship, becomes feasible. We then developed a classification of possible interactional patterns. The first major subdivision is between positive and negative effects. Therefore, experiential techniques can either cause a relational rupture or improve the quality of the relationship.

In reasoning about possible ruptures and improvements, we focus on the most operationalized element of the therapeutic relationship, namely, the alliance. The alliance has three components: bond quality, agreement on goals, and agreement on tasks (Bordin, 1979). On this basis, Safran and Muran (2000) distinguished alliance ruptures into *withdrawal* and *confrontation*.

The patient shows signs of withdrawal breakdown when, for example, he shuts down emotionally, remains silent, or responds dryly without articulating the discourse, arrives late, or changes the subject when relevant issues are addressed. Regarding techniques, he does not engage in homework or emotionally participate in experiential interventions in sessions even though he has formally accepted them.

The patient shows signs of confrontation breakdown when, for example, she criticizes the therapist or the rationale for therapy, responds with irony and sarcasm, and explicitly rejects techniques by questioning their usefulness or appropriateness. In contrast, when improvements occur, the patient may respond to the proposal to use a technique by showing verbal and non-verbal signals of curiosity, involvement, playfulness, confidence, hope, and feeling the therapist closer and encouraging at the same time.

From this distinction between the positive and negative effects of techniques on the relationship, we propose a taxonomy of five patterns of interaction between techniques and alliance.

1. The very proposal to use a technique or its initiation generates a deep and prolonged rupture in the relationship to which the therapist must pay attention until repaired.

    In this case, the patient already feels hurt by the suggestion to involve themselves in guided imagery, chairwork, or enact homework. For example, one may feel disrespected because he would like to continue talking about his problems instead of interrupting this to begin the two-chairwork. He might become angry because he imagines in advance that the therapist will force him to perform the technique and won't respect his possible refusal. He may be flushed with shame at the idea of starting a role-play, or he may become frightened at the idea of closing his eyes and reliving a painful scene.

In the face of these reactions, the therapist may, in turn, react problematically, contributing to an interpersonal cycle (Safran & Muran, 2000). An *interpersonal cycle is* when both components contribute to the deterioration of the relationship by reinforcing each other's negative attitudes. The therapist may feel guilty for causing pain, ashamed at the idea of having made a mistake, and worried about causing harm. On the other hand, she may feel frustrated because she judges the patient's reaction to be unmotivated and counterproductive. She may also become irritated or angry because she feels disrespected. If the therapist is not quickly aware of these internal signals and does not modulate them, the rupture is likely to extend. We suggest that, in such cases, the therapist should immediately give up continuing with the technique and move on, after modulating her reaction, to jointly reflect on the relationship. Only after repairing the relationship can she return to seeking avenues with the patient to further therapeutic progress.

2. The patient accepts the technique and prepares to practice or initiates it but experiences negative effects.

In this situation, painful memories or intrusive thoughts may surface that patients would tend to avoid and now cannot push away. They may experience unpleasant emotions associated either with the surfaced memories or related to the practice they are performing. Emotions or somatic sensations may also emerge in a nonintegrated way, whereby patients experience disturbing arousal for which they do not recognize the cause. These negative reactions can create a rupture because patients fear the therapist's intervention, consider it dangerous, or find the work simply too painful. Again, it is necessary for the therapist to stop the exercise and move on to regulate the patient's negative effects and reflect on what has happened until he or she feels that the therapeutic relationship is repaired.

3. The proposal of the technique or its execution generates negative emotions and thoughts that are transient and do not prevent one from continuing.

On some occasions, patients construct the therapist as harmful, critical, distant, or dominant. However, they tolerate these negative reactions and agree to begin and continue the experiential practice until they discover that the effects are positive and helpful. The therapist should not stop the process but rather notice any problems, explore them, and check that these patients are comfortable continuing. The therapist maintains an attitude of encouragement and trust. Very often, these momentary negative reactions flow unnoticed and emerge if the therapist asks patients how they feel after the exercise. During the practice, patients' perception of the therapist changes, and they come to see her as solid, supportive, validating, and able to stand by them even during an emotionally intense transition. We then witness the sequence: micro-fracture of the relationship, followed by consolidation.

4. The experiential technique immediately reinforces the therapeutic relationship, either from the proposal itself or during its execution.

This is an overlooked element. In our experience, it is common for patients to experience the proposed technique as something that promises efficacy and allows them to relive painful memories without being overwhelmed by them, to face relational scenes they feared were unmanageable with new confidence, and to experience painful emotions hoping to keep them under control. They may also be curious, transiting from the problematic mental state they were trapped in to a state of playfulness and surprise, in an attitude of discovery. It also happens that seeing the therapist solid, confident, and willing to enter painful scenes where intense affections will emerge is a welcome novelty to patients, especially if they come from histories of neglect or where reference figures have been preoccupied or fragile. Imagine one of the first sessions with a woman with a dependent PD who grew up with an anxious mother and an emotionally distant father. She comes into the session worried because of an argument with her partner; she has a fear of abandonment, and the argument has triggered a panic attack. She would like to be helped but fears that the therapist might scare her, like her mother, or be distant like her father. She describes the tension between the anxiety of abandonment and the fear that the therapist will react negatively. Instead, the therapist remains calm and proposes a body regulation exercise to calm the psychomotor agitation. Experiencing the therapist as firm, present, and purposeful in asking her to engage in active work surprises her and can serve as a corrective emotional experience (Alexander & French, 1946).

5. The technique generates benefits after the session, and this reinforces trust in the therapist.

Experiential techniques can also have a positive impact on the therapeutic relationship through this delayed mechanism, whereby patients discover that these techniques are effective in reducing symptoms and problems. This is a different case from the previous one. In the first part of the work, patients experience a level of relational alliance and trust that allows them to accept and perform a guided imagery or role-play. Patients might also accept it and carry it out while simultaneously maintaining a degree of skepticism and concern and may experience a degree of emotional pain during the exercise. However, at the end of the practice, or during the week that follows, they discover that thanks to the technique, they feel better, their symptoms have reduced, and they have dealt with relational situations in a new way. Thus, one of the known elements of the change process is realized: the effectiveness of the therapeutic intervention, in this case, its experiential component, improves the alliance. Finding that therapy works consolidates the bond.

In the remainder of this volume, we will keep this taxonomy as a guide for analyzing the therapeutic process in the clinical examples we will describe. We will proceed in the following chapters to provide the theoretical and procedural benchmarks for combining attention to the therapeutic relationship with the active use of a wide arc of experiential techniques.

We will begin with a description of how MIT understands both personality disorders and case formulation. We will make clear that an effective formulation needs to be shared. Next, we will describe intervention procedures and the use of techniques and intertwine them with work on the therapeutic relationship. We then describe how we work through the therapeutic relationship. Subsequent chapters get into the nitty-gritty of how technical and relational work are intertwined in each moment of treatment.

Throughout these passages, we will show how, to be effective, continuous and manic attention to the explicit renegotiation of goals and the constant reformulation of the therapeutic contract is necessary. We work at the level of automatic procedures and subconscious processes and attempt to promote changes that start with cognition and modify behavior patterns, as well as changes that modify somatic states and behavior patterns to modify cognitions about self and others. But, throughout this process, we always take care that therapists rely as little as possible on their own clinical intuition or instinctive assumptions about what the patient is thinking and feeling, or what the patient may benefit from or suffer from.

MIT works to take territories out of the realm of the implicit and unspoken and annex them to the lands of the explicit so that each step of change is based on decisions that the patient and therapist have visualized and chosen together.

Chapter 2

Personality psychopathology in metacognitive interpersonal therapy

Experiential techniques are exposure-based. We ask patients to face painful emotions and confront negative images of themselves that they often keep at bay. We ask them to immerse themselves in intense scenes, firstly to better understand their inner world and then to find a new way forward. Doing so requires attention to the therapeutic relationship, attention that, let us be clear, means neither caregiving nor protection.

The success of a technique rests on a pillar: the shared formulation of the patient's functioning. The technique can be successful and bring the desired benefits as long as clinicians predict how the patient will react right from the moment they propose a guided imagery or body intervention and are able to update that prediction based on the patient's response. In other words, therapy works from a precise and sharp formulation of the patient's functioning, especially when that formulation is shared.

To be effective, therapists need accurate and continually updated hypotheses about a) the wish, especially the healthy wish, that the patient would like to pursue, b) the maladaptive interpersonal patterns that drive the patient, and c) the protective mechanisms or coping strategies that the patients use that hinder their ability to fulfill their wishes. In addition, it is necessary that therapists ensure their hypotheses correspond to the model that patients have of their own minds. Indeed, it is the moment in the patients' minds, not the therapist's, that will actually enable or hinder the operations of change.

We are going to summarize personality disorder (PD) psychopathology, which remains our main target. Throughout the book, we will use the categorical classification of DSM-5 for PD, given the power that categories have to help clinicians visualize the main aspects of a person's malfunctioning. In the background, however, we are accompanied by the proposal to name PD *interpersonal disorders* (Wright et al., 2022). This proposal has three advantages: the first is that it puts the relational element, the most characteristic aspect of PD pathology, at the center of the diagnosis. The second advantage is that it starts from a model of human functioning (Pincus et al., 2020). According to this model, people suffer because they fail to realize basic motivations such as *agency*, which corresponds largely to the

DOI: 10.4324/9781003570967-2

social rank system, and *communion*, which covers many other motivations, such as attachment, caretaking, and group membership. The third point is that talking about "*interpersonal disorder*" helps in destigmatizing the condition, that is, to separate the person from his or her pathology. *Personality disorder*, on the other hand, even with all the attention we pay, suggests that the person as a whole is ill and dysfunctional. By saying, "That *person* has an *interpersonal disorder*," it is more intuitive we are not referring to the wholeness of his or her being.

We will now describe the nuclear elements of PD psychopathology that require more attention during treatment. Having these elements in mind helps in the fundamental operation: helping patients form a model of their own mind, including what they know and what they do not know about themselves, their ideas, emotions, reactions, and the degree of conviction they have in their appraisal of the social world.

Core elements of psychopathology

We will deal specifically with *narrative dysfunction*, some aspects of *metacognitive difficulties*, *maladaptive interpersonal schemas*, and various forms of *coping*, that is, the dysfunctional ways in which patients regulate emotional suffering and deal with the failure of their core wishes to be fulfilled.

Narrative dysfunction

The first element is a poor and abstract narrative. Patients struggle to narrate their experiences autobiographically and use semantic codes more frequently, which lead to broader generalizations and abstractions. This limits the therapist's ability to access the mental states that motivate dysfunctional actions and, at the same time, to recognize the healthy aspects, which can be easily obscured. In practice, if a man describes himself in terms of "I'm too shy, awkward, I don't know how to get out of it," the therapist has little power. If, on the other hand, he narrates a specific autobiographical episode, what may emerge is an impetus to act and expressions of hope and curiosity that he has not previously noticed and included in his self-image. Of course, the patient is always dominated by the core idea of self-as-inferior self and the other-as-spiteful other. However, the therapist has access to more specific negative cognitions and emotions and to the healthier parts of the self that can be brought to light.

The second type is the chaotic and disorganized narrative. In this case, a patient may also report autobiographical episodes, but the narrative is disordered; confused, exchanges that took place in different places and times are lumped together, and the patient opens parentheses upon parentheses that prevent the therapist from distinguishing the main thought themes from the secondary ones. In this second case, before intervening, the therapist will have to help the patient put the discourse in order, making the contents more intelligible.

Metacognitive difficulties

Patients with various pathologies have difficulty describing their internal world; that is, they have poor *metacognitive monitoring* (Semerari et al., 2003). Instead of naming specific emotions, they use generic expressions that describe most physical states or changes in arousal: tension, discomfort, annoyance, fatigue, and tiredness. Once they become aware of the emotions they experience and the ideas that guide them, a more complex step is to become aware of the cause-and-effect links between events, thoughts, emotions, and behaviors. This element, the *relationship between variables* (Carcione et al., 2010), is one that is most lacking in sessions. Patients, in fact, respond to triggers of which they are unaware and react by following automatisms that they do not know are driven by cognitions.

Patients are convinced that the causes of their suffering depend on external realities, especially on the way others treat them or on their being flawed in some way. They lack the awareness that the reasons why they suffer and act in ways that take them away from their goals lie in their predictions that their desires will meet an adverse fate. That is, they lack the awareness that they are driven by patterns, and this issue, in metacognitive language, is called poor *differentiation.*

Note that the concepts of monitoring and differentiation are distinct (Semerari et al., 2003). Monitoring refers to the ability to describe internal states in varying degrees of richness, articulation, and integration (Carcione et al., 2010). Differentiation indicates the ability to consider one's ideas about oneself, others, and the world as viewpoints, subjective perspectives, and assumptions, which may be plausible but not necessarily true. A sign of good monitoring is,

> When the girl didn't text me back, I thought I was a loser and I felt ashamed. I decided not to leave the house, because I would have to tell my friends about the rejection, and I didn't feel like putting up with their jokes.

Differentiation, on the other hand, requires the patient to add to the chain of thoughts, emotions, and behaviors. An example of differentiation is, "I realize that it is my idea that I am worthless that has resurfaced and once again I have taken it as the truth."

As we shall see in the intervention procedures, therapists often make this mistake: they exchange high levels of monitoring for the onset of differentiation. The result is that they work to promote change when patients are still fully convinced of their own pathogenic beliefs. Therapists think that an articulate description of the internal world is a sign of the patients' awareness that they are schema-driven. Patients, however, are only describing their own thought process but are being guided by a schema that they have no awareness of!

Helping patients improve their theory of mind and their capacity to see others from a decentered perspective is something that MIT does only after patients have begun to differentiate, that is, to consider their own schemas as schemas and not to still consider their ideas about themselves and others as mirroring the truth. Of the theory of mind, we are interested in the patients' describing, with some clarity, what the other person thinks and feels and formulating hypotheses about why he or she acts in a certain way. Again, beware: we are only interested to a certain extent in whether the description of the other's mind matches the truth. We do mind that the descriptions are reasonable and realistic and that the interpretations patients advance about why the other acted like that are plausible. But beyond the reality principle, for much of the treatment, we consider the other as a figure of the internal scenario: not the *real* other, but the *representation of the other*. Thus, we promote patients' ability to describe and articulate three-dimensional characters. Only in advanced therapy will we reflect on the patients' relationships with the, so to speak, *real* others.

The reason for this is that as long as patients do not differentiate, they are not describing flesh-and-blood people; they are simply telling stories woven around schemas. Descriptions of the unfaithful husband, the hypercritical wife, the apprehensive mother, and the distant father do not interest us because they are really like that. In reality, as therapists, we do not know. They interest us because patients include figures or characters with those characteristics in the discourse constantly, repetitively, and patients always relate to them in the same way: a way that paralyzes them and causes them suffering.

Consequently, we will guide patients to a more decentered perspective – that is, to understand that others have a view of the world that is not usually centered around us and that they see the world differently from us – only after they have distanced themselves from their own tendency to construct others in a schema-dependent way. Only then will it be possible to distinguish the other in the narrative – judgmental, abusive, critical, neglectful, controlling, and dominant – from the flesh-and-blood person the patient is talking about.

Mastery is a crucial component of the metacognitive system. It is the ability to use knowledge about mental states as nourishment for strategies aimed at regulating suffering, solving relational problems, and moving toward the realization of one's goals (Carcione et al., 2011). The trunk from which it branches is the sense of *agency over mental states*, without which there is no possible strategy. It consists of the idea that one can act on a problem, accompanied by the intention to take steps to that end and the embodied sense that this is possible (Dimaggio et al., 2009). The therapist must continually assess the presence of this intention; without agency, the therapy does not begin, and the session itself is not really operative.

Mastery has, therefore, two components: knowledge about mental states and planning. The former constitutes the information needed to devise problem-solving strategies and the pursuit of desires. Good mastery is characterized by its potential effectiveness. It is not necessary for a strategy to be metacognitively sophisticated; what matters is that it serves the purpose. A sign of health is the use of more complex, metacognitively articulated strategies when simple ones, which require minimal knowledge about mental states, fail.

Mastery strategies, then, are divided based on the increasing levels of mentalistic knowledge on which they feed. The yardstick for evaluating these strategies is whether they help persons reduce pain and increase their ability to successfully pursue their goals.

Patients with PD, eating disorders, post-traumatic disorders, psychosis, and numerous other conditions have a reduced repertoire of mastery strategies. When faced with pain and interpersonal difficulties, they adopt solutions that, instead of solving the problems, make things worse. We will address these problematic coping strategies later in this chapter. We now describe mastery strategies, but not systematically, as they have been analyzed extensively elsewhere (Carcione et al., 2011, 2021; Dimaggio et al., 2015, 2020).

The simplest of mastery strategies require minimal knowledge of the internal world: it is enough that, in addition to the necessary agency, the person describes an internal pain on which he or she intends to work. The patient can say, "I am tense, agitated, nervous, restless," and on that basis decide to do something. The strategy can be simple, the most basic being behavioral activation: "When I'm tense, or agitated, I get out of the house and take a walk or do some exercise because it calms me down." Deliberate avoidance also helps reduce tension or conflict: "You know, what's new? Let them have it! I just pull my head in and go watch the game."

People may seek out relationships for the sole purpose of interrupting a painful state of mind, without much articulation of either their own or others' internal worlds: "I'm down on my luck with work. I'll call a couple of friends to go to the pub because I know we'll have a laugh, and I'll feel fine afterwards."

The same strategies can be used with greater mentalistic awareness of the problem to be solved:

I feel like crap, incapable, a failure, I can't find a girl I like, who attracts me and in whom I don't find some flaw. If I stay home, I get into a crazy spiral and eventually risk getting drunk, better to call a friend to vent to.

Or,

I'm obsessing over what my lover is doing with his wife this weekend. If I keep this up, my jealousy and anger will mount and I'll end up losing control and storm him with text messages. I'd be better off putting on sweatpants and sneakers and going for a run in the park.

At higher levels of mastery, we find strategies in which articulated awareness of one's internal world and that of others is coupled with problem-solving strategies that can be either simple or socially refined. Let us look at an example in which an articulated self-understanding is coupled with a simple strategy:

I realize that when I receive a rejection, the usual way of thinking is activated. On the one hand, I am convinced that I am worthless, and I break down. At the same time, however, it gnaws at me because the criticism seems unfair, I get angry and mull it over. As a result, I get stuck. I have realized that in such cases,

I simply have to persist in what I do despite being in a bad mood, or else things will get worse.

In the following example, articulate understanding is coupled with a socially refined strategy:

My wife often accuses me of being untrustworthy and unfaithful because, in the past, I had an affair at a time when we had broken up. In those moments I, on the one hand, feel guilty and justify myself, and on the other hand, I react very badly and yell at her because the accusations are unfair, and I can't take it anymore. It really irritates me when she does that, and I often snap because it's exactly the same way my father treated me, with unfair and unfounded accusations. When I realize that my intense reactions stem from my past experiences, I tell my wife to stop because it hurts me, and I can't bear to continue the discussion. If she persists, I go for a walk, and I explain that it's not because of her, but it helps me. I know that after a while, she comes to realize there was nothing to worry about and is sorry for attacking me.

Maladaptive Interpersonal Schemas explained – hopefully – with clarity

The backbone of personality pathology is the interpersonal schema: we are consistent here with the idea that it is more helpful to speak of *interpersonal disorders* than personality disorders (Wright et al., 2022). Interpersonal schemas are systems of thoughts and emotions that individuals adopt to predict whether their wishes will be fulfilled (Luborsky & Crits-Christoph, 1990). For example, a patient wishes to be liked and hopes to be liked but fears that if he exposes his actions, he will face criticism. Any minimal hint of actual criticism, even if it is just imagined, confirms his core self-image of being inferior and incapable and makes the alternative image of being worthy and skilled, an idea that he harbors somewhere, even less credible.

Interpersonal schemas are systems of predictions, interpretations of the reasons underlying others' behaviors, and guidance to action (Leahy, 2019) that revolve around a set of goals we call evolutionarily selected *wishes*. We repeat: we do not offer a systematic treatment here; instead, we distill the main concepts to show their impact in the patients' lives and in the therapy room.

The motivations at the root of the schema

Human behavior has been shaped under environmental demands, and psychopathology can be understood through the lenses of an evolutionary analysis (Del Giudice, 2014). Humans need to know that certain motivations selected for the sake of survival, reproduction, and adaptation to the ecological niche will be, at least in part, satisfied, and if this does not happen, they experience suffering (Liotti &

Gilbert, 2011). These include attachment, social rank/competition, autonomy/exploration, group inclusion, caregiving, sexuality, and peer cooperation.

The wishes that are most likely to be found at the root of suffering in PD are attachment, social rank, autonomy/exploration, and group inclusion. People suffer when they fear that they will remain uncared for, devalued, blocked and limited, excluded, and rejected.

However, are sexuality, caregiving, and cooperation less important? They are fundamental, but they should attract less of a clinician's eye. The reason is that caregiving is a source of distress in itself only when persons motivated by caregiving find themselves caring for a loved one, usually a child or spouse, suffering from pain and problems that will not go away: illness, economic collapse, social problems. In these situations, the caregiving system activates, generating stress that does not shut down, and missing the one signal that would turn it off: when the other is okay again.

In all other cases, if patients bring the suffering of the other to the center of their discourse, they are driven not by healthy caregiving but by inverted attachment. In other words, they need to care for the caregiver, the very figure from whom they would like to receive care and attention. This is, therefore, a pathological form of caregiving that should not be encouraged at all; on the contrary, it is a particularly harmful coping mechanism.

What about sexuality? Certainly, if our sex life is not at least satisfying, if it is not rich and fulfilling, we suffer and may experience depression or anxiety. But if we talk about personality, the sexual system is less relevant in itself. The negative impact of sexual frustration is to provide information about the failure of other motivations. Simply put, patients with sexual dysfunctions or an unsatisfactory sex life are worried that because of their problem, others will abandon them – the frustration of attachment, judging them – the frustration of social rank, excluding them from the group – the frustration of belonging. When faced with a patient who brings a sexual problem, therefore, in addition to acting specifically, the therapist will turn attention to the other motivations because interpersonal schemas will revolve around the latter.

And then the cooperative system. Clinicians beware! Patients do not come to therapy because of failure to cooperate! The goal of cooperation is to achieve a joint end. We cooperate to feed ourselves, explore, defeat the opposing team, and defend ourselves from danger. Thus, the compromised goal is never cooperation per se. It is the joint goal that seems unattainable. From there, suffering arises.

Another more basic motivation, however, is very relevant in psychopathology: the search for security, also named threat detection or the precaution system (Cosmides & Tooby, 2013). It is an evolutionary drive that precedes attachment. In the face of environmental dangers, human and nonhuman, people react in known ways: *fight, flight, freeze,* and, indeed, search for care from others. Many patients tell episodes that seem to start from a failure in attachment, autonomy, or rank. But fear surfaces. In those cases, it is almost inevitable that at the root are stories in which they have experienced violence or threats that go beyond abandonment or humiliation. The emotion of fear must lead the clinician to search for memories that have to do with concrete dangers to the integrity of the body, such as physical violence, sexual abuse, threats, or states of neglect that put health at risk.

Therapists often make another common mistake, which is to think that patients are driven by the motivation "to be seen." Let us be clear: such motivation does not exist! It is a language, metacognitively poor, with which, unknowingly, patients refer to other frustrated motivations. "The other doesn't see that I am hungry" indicates a failure in attachment and in the regulation of homeostasis, which a good dish of Italian-style cooked pasta with tomato sauce is capable of satisfying. "The other does not see what I am worth," and it is here the rank system fails. "She does not see that I desire her" indicates that sexual drive is likely to remain unfulfilled. "He doesn't see that this trip is really important to me" indicates the worry that the exploratory system will remain unmet, that is, that we will not go on vacation. In short, when patients tell us that they suffer because the others do not see them, we must always ask, "What exactly do they not see about who you are and what you desire?"

There is a case where "not being seen" represents a primary failure: the inability to get the other person's attention. Some patients really suffer when others do not look at them, literally. Why is that look so important to them? The mind functions through connection with other minds – this is primary intersubjectivity (Trevarthen, 1987) – and if this is missed during development, the outcome is dissociation (Liotti, 2006).

The paradigmatic experiment that shows the consequences of failure to build relational contact through shared attention is the *still face experiment* (Trevarthen, 1979). In this experiment, when the child does not receive signals from the mother, and the mother remains inexpressive, the child experiences increasing stress to the point of shutdown, and consciousness is dulled. In this situation, the child's problem is in reality about not being seen and mirrored. The current problem is rooted in a historical frustration of intersubjective connection in patients who come from histories of abuse, violence, and neglect. Their caregivers were dramatically incapable of attunement. The outcome is usually severe psychopathology, such as dissociation, self-harm, substance use, and the like. In short, in the absence of such histories and their psychopathological manifestations, to say that patients suffer because they do not feel seen is a mistake.

Let us now look at the structure of maladaptive interpersonal schemas. It is, we repeat, a system of predictions about the fate of wishes in the relational world, and it is also a guide to action. In its healthy aspect, an interpersonal schema is a quick and indispensable tool that helps us assess how others will respond in the face of our drives, plans, and projects. Based on these predictions, people develop maps for action that will help them make quick decisions, navigate the complexity of the social world, guided by quick strategies whose effects will, to some extent, be predictable.

Let's take an example. Driven by a desire to explore, I ask my parents for a ride to a party, confident that despite some protest about the return time, they will eventually offer it to me. The script requires that the request be made calmly and with humility, to avoid any adverse reactions, predictable by the way, of rebuke and, at the extreme, rejection.

In PD, the patterns predict that the desire will remain unfulfilled. The reason is that at their root lies a negative self-image believed to be almost completely true. If I desire appreciation, I start out guided by an affectively charged nuclear image, coupled with somatic sensations, of myself as inferior and inadequate. This image is coupled with an image of the other as critical and contemptuous. It goes without saying that if I think of myself as inferior in the face of a contemptuous other, the hope of hearing my dear ones say, "well done" on the day of the dance recital or exam is minimal.

In addition to predicting, patterns guide the reading of the other person's intentions (Leahy, 2019): if he openly criticizes me, then he is definitely criticizing me; so far, nothing surprising. But if he has a neutral expression or he delays expressing his opinion, I automatically assume he is still criticizing me. This is evident, for example, in borderline PD, which reads hostility in neutral faces (Seitz et al., 2021). Note that the schema-dependent nature of actions is evident in another study, also on borderline PD (Bertsch et al., 2022): patients read hostility in neutral facial expressions. Further, they tended to attack and not back away. Schema-dependent reading of the event and action tendency go together.

Another example comes from patients in remission from depression who are slower than a healthy control group to detach attention from facial expressions of disgust. It is a sign that they have a schema-driven bias that captures their attention and keeps it tied to the other person's face when it indicates that they are disgusting (von Koch et al., 2023).

Patterns guide action in automatic, quick, and dysfunctional ways. If I hope to be liked but believe I am worthless and imagine that the others will regard me as poor, my actions will be hesitant, clumsy, and awkward.

We summarize the elements of the schema in our formulation, which is an elaboration of the Core Conflictual Relationship Theme (Luborsky & Crits-Christoph, 1990).

The wish corresponds to one of the interpersonal motivations, usually one among attachment, rank, autonomy/exploration, and group inclusion. If patients express fear, explore the possibility that the schema revolves around the safety/threat detection system.

• *Nuclear representations of self.* These are the patients' ideas of themselves, and it is important to pay attention to them. As we will discuss later, to bring these ideas to the surface, explicit questions must be asked about the patient's cognition about the self: "What do you think of yourself now that the other person has answered you this way?" There are at least two images: negative and positive. For example, in the rank system, we will look for ideas such as inferior/valid. In the exploratory system, active-free/paralyzed-constrained.

- *Adaptive "if . . . then . . ." procedure.* These are the actions that the person plans to elicit the other's hoped-for response. Frequently, the therapist confuses these actions with other procedures, again of the *if-then* type that characterizes coping. Instead, these actions are distinct. Those designed to elicit the other's hoped-for response are functional and almost never surface; the therapist needs to elicit and construct them. Some examples are given here:

  - **Attachment**: "I need care. *If* I show that I am sick, *then I* hope the other person will take care of me."
  - **Social rank**: "I did my homework diligently. *If* I tell my father, *then* he will realize that I am responsible" (not to be confused with a perfectionist procedure).
  - **Exploration and group inclusion**: "My friend is holding a wonderful party, but it is far from home. *If I* ask my parents nicely, *then they will either* give me a ride there and back or arrange for other parents to share the jouneys."

As you may have noticed, these procedures include a realistic aspect. It is not a matter of "if I ask, then I get." We have described actions based on learnings of relational procedures that have the power to elicit realistic satisfactory responses.

- *Other's responses.* As with nuclear representations of self, the other's responses can be multiple. The dominant response in PD is naturally negative. Alongside the negative, however, patients harbor hope that a different, more benevolent response will emerge. Here are some examples:

  - **Attachment**: "If I ask for care, my mother neglects me or gets angry or tells me I am a nuisance and have ruined her life." The other neglects, criticizes, or suffers.
  - **Social rank**: "If I tell my parents that I got a B they will say I'm not trying hard, I haven't done enough, and my life will be a failure." The other criticizes, despises.
  - **Autonomy/exploration**:

If I tell my parents that I want to take electric guitar lessons, they will tell me that it's nonsense and useless, and that I have my head in the clouds, so no chance they will buy me a guitar.

The other inhibits, offers no support, hinders.

To be clear, the other's response is a contingency, something that happens within the autobiographical memory. The others' responses, however, appearing in similar ways in multiple episodes and in the therapeutic relationship, allow for the distillation of the *representation of the other*, that is, how the patient constructs the others in a schema-driven way. Thus, it is not the description of a real person but the construction of an internalized figure. Remember that the other can also be the person himself. What does this mean? Let's think of when, while ruminating or simply during his own inner speech, the person criticizes himself. Here, he is applying an interpersonal pattern! Simply put, in place of the other is a part of the self. So, if a young man with avoidant PD says, "I think I am worthless, I am a jerk," the pattern is, "I wish to be liked, but if I show what I do, the other (internalized) person thinks I am a jerk."

The responses of the self to the responses of the other

Here, we find information that will allow us to access the person's core self-image in the narratives. When the patient has decided that the other has reacted in a certain way, usually negatively, a sequence of cognitions, affects, behaviors, and somatic reactions begins. The other's response acts as the A of a cognitive therapy antecedents-beliefs-consequences (ABC). Thus, in the response of the self, we will have to look for cognition (B) and emotions and behaviors, along with bodily reactions (C). Again, beware: cognition is not of the "the other thinks that" type; this is still part of the other's response. Cognition must be an idea about oneself and must be investigated explicitly through questions that elicit the dimension of, precisely, beliefs.

A valid cognition sounds like, "If the other person criticizes me, they are right; I deserve it," which is a plausible antecedent of emotions such as shame or sadness. The cognition may also be different: "The other has criticized me unfairly!" which is a likely antecedent of anger. By carefully exploring these cognitions and emotions, clinicians will be able to identify multiple self-representations emerging in parallel. In the face of the critical other, the patient may indeed oscillate between "She is right, and I am ashamed" and "She is wrong, he is unfair, and I am angry." The nuclear representations, consequently, are *inferior* in the former case and *valid but mistreated* in the latter.

It is also important to explore the somatic component: what level of arousal did the patient have in the episode? What somatic sensations are associated with core cognitions about self and emotions? The therapist may ask "You think you are inept and feel ashamed. Well, in what parts of the body do you feel these ideas and emotions are located?" Figure 2.1 shows the structure of maladaptive interpersonal schemas. The example revolves around the social rank motivation.

The schema is a dynamic structure, which is set up as a relational test (Figure 2.2), following the principles expressed by Control Mastery Theory (Gazzillo, 2023; Weiss, 1993). We describe the steps of the testing process in a way that, hopefully, helps clinicians share their understanding of the schema with the patients.

The starting point is, we repeat, the wish. Usually, motivations are turned on by environmental triggers. A motivation is, by definition, healthy; the beginning of the dynamic is still outside psychopathology. The person now faces a dilemma: with respect to that motivation, she has at least two nuclear images of herself, one negative and one positive, with the former having more power in the case of PD. The negative image is believed to be true, surfacing to consciousness more quickly, and generates bias in reading the others' intentions. The positive image is in the

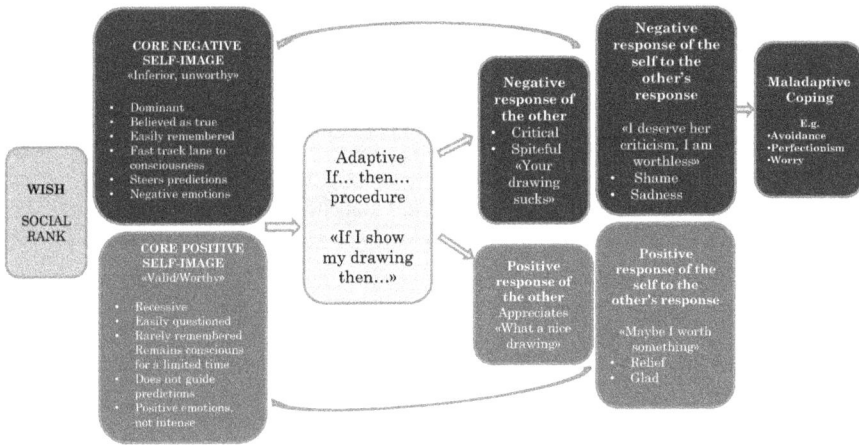

Figure 2.1 The maladaptive interpersonal schema

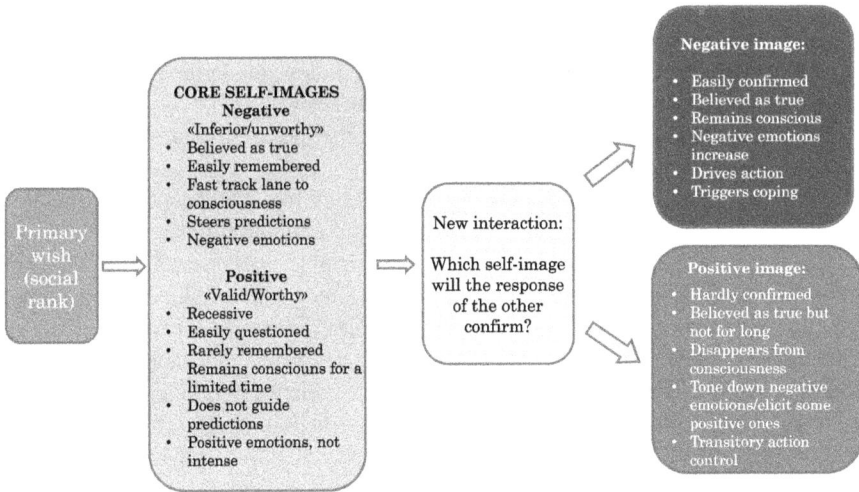

Figure 2.2 Schemas as relational tests

background; without it, the person would be hopeless. Faced with the activation of motivation, she would give up before even exposing herself to the other's response.

At this point, a relational test begins (Figure 2.2). The person exposes the request to the other in reality or, anticipatively, in fantasy. She now assesses whether the other will respond negatively, as she fears, or positively, as she hopes in her heart, even if she believes it little.

When, by a series of signals from the other, or attributional bias, or simply after an internal decision process, the person determines that the response is negative, the test fails. At that point, the negative nuclear self-image is confirmed, and a series of thoughts, emotions, and somatic states surface. Here is the self's response to the other's response! In this cognitive-affective-somatic process lies the material that will allow the patient's nuclear self-image to be inferred. When the patient responds to the other in reality, she is reacting contingently: "He criticized me, I am ashamed, and I shut down." But upon the recurrence of similar responses in various episodes, we find that the response of the self is only the confirmation of something the person believed beforehand, namely the core idea of self: "He criticized me, and he is right; I am worthless, I am ashamed, and I shut down."

The transition to coping and the secondary schema

The cascade of thoughts, emotions, and somatic states that constitute the self's response to the other's response sets in motion a series of reactions. These serve two purposes: a) to attempt to elicit a different response from the other once the initial request "Appreciate me, take care of me, accept me into the group, support me when I explore the environment" has been frustrated; b) to regulate the pain associated with the nuclear self-image and related emotions. In both cases, these activate maladaptive coping strategies that we will describe in the next section.

We focus here only on one type of reaction: the activation of a secondary schema that we call, precisely, *coping schema*. Usually, the therapist notices only this and neglects the schema that arose from a primary, healthy wish. As we described in *Body, Imagery and Change* (Dimaggio et al., 2020), the secondary or coping schema can arise from the same wish or start from a different wish.

To illustrate, here is an example where the primary wish was social rank: the patient wished to be appreciated by the gym teacher for how she performed a figure, but the response was dismissive. This, in turn, generated a response such as, "She is right; I am sloppy and this makes me feel ashamed." The confirmed nuclear image is *incapable* and *inferior*. At this point, the patient can remain in the domain of social rank and activate a secondary perfectionistic schema. The wish is then always to be liked. The "if . . . then . . ." coping procedure is "If I try my hardest and don't make any mistakes, maybe then the teacher will appreciate me." Usually, the other's response remains dismissive, which leads to the crystallization of the nuclear self-image.

Let us repeat: to avoid errors in the case formulation, usually this "if . . . then . . ." procedure is the one that most easily surfaces in narratives and clinicians mistake it for the initial "if . . . then . . ." procedure, which is healthy and adaptive. Here, a secondary "if . . . then . . ." procedure is activated after the primary wish has been frustrated. This secondary procedure is, by definition, maladaptive. Why?

Let us assume that the other's response is positive: that the teacher offers a half-smile of appreciation or at least no criticism in the face of the perfectionist efforts of the child in our example. What is the effect? The child's nuclear self-image remains negative: "I remain inadequate at the core, but if I don't make any mistakes, if I become perfect, at least I will get some appreciation." When the patient fulfills the secondary coping schema, she accepts that the primary wish cannot be fulfilled, or at least not in a healthy way. This child will no longer believe that she will receive a benevolent smile when she plays, jokes, or studies with a sustainable degree of effort. She will learn that to gain some form of acceptance and secure the closeness of the other requires titanic efforts.

We focus now on a very harmful element: dysfunctional strategies for regulating painful emotions associated with contact with negative nuclear self-concepts.

Coping

The contents of maladaptive schemas tell us *what causes* the patients to suffer and what issues lead them to see themselves and the world as a source of frustration and pain. However, the suffering and problems that arise at the time a schema is activated are not intended to remain in consciousness for long. A substantial part related to the maintenance of personality and symptomatic disorders can be attributed to the ways in which people react to suffering.

We call *coping* (Carver et al., 1989; Lazarus & Folkman, 1984) the set of responses to psychic pain, the effect of which is a worsening or maintenance of problems; by definition, we refer to *dysfunctional responses*, with a vast body of literature noting they are strongly related to psychopathology (Zimmer-Gembeck & Skinner, 2016).

Coping takes various forms. Some are reactive, almost immediate behaviors. Others, however, are chains of responses to emotional distress, sequences of cognitions, emotions, and behaviors that unfold over a time interval, ranging from short to wide. The repertoire of coping strategies is vast (Skinner et al., 2003), and we do not draw up an exhaustive catalog here. For orientation, we will subdivide the many strategies into classes, categories, and types in the next section.

Behavioral vs. cognitive-attentive strategies

Procrastination, binge eating, drinking alcohol, smoking cannabis, verbal aggression, writing rancorous comments on social media, and working to exhaustion belong to the class of behavioral coping. A typical example is perfectionism (Dimaggio et al., 2018; Hewitt et al., 2017). Other relevant coping strategies include obsessive rituals, self-injurious acts, compulsive seduction and sexuality, video gaming, gambling, and so on. Forms of behavioral coping vary according to context, culture, and what is available (Moos, 2002; Skinner et al., 2003).

Cognitive-attentive strategies instead take on limited and recognizable modalities. They are transdiagnostic, thus requiring treatment across all forms of psychopathology (Kaplan et al., 2018). Research has highlighted that dysfunctional cognitive processes such as repetitive thinking play a central role in the maintenance of a variety of symptoms and syndromes (Ehring & Watkins, 2008; Wahl et al., 2019). Recent evidence noted how repetitive thinking is present across all cluster B PD, for example, borderline and narcissism (Kelley et al., 2024).

We briefly describe the ones that are most frequent and most damaging in PDs. First is rumination, an iterative and inconclusive mechanism of reevaluating past episodes or the subject's current condition. The effect of rumination is always the same: mood deterioration. The best-known form is *depressive rumination* (Nolen-Hoeksema, 2000), in which persons negatively reevaluate their current condition; for example, they grieve for not having been able to find a stable partner. *Angry rumination* is common (Sukhodolsky et al., 2001), where individuals think back to episodes in which they were subjugated, humiliated, or suffered injustice. They now try to write in their mind a different ending, imagining getting revenge or retaliating brilliantly by defeating the opponent. Frequent is *counterfactual rumination* (Broomhall et al., 2017) with themes of guilt, in which persons imagine actions they could have taken to change past situations that, in their mind, have caused harm to others. One patient often went back to the day he chose the clinic where his father was hospitalized and then died; he fantasized about choosing another clinic where he would have been saved. *Self-critical* rumination is very frequent (Ehret et al., 2015): that is, thinking back on one's qualities and actions in a negative way without restraint. This is a process that feeds shame, guilt, and anger toward oneself and promotes depression.

Another type of perseverative thinking is *worrying*. Unlike rumination, which easily fuels depression and anger, worrying tends to fuel anxiety. It is a constant preoccupation focused on situations whose outcome is uncertain (Sibrava & Borkovec, 2006). Interpersonal worry leads to constantly anticipating the worst outcome of a relationship in mind: one patient with dependent PD worried about every autonomous action of her partner and every conflict they experienced; to her, they were all premonitory signs of impending abandonment.

Less mentioned in the literature is *desire thinking* (Caselli & Spada, 2015). It consists of focusing on a dreamed relational scenario while doing something else. It is a thought that tends to result in two negative consequences: a) it deflects mood because persons lose touch with the fulfilling aspects they are experiencing in the here and now, while focusing on what they want but do not have at the moment; b) they believe that only by getting what they want will their suffering end and they will be happy. Thus, it activates the urgency to act without evaluating the consequences on oneself and the other person. One patient had just ended a love affair. At every moment when she found herself feeling better, she engaged in desire thinking. She fantasized about how good it would be to be there with her ex. At that point, a mixture of longing, jealousy, and anxiety increased to the point where she would send him a message. He would not respond, and she would get sad, losing touch with the positive emotions she was previously experiencing.

The cognitive and attentional processes we have described so far are all perseverative and repetitive. They often alternate with a different, non-perseverative strategy, namely *cognitive avoidance* (Sagui-Henson, 2017), in its various forms: distraction, denial, and thought suppression. Cognitive avoidance also maintains psychopathology and social dysfunction; trying to suppress an unwelcome thought makes it appear more frequently in consciousness (Wegner & Erber, 1992). Avoiding thinking about a feared event, for example, delivering a speech at a business meeting, leads to forgetting the reasons why we fear the event. As a result, emotional arousal remains high, and, at the same time, we no longer know what cognitions to work on to deal with the problem effectively. In summary, patients engaged in avoidance may say "I don't know, I got distracted, time passed, and I didn't do anything." However, the actual cognitive-affective process was "I was afraid of being judged, and I tried not to think about it because, at the mere idea, I felt unable to cope with it and ashamed," but they no longer recognize this process.

Coping and arousal: diverting attention from suffering

All coping aims to reduce suffering. Some strategies are aimed at toning it down, for example, binge eating, vomiting, and especially avoidance. Other strategies increase arousal, for example, extreme, dangerous behaviors, risky sports, and so on. Some strategies are then aimed at experiencing pleasurable states and succeed in short-term pain reduction: alcohol and substance use, behavioral addictions, gambling, video gaming, and pornography. Some behavioral strategies may have mixed effects on arousal; for example, self-harm may either reduce distress or exit from dissociation through an increase in pain.

Coping and arousal: focusing attention on the problem

Other strategies start from the need to reduce suffering and do so but pay more attention to the possible reasons underlying a problem, with the result of escalating suffering. The main ones are the various forms of repetitive thinking we have illustrated above, such as rumination, worry, desire thinking, and threat monitoring.

Interpersonal Repetitive Thinking

We now turn to the relational component of cognitive-attentive strategies, and for the rest of this volume, we will call these strategies Interpersonal Repetitive Thinking (IRT). The main characteristics of IRT are a) it arises in response to present or feared painful mental states; b) it is voluntary, although adopted with varying degrees of awareness; c) it is goal-driven, for example: reducing suffering, reassurance, or controlling events – and is sustained by specific beliefs (Nordahl et al., 2022); d) it is applied repetitively; and e) it focuses on interpersonal relationships. People adopt it because, guided by maladaptive interpersonal patterns, they expect the other person to criticize them, abandon them, attack them, humiliate them, betray them, and so on.

IRT has various negative effects: a) it increases negative emotions; b) it slows down or blocks healthy and effective behaviors (those who ruminate or worry tend to take less action and do not implement effective problem-solving strategies); c) it reinforces the negative nuclear images about themselves and others; d) it paves the way to behavioral coping, which then deteriorates the quality of interpersonal relationships. For example, the person first thinks incessantly about being wronged and then takes action: offends, provokes, controls, and inquires until the other person reacts badly, thus confirming the original negative prediction.

What are the maintenance factors of IRT? First, some typical beliefs, *meta-beliefs* (Wells, 2009). *Positive meta-beliefs* motivate repetitive thinking or paying attention to certain stimuli such as relational threats: "I can only stop suffering if I understand for sure why my partner left me"; "If I scan the environment carefully, I reduce the risk of being humiliated." *Negative meta-beliefs* concern the uncontrollability of IRT: "I always tend to think my partner is insincere; he says he loves me, but in reality, he is having an affair with someone. I can't control this thought; it settles in my mind and doesn't go away." Driven by this meta-belief, the patient does not even try to stop worrying.

Poor metacognition, particularly poor awareness of the connections between thoughts and emotions, maintains IRT. Patients are not aware of how perseverative thinking and attentional strategies fuel emotional distress and thus underestimate how important it is to try to interrupt them.

Given that both activating and deactivating strategies are goal-driven, for example, reducing suffering or preventing future risks, when we invite our patients to let them go, we are asking them to pay a price: they may transiently experience pain and take risks. We will see how to address this issue in chapters 8 and 13.

Coping in case formulation

A key issue in case formulation is to distinguish suffering produced directly by the activation of maladaptive patterns from suffering resulting from coping. Psychological suffering has three different moments. Let us imagine a patient with borderline PD and bulimia nervosa. She suffers at three levels.

The first is congruous and contextual: her partner neglects her, and it is normal for her to feel hurt. Here, the clinician performs *validation* and *normalization* operations.

The second level is schema-dependent: the patient sees herself as unlovable in the eyes of a distant, critical other and feels ashamed because she believes the reason for the abandonment is her inadequacy. In parallel, a part of her feels that being neglected is unfair and becomes angry, experiencing further distress. This suffering, therefore, goes beyond the plane of reality; it is related more to the activation of the schema.

The third level of suffering depends on coping: our patient activates a chain of IRT – ruminates oscillating between a sense of nuclear unlovability and the idea that the other is unfair because a part of her deserves to be loved. In the face of these thoughts, shame mounts, sadness and forlornness at having been abandoned, anger and helplessness. To quell the now exhausting suffering and rumination, she gives in to hunger, breaking the restrictive rules she has imposed on herself, and binges. At that point, she is ashamed of her behavior, considers herself weak, and fears she has gained weight. She is now driven by social rank: she fears that her partner will find her ugly and thus abandon her, and her merciless inner gaze confirms she is worthless. Consequently, she self-induces vomiting to compensate for the effects of binge eating. The final outcome of this chain is depression. In this case, symptoms of depression and bulimia are the outcomes of a chain of coping.

Working on coping is essential but not conclusive. In our example, it is necessary to first regularize the eating behaviors; then the heart of therapy is to explore the underlying level of distress related to maladaptive nuclear schemas, as we do in MIT for Eating Disorders (MIT-ED; Fioravanti et al., 2023, 2025). If patients have reduced coping but do not change their schemas, it creates breeding grounds for the resurfacing of pain, which, in turn, will trigger coping again.

Clinical practice based on the psychopathology model

How will clinicians implement the model we have described? Above all, how will they work experientially and constantly immersed in the construction and repair of the therapeutic relationship? The rest of this volume aims to address these questions. Below, we outline a guide as to what operations we are aiming for and the order in which we perform them.

Therapy starts with helping patients recount clear autobiographical episodes that are rich in psychological knowledge. Where autobiographical memory is lacking, therapists invite patients to collect episodes week after week so that they have first-hand material that sees them immersed in the network of relationships.

These autobiographical narratives will be the first in a series of what we metaphorically call *lakes*, that is, areas where we identify mental states: cognitions, emotions, and body states that color subjective painful experiences. Sustained attention to autobiographical narratives is also necessary for identifying aspects of health and positive functioning. We refer to these, for simplicity's sake, as *healthy parts*. The second lake in which we look for subjective experience is non-verbal language, usually a privileged source of information. The therapeutic relationship, the third lake, is also rich in valuable knowledge about patients' patterns once therapists have recognized and regulated their own possible contributions. If the first lake is natural, the last is an *artificial* lake: that is, therapists search for mental states while actively working to modify patients' subjective experience. For example, they may use bodily exercises and explore with the patient how changes in their posture impact their beliefs and emotions.

The next step will be to help patients discover how their minds are partly activated after relational triggers and partly driven by intrapsychic automatisms. This is the relationship between variables, that is, the discovery of psychological cause-and-effect links among events, thoughts, emotions, behaviors, and body states.

When the patient and therapist have gathered rich and articulate information about the former's inner world, the therapist helps the patient discover how dysfunctional behaviors and suffering are driven by dysfunctional interpersonal patterns and then reinforced by coping.

Once patients become aware of how patterns, rather than reality, are the source of psychic suffering, it is time to guide them toward structural change. The goals are intertwined and are (a) reduction of suffering, (b) adoption of modes of meaning attribution and behaviors that lead toward well-being and social fulfillment, and (c) disruption of schema-driven coping behaviors. MIT therapists promote all of this by working through dialogue, primarily, but also through a continuous interweaving of experiential work and attention to the relationship.

We want clinicians to carry one concept in mind at all times during the session: *the real driver of change is not the therapist's ability to formulate the case correctly and help the patient act accordingly. The idea that guides us is that therapy is effective if therapists can first help patients form a mental model of their own functioning.* In other words, to help them realize that they are guided by patterns and that it is those patterns, rather than reality, that generate symptoms and relational dysfunction. At that point, therapists need to support patients to become agents of change. That is, they must show them that to get better, to heal, they must use their understanding of how they function in a voluntary, conscious, and deliberate way, to try and see things from another point of view and move day by day in the direction of health. Therapists must ensure that patients clearly agree and ask them to vocalize their agreement.

Therapy becomes really transformative when patients say

Okay, I realized that I suffer because I've become accustomed to thinking I'm worthless, that others will criticize me, and that, at that point, the best thing I can do is to give up, to withdraw. I've realized that this is not necessarily true; instead, it's an idea that I've developed over the course of my life or that I believed to be true anyway, and today, it's just causing me pain. Changing it is difficult, behaving differently is difficult, but I'm going to actively try.

Do not think our clarification is unnecessary. A great many of the colleagues we train show difficulties at exactly this level: they pay attention to the accuracy of their own formulation and then try to push patients toward health. Instead, they neglect the most important step, precisely making sure that patients have made the model of functioning their own and have decided and explicitly communicated that they intend to use that model as a guide to act differently. If therapists pay attention to this dimension of collaboration and do so within a careful relational modulation, experiential techniques can achieve their full potential.

Chapter 3

The therapeutic relationship in MIT

General principles and interaction with techniques

PART I

MIT procedures flow along two parallel tracks: on the first, the operations and techniques aimed at arriving at the shared formulation and promoting change; on the second, the therapeutic relationship. In PD, it is necessary to be active to dismantle the various aspects of psychopathology. For the patient to get involved in the necessary actions, the relationship must be good and ready to support the intense emotions that will emerge. A good relationship, moreover, is the ideal ground for metacognition to improve (Semerari et al., 2003). The idea is to bring the patient to experience therapy guided as much as possible by the cooperative system (Liotti & Gilbert, 2011), which supports the working alliance, and by exploration, which supports curiosity about one's inner world and seeking new avenues to fulfill one's own wishes, after having deprived schemas of their power (Dimaggio et al., 2020). When assessing in-session activation of attachment and cooperation, only the latter was correlated with improved metacognition (Farina et al., 2023), a result consistent with work showing that when patients and therapists are coordinated in various ways – verbal, physiological, movements – therapy outcomes are better (Wiltshire et al., 2020).

Consequently, therapy must also follow procedures to regulate relationships and therapeutic alliances, which we discuss in this chapter. As we move on the first track, we constantly monitor the second, and as soon as problems or ruptures arise, we leave the technical work aside and focus on the relationship (Dimaggio et al., 2020).

Let's bring in an example. A patient is talking about problems in her relationship with her mother and some schoolmates. The therapist asks her about a specific episode, but the patient huffs, assumes an uncomfortable posture, and changes the subject: "No, it's just that the problem is all these tasks; I just don't feel like it." The therapist thinks, "She seems listless, slumped, unhinged."

How should the therapist act? Follow up on the new topic, that is, lack of desire to do homework? Insist on asking for a relational episode with the mother

DOI: 10.4324/9781003570967-3

or friends? No, because it would ignore verbal and non-verbal signals of possible problems in the alliance. Rather, the therapist should ask,

> What does this attitude mean? You already seemed bored, but after I asked you for episodes, you looked annoyed, probably by me. While exploring your internal world, did I evoke something in you? Could you perceive me as intrusive and dominant? And are you protecting yourself from being subjugated, a slave without freedom? Or are you afraid that if I found out what you think, I would criticize you?

The reasons could be others: the girl fears that she will bore the therapist or that she is not "good" at finding specific episodes and will thus disappoint her. Or, again, she assumes that the therapist will not welcome the suffering she experiences when reporting episodes.

How does the therapist solve the dilemma? Here is the point: she cannot know a priori, and, more importantly, she should not give herself the task of discovering it herself! Meanwhile, the lack of desire to do homework must be investigated. In doing so, the therapist will find herself in an uncomfortable role because the patient is constructing her in a negative way. What do we do when problems like this arise? The answer is simple: when a patient emits signals, verbal and non-verbal, that might indicate either that she is becoming detached or hostile toward therapy, the therapist temporarily sets aside the patient's problem – in the example of the girl, both her relationships with her friends and her mother and her overdoing of homework – and deals with the here and now of the relationship.

The therapist will point out to the girl that her face and speech changed and she did not respond to the request for an autobiographical episode. She will form hypotheses about the underlying action tendency: "It's as if you want to change topic, could it be? How come?"; on the mental states surfacing: "It seemed to me from your face you were irritated (or worried)"; and ask for feedback, "Did you feel the way it seems to me, or in another way I didn't catch?"

We will see in what situations it is convenient to move to the second track to deal with possible therapeutic alliance ruptures. We will describe the tools for repairing minor and major ruptures and the operations that will enable us to return to formulating functioning and promoting change.

Reasons for monitoring the therapeutic relationship

Identify the presence of interpersonal patterns

The relationship informs us about patients' interpersonal schemas and the coping strategies they use (Leahy, 2008; Luborsky & Crits-Christoph, 1990). Maladaptive schemas are predictive and organizing structures of behavior, directing attention and imposing a rigid, often negative, reading of the relational situation in which one is engaged (Chapter 2). Not surprisingly, they are activated in relation to the therapist, in PD. For example, borderline PD patients often do not trust their therapist, so there is the need for active work in restoring trust and making therapy work (Choi-Kain et al., 2023).

Sal, 28, suffers from narcissistic PD; his pattern is related to attachment and is activated when he feels fragile and needy. He shows himself to be gentle, bright, and outgoing. He talks about the stop in his university studies for which he asked for help with calmness and self-deprecation, but he intellectualizes, and recounts episodes but shows no pain. When the therapist asks him about his own internal states, he becomes laconic and elusive. After a few attempts, our colleague notes that he appears irritated and becomes detached, his face expressionless. The therapist, at this point, talks about the relationship:

> Sal, excuse me, have you noticed that when I ask you to describe the details of your experience in an episode, you change your posture and attitude, shift topic and get fed up. I wonder what happens to you. Do my questions bother you in any way?

This is the first operation in metacommunication, a topic we discuss later.

Sal does not find these questions "comfortable." The therapist tells him that he cannot answer but that it is interesting to understand what the psychological inquiry elicits in him. The two understand that the therapist's questions ignite painful emotions and self-images. Sal fears that if he shows pain, the therapist might think he is weak; when she asks him, "How did you feel at that moment" she looks dismissive to him, so that he feels angry and humiliated. But he at the same time feels ashamed and lonely.

These are typical steps at the beginning of therapy with narcissistic PDs: even simple questions can activate the negative schemas that include the therapist. If instead of continuing to travel along the first track, in accordance with the decision-making procedures (we describe them in chapters 4 and 5), the therapist switches to reflecting on the relationship, the schemas become readable in the relationship for both therapist and patient. Conversely, insisting on working without overcoming the relational rupture accentuates the latter and makes therapy fruitless.

In short, the therapeutic relationship is not only the terrain where conflicts are narrated but also where they are acted out, sometimes in ways that are disturbing to both. Focusing on the relationship is difficult but offers a unique opportunity to observe interpersonal patterns in action, to unravel them, to reflect on them jointly, and even to modulate them. Above all, it saves from the frustrations of unproductive, unsuccessful work.

Assess the agreement on goals

Psychotherapy is different from other professions. If one goes to the doctor, one wants to be treated; if one goes to the lawyer, one wants to be defended; if one goes to the mechanic, one wants one's car fixed. In our profession, patients' purposes do not always coincide with those of psychotherapy. Usually, a care motivation is present, more or less consciously, but often, especially in the case of PD, it is not enough.

Psychotherapy sometimes directly heals wounds; at other times, it requires going through painful emotions to live a full life free of blocks and frustrations. Some people go to a psychotherapist to get help to change those aspects of themselves that prevent them from overcoming problems. This is the ideal motivation for setting up work because it aligns with the mission of psychotherapy. Others go to therapy to be understood; others expect the therapist to solve the problem for them, which is not a good therapy start! Others seek an ally in a conflict; others seem to have no purpose other than to please their parents and partners and comply with others' expectations. A patient with narcissistic PD in therapy with one of us said, "I don't know, I'm curious; my wife claims I might need it." The list could go on and on. More frequently, the reasons and purposes for which a patient approaches psychotherapy are multiple and alternating.

Donatella is 50 years old and suffers from dependent PD. Her initial claim seems congruous: she is depressed because the man with whom she thought she was in a romantic relationship for a year left her for another woman, denying he ever intended to establish a lasting bond with her. Since then, she has been paralyzed, ruminating about the incident and would like to "get out of this tunnel." However, she feels unable to move on and search for new friendships and interests, and, why not, even a new partner. The problem thus stems from reduced autonomy.

As long as the therapist merely explores episodes, Donatella cooperates: she narrates, tries to understand what emotions she has experienced, expresses them, and reasons about them. She allows the therapist to act on emotional regulation: she willingly agrees to mindfulness exercises to calm herself. The relationship is good.

However, when the therapist suggests actions and tasks for her to change in real life – for example, to go Salsa dancing, an old passion of hers – or when he spurs and encourages her by telling her that she can get better and that it is necessary to act outside the therapy room as well, Donatella gets irritated. She protests and rejects all the proposals saying, "Yes, I might as well do it, but what good would it do me? I'm 50 years old, I'd be ridiculous"; "Yes, okay, but in the end I am always alone, why does no one invite me?"; "Yes, but why do only I have to do these things? My friends have partners who take them dancing, on trips and all that. Why does it have to instead be a task for me?"

The therapist encourages her, and in response, Donatella protests more. She also gradually lowers her shoulders, slumps like an empty sack, and becomes sadder. What is happening? Through reflection on the relationship, they come to understand that Donatella is now driven by the schema-related prediction that she will fail and cannot succeed as she is powerless. Her purpose has now changed; her expectation structure is of the "I have no power, and the other person has power over me" type. It is as if she thinks, "I can't cure myself, I will be better off if the therapist solves the problems for me." The task agreement is absent, and cooperation is absent. She is now driven by attachment but passively. When she sees the therapist does not solve her problems as she expects and demands, she constructs him as distant, cold, and insensitive. The agreement on the goal is gone; the working alliance is broken. In the section on metacommunications, we will see how the therapist worked to overcome this difficulty.

Evaluate the agreement on tasks

Bernard is 28 years old and suffers from avoidant PD and generalized anxiety. He avoids anxiety-provoking situations: elevators, cable cars, subways, and buses. He also avoids, in general, exposing himself to strong emotions; he no longer watches dramatic movies or the news. All of these avoidances carry a high social cost: he feels different from his friends, and the difficulty in traveling reduces the chances of having relationships. He would like a normal life.

In therapy, he seems cooperative, but only if the therapist just does small talk. The problem is that his ability to describe internal states is minimal, so the therapist asks him to recall an episode in his imagery to increase metacognitive monitoring. Bernard initially seems to agree, closes his eyes but reopens them frequently, seems listless, more compliant than involved. The therapist interrupts the procedure and explores the reason for these behaviors. Bernard answers, "I don't believe in these things, what do I need them for? . . . It sounds like sorcerer's stuff to me."

The therapist does not feel scorned; Bernard is skeptical only about the experiential procedures. Exploring the problem, the therapist realizes that Bernard has poor mastery over his own mental states: he fears painful emotions as he believes he cannot handle them, and if they appear, they will spiral out of control. For this reason, he is anxious about having to look inside and experience them. In contrast, during the therapeutic conversation, Bernard can control himself and enact subtle emotional avoidance mechanisms. But in protecting himself, he prevents the therapist from intervening.

He recounts an incident of bullying he suffered in middle school. He comes close to describing the pain; the therapist guesses that it is related to a nuclear idea of himself as inferior and submissive, but . . . Bernard shifts topic and arousal drops. The therapist asks him to stop on the previous scene, and he gets irritated and criticizes the therapy.

B: "Look, I realize that maybe I need a different kind of therapy. I am a creative guy; I like to space and connect things in my own way, whereas you force me to stay on episodes that have exhausted their evocative potential for me."

T: "Like they bore you?"

B: "Exactly."

T: "Are you sure it was boredom that you felt when you were recalling the harassment you suffered in middle school?"

B: "Well, not really, I would say discomfort."

T: "So you felt an uncomfortable emotion. Could you say which one? From your account, it sounded like a particularly humiliating situation."

B: "Yes, it was very humiliating, even now just thinking about it. But I don't understand why you want to keep me there."

Bernard is irritated because the therapist pushes him to dwell on emotionally painful memories. He has the same reaction when the therapist asks him to remember his grandfather's funeral two years earlier, where he had an anxiety crisis that triggered avoidance.

Exploring the therapeutic relationship, we see how the proposed imagery work triggers a relational rupture; it is a type 1 technique-relationship interaction pattern. If the therapist had insisted, it would have made the rupture deeper. Again, reflecting on the relationship made it possible to discover that the agreement on the task – that is, guided imagery aimed at better understanding internal states – had failed. In subsequent sessions, the therapist would work to repair the rupture, and only then would she again propose to explore the internal world in imagery, this time successfully.

Assess whether patients are testing the therapist

Problems in sessions happen when patients test the therapist, as explained by Control Mastery Theory (CMT; Weiss, 1993). The idea is that patients are driven by *healthy desires* but blocked by *pathogenic beliefs* – for example, "If I leave the other, I will destroy him." They enact plans, that is, sequences of predictions and behaviors, that are often unconscious, hoping to disconfirm these beliefs and discover that the outcome will be positive as opposed to feared (Gazzillo et al., 2022). For example, a patient with the attachment-related belief "If I show my problems, I am a burden for the other" will act out tests in multiple ways. Possible scenarios, according to CMT, are as follows: a) the patient tries to behave contrary to his own desire – for example, he describes problems with irony and avoids complaining; b) the patient protests if the therapist does not pay absolute attention to him and complains all the time; c) another way is role reversal, that is, it is the patient who emphasizes how intolerant the therapist is when he asks for something. At that point, he considers whether the therapist succumbs to his complaints or reacts without being destroyed; or d) the patient tries to please the therapist and give her what he himself would always have wanted, hoping that the therapist will sooner or later reciprocate.

Passive-into-active shifts are frequent. A patient has a rank-based maladaptive pattern: in the context of wanting to be liked, she has poor self-esteem, and she predicts that if she shows her skills, others will criticize her or be disappointed. Passive-into-active tests consist of attacking the therapist for even a slight inaccuracy, telling her that she has deeply disappointed her. The patient thus goes from defendant to ruthless judge, from feeling attacked to being the aggressor (Gazzillo, 2023). In this case, the therapist passes the test by not allowing herself to be disappointed and by voicing, in a modulated way, her feelings in the face of harsh criticism. In this way, she can become a kind of model showing how one can defend oneself calmly and proudly without being ashamed or overreacting angrily.

MIT therapists almost never let the test take place without identifying and describing it in a way that is clear to both patients and therapists so that they are fully aware. Do we notice a rupture marker in the working alliance? Do we assume there is a test in place? If so, we first adjust our mental state and then formulate hypotheses based on our knowledge of the patient and his or her patterns. Finally, we share these hypotheses with the patient and engage him or her in reasoning about the relationship in the most cooperative way possible. We do not hope our answer will let us successfully pass any test; more reasonably, we try to bring it to the surface, investigate it, and make sense of it considering the maladaptive pattern active in the patient.

Attempts at problem-solving in the therapeutic relationship

We now describe how to solve problems in the therapeutic relationship. We show how to act when we notice a rupture marker in the working alliance. We see two different situations: in the first, the rupture depends on an error in the formulation of functioning that was evidently incomplete or incorrect; in the second, the problem arises from the schema-dependent way in which the patient constructs the therapist, and the latter loses regulation over her own mental state and contributes to the negative interpersonal cycle (Safran & Muran, 2000).

Relational breakdown is due to an error in wording: correct the formulation

Not all relational breakdowns can be attributed to patients' "defenses" or relational problems. Often, the reason is that the case formulation is wrong! If we do not accurately grasp the wish and structure of the schema, we risk pushing the patient in the wrong direction, and the consequence is that she feels misunderstood and does not agree with goals and tasks, and therapy stalls.

Ester is 26 years old, sunny, smiling, and curious. She gets gloomy, and tears flow as soon as she starts talking about the problem with her partner. She comes from a long psychotherapy, but the grip of gloom is still there. She talks about seemingly trivial situations of which she is a little ashamed, for example, the fact that her partner did not clear the table after dinner: "Yet he knows well that I care about these things." Sadness is evident, and the therapist explores the episode: Ester is not hypersensitive to disgust, nor did she feel compelled to compulsively clean up with a sense of sacrifice. Moreover, when she saw the mess, she angrily called her partner, scolded him, and he cleared up. She achieved her goal, albeit through scolding, but suffering remained, which seemed strange. It is a sign that the formulation is incomplete. The therapist asks her what she feels besides anger. Ester replies, "I'm sad; I don't feel seen."

Not seen, not considered, and such statements are pseudo-images that do not disclose what frustrated wish they refer to: does she want to be seen as an object of care and protection? Or as a valuable and appreciable person? Or sexually desirable? The therapist must explore what "to feel seen" means.

Ester explains that this is an attachment-related problem. She has mentioned it dozens of times in previous psychotherapy, and the current therapist is also convinced that it is so. In the third session, however, the alliance breaks down: every time the therapist intervenes, Ester is discouraged and annoyed.

E: "It's just that I know these things; I know very well that I demand that the other person is always tuned in to me, but they don't satisfy me, or I feel like I don't grasp it. I mean, what have I solved now?"

The therapist explores episodes related to attachment with her partner, who, however, offers her tons of care, affection, attention, and protection, and so do her parents. But then, where does her sensitivity to the alleged lack of care come from? The therapist seeks to understand more and asks for other associated memories (we will see their role in the next chapter); she needs episodes that lead her to the correct formulation. Ester brings back stories involving her mother, who, like her partner, is extremely loving and caring but, on many occasions, has caused her suffering. She remembers being 14 years old when her mother entered the bathroom without knocking, despite knowing how much she valued intimacy. Another incident: her mother peels posters of singers Ester loved off the walls of her room. Ester became angry, but to no avail. Ester acknowledges it feels like seeing the table covered with dirty dishes and cutlery.

The pattern takes shape, and Ester is surprised: her distress arises when she perceives the other as *overbearing* and *intrusive*, disregarding her needs. The wish is not attachment – she has never lacked care – but to have her boundaries respected. Thus, the dominant motivation is autonomy, invalidated by maternal intrusiveness. At this point, Ester moves to social rank and protests with her mother, demanding respect. The self-image underlying the primary wish for autonomy is *victim and powerless*. This is why today she easily perceives a gesture, or lack of it, by the other as a prevarication. They return to the episode of the dirty table, and it surfaces that Ester's desire was to lie on the couch and watch a TV series. The companion, then, was not uncaring but an obstacle! At this point, Ester shifts into social rank and sees the other as overbearing and arrogant. She realizes her self-image is *powerless* but also *submissive* and then counterattacks: she gets angry, resulting in reversing roles and dominating. *If you don't respect my autonomy, I will subjugate you, so I will do what I want.*

The new formulation has an immediate effect: Ester relaxes and says she understands herself thoroughly for the first time. But she is left with a doubt: "In what you told me, what does sadness have to do with it? I get tears just thinking about it and every time I remember those moments." Non-verbal signals are now good. By correcting the formulation, the therapist has repaired the relationship. From now on, Ester and the therapist work together to understand where sadness came from and overcome it.

The problem arises from patients' or therapists' schemas: therapists' internal state regulation

Interventions in the relationship require reflection on the part of the therapist: what is happening in the midst of the ongoing transaction with the patient? This reflection takes place *while* one is actively involved in the therapeutic relationship and a fracture of the alliance is taking place. In fact, in PD treatment, it is common for the therapist to become involved in dysfunctional interpersonal cycles, to be driven by ideas and emotions that would lead him or her to act in a way that would hinder treatment. Anger, guilt, helplessness, anxiety, alarm, humiliation, or shame are emotions well known to psychotherapists, and it is natural that they are also activated in front of patients.

In most cases, they are the consequence of patients' dysfunctional behavior. In the face of some behaviors, it is almost inevitable that the therapist will react in an unmodulated manner (Kiesler, 1996). For example, a patient with borderline PD is agitated, going from one emergency to another and demanding an immediate solution. Can the therapist avoid reacting with alarm, worry, guilt, or irritation? Of course not; these are human, instinctive reactions. A patient with narcissistic PD criticizes and devalues the therapist and emphasizes her interventions with subtle grimaces of disgust and impatience. The therapist feels anger and would like to tell the patient to be more respectful and behave! The previous therapist of the same patient, faced with the same behaviors, felt anxiety, perceived herself as fragile and inadequate, and tried anxiously to settle things down but without any success. Do the two therapists deserve our blame? Should we expect them to maintain calm, approaching superhuman wisdom? Of course not.

At other times, therapists find themselves involved in interpersonal cycles not so much because of how patients relate to them but because of their own patterns. For example, an inexperienced therapist may think of himself as inadequate and thus feel anxious, constructing the patient as critical but in the absence of signals. Or, listening to a story in which the patient has become very angry, the therapist may become afraid or take the side of the spouse the patient is talking about. Driven by these reactions, the therapist tends to act incongruously with the formulation or relate to the patient in an emotionally unmodulated way. The patient, in turn, reacts negatively; the interpersonal cycle is activated.

How do we address these problems related to the activation of interpersonal patterns of the patient, the therapist, or, as is often the case, both?

Therapists need to

a) have achieved a good awareness of the mental state that patients' behavior has evoked in them;
b) have regulated, at least in part, negative emotions and assumed critical distance from the nuclear self-ideas active at that time;
c) regain empathy, at least in part, for the patient;
d) find within themselves a cooperative and exploratory motivation;
e) make assumptions about why the patient has broken the alliance;
f) connect back, after repairing the rupture, the reasons for the relational issue to the shared formulation of the patient's functioning.

Safran and Segal (1990) termed some of the therapist's internal self-regulatory operations *inner discipline*. In MIT, we have absorbed the essential aspects of this practice but have added specific elements. In the rest of the chapter, we will therefore use the expressions *inner discipline* and *therapist self-regulation* interchangeably to define the set of practices aimed at regulating one's problematic mental states and antitherapeutic tendencies.

Inner discipline takes place in three steps: 1) the therapist recognizes that his or her own state is problematic and decides to try to regulate it; 2) the therapist tries to understand the elements of his or her own problematic mental state:

What do I think and feel about myself and the patient and for what reasons? How much of what I feel depends on my personal history, my patterns, and my values? What are the patient's words, behaviors, and non-verbal cues that have elicited this mental state of mine?

This is a stage centered on self-reflection, but it does not mean that the therapist necessarily has to reflect on his or her whole life. Of course, sometimes it may be necessary if the therapist's schemas are active outside the room as well. To this end, the therapist can turn to his or her supervisor or own therapist. What is needed at this moment is a sufficient level of self-reflexivity to understand what is going on, achieving the awareness that allows release from the ongoing interpersonal cycle (Kiesler, 1996); 3) the therapist focuses on the patient and a) formulates hypotheses about the mental states active at that moment; b) wonders if there is similarity or complementarity with his or her own; c) formulates hypotheses about the reasons that may have prompted the patient to act in that way; d) tries to attune to aspects of the patient that he or she can appreciate and validate, to re-establish respect and empathy.

The operations described above occur within the therapist: they are done *for the* patient but not *with* the patient. However, they place the therapist in an optimal position for proceeding with other relational interventions, such as metacommunication or reformulation of the therapeutic contract, aimed at repairing the relational rupture and restoring a working alliance with explicit and shared goals and tasks.

What did the therapist achieve by modulating herself? First, already at this level, she was able to disengage internally from the interpersonal cycle into which the patient had drawn her and/or from her own pattern that surfaced during the interaction. By adjusting her internal state, she also recovered a more positive image of the patient, restored her own inclination towards cooperating and exploring, and regained confidence in therapy. Not least, she has formulated new hypotheses about the patient's mental state and the reasons behind the alliance breakdown. She now possesses the material needed to reformulate the case after the rupture has been repaired.

It sounds clear and simple to describe. It is much less so to put into practice. One difficulty is contextual: the therapist finds herself performing these tasks in the midst of a problematic transaction with the patient, in the presence of sometimes intense negative emotions and feels the urge to act in an antitherapeutic manner.

An example helps us appreciate how self-regulatory operations enable therapy to continue successfully even after problematic relational moments. We show here where the relational breakdown begins and how the therapist works on herself to overcome it. In the section on metacommunication, we will tell the sequel to the episode when the therapist, after modulating herself, reflected together with the patient on the relational problem until a new agreement on goals and tasks was found.

Therapists work on their inner world: deliberate practice

Entering the session in a self-regulated state may require dedicated work. Therapists often react guided by their own patterns. The patient in front of them is not the patient but embodies a ghost and represents problematic figures from their history. They experience memories of grief and helplessness, of humiliation and abandonment, of injustice and missed rebellion, and, captive to these scenes, they fail to keep to procedures. Sometimes, they do not see the way, lose clarity, and cannot discern the patients' patterns. Or they visualize the correct step to take but remain paralyzed in a kind of fog; they understand on the surface but remain confused, especially when patients do not move forward. In the face of these signs, active work on the self is needed to break out of the fog and return to technically oriented action. Newer orientations do not require therapists to know every rivulet of their problematic past or to have explored it over long periods of personal therapy. Sometimes this is indispensable, but our goal here is only to help the therapist get rid of his or her own ghosts in the next session with that specific patient and then return to the procedures.

These are so-called *deliberate practice* strategies (Rousmaniere et al., 2017). It is an approach based on the principle that skills develop through training with guidance: a violinist learns from the teacher, a tennis player from the coach, and a young surgeon from the experienced surgeon. Psychotherapy is no different. The idea is that if therapists identify their weaknesses and work to overcome them, they will become more effective (Bennett-Levy, 2019; Chow et al., 2015). Some data show how therapists who adopt this benefit, and this helps them view the therapeutic relationship more positively (Hill et al., 2020). Although research is just beginning, it appears that deliberate practice is a more effective way than others to teach and develop therapeutic skills (Mahon, 2023).

Here, we focus on one aspect of deliberate practice, which is to help the therapist work under pressure (Muran & Eubanks, 2020). As we have seen, it is common for the therapist to be overwhelmed by negative emotions, which are usually a sign of schema reactivation. We want to help him go into the next session aware that his internal difficulty will reoccur with the patient. At this point, we provide him with tools to enter the session already adjusted, ready to work through adverse conditions, or to notice in time when he loses his balance so that he then recovers it (Goldman et al., 2021).

Let us look at the steps in sequence, in line with the guidelines for deliberate practice (Rousmaniere, 2019). The first step takes place in supervision (Sacks & Vaz, 2023) and consists of leading the therapist to recognize the precise moment when he loses balance in front of the patient. This is followed by an exploration of the cognitive-affective processes that lead the therapist to see himself as incapable, guilty, inadequate, and powerless in the face of a patient perceived as incurable, hostile, judgmental, humiliating, or in grave danger. It is now necessary for the therapist to recognize that his reaction is not necessarily based on reality or, if it is, it is, in any case, a reaction that causes him to lose clarity. We often lead therapists to recognize that they are haunted by specters of their history. We do not ask them to tell us the details; it is enough for the internal spark – insight, if you will – to be lit and for the therapist to say, "I understand what is triggering me; now I know whom I am really dealing with." Now, the therapist is ready to recover self-regulation.

It involves planning individualized exercises. We ask for the therapist's willingness to expose himself to the painful state again in the patient's absence. He thus has to retrieve scenes in which he sees himself, for example, accused, humiliated, harmed, or a failure, and feels intense negative emotions.

The next step is to design the exercises and agree on the timing of the training. For example, the therapist can reenact the emotion of guilt and shame at home for a few days and let it slip away during a short meditation. Or he can get in touch with feelings of inferiority, fear, humiliation, and helplessness, at which point he will adopt tonic postures until he overcomes the state. If the therapist practices sports, dance, yoga, or any structured activity involving the body, we ask him to use exercises taken from his own area of interest, knowing that they will help him regulate the negative state.

We may, in some cases, ask him to reenact a painful scene, either with figures from his own life or with the patient himself, and engage in an internal dialogue using guided imagery until he is able to overcome the problematic emotions or gain critical distance from the pattern. We may still ask him to identify a peer of his own with whom to carry out the same exercises.

Very often, it is sufficient to do the exercises on the day of the session with the patient who has challenged him. The precise time depends on the therapist's schedule. It may be at the beginning of the working day or in the interval soon before a likely problematic session. The common element is that the therapist chooses to train, voluntarily expose himself to the painful state, and practice overcoming it.

We illustrate the application of deliberate practice with the example of a colleague who, in supervision, reported difficulties in working with Marcello, a 37-year-old patient with obsessive-compulsive PD. The patient had cheated on his girlfriend and was ruminating in a session about his own moral guilt: "Should I go back to my ex and atone or stay with my new lover?" He would prevent the therapist from stopping his rumination or ask him for help but in a desperate and completely passive way, "You have to help me decide." The therapist reacted driven by the need to be effective and, in the face of the unassailability of Marcello's interpersonal repetitive thinking (IRT, see chapter 2), he himself began ruminating about his own defects. He was preoccupied with the idea of being worthless, saw himself as harmful, and felt guilt and shame. Guided by this state, he could let Marcello's endless ruminations flow or try to bring him back to the plane of reality to help him remember that he had betrayed his partner for understandable reasons. All this was useless; Marcello would immediately resume his self-critical ruminations from where he had left off.

The correct intervention, as we will see in chapter 8, would have been to stop the patient and make him realize he was ruminating and place the goal of interrupting this process at the center of therapy. If he does not accomplish this first step, the patient cannot be helped. However, the therapist does not do this and does not imagine it is possible. The supervisor asks the therapist to think about what personal scenes Marcello conjures up for him, and the therapist realizes that he is looking at his father, who is, on the one hand, warm and caring and, on the other hand, suffering. This has always evoked in him a sense of sorrow and helplessness that he tries to remedy by compulsive caregiving: "Dad, don't worry, I swear I'll find the money to help you solve the problems."

On the one hand, the therapist realizes that he will be able to process this image in his own ongoing therapy; on the other hand, he agrees with the supervisor on a deliberate practice exercise. Immediately before the next session with Marcello, he imagines that he is faced with him in full rumination, to the point of feeling useless and powerless. At this point, he assumes a toned posture, standing with legs spread wide and firmly planted, arms outstretched like a hug towards Marcello. Having reached this posture, the therapist repeats to himself, "How difficult it is to help him. I'm sorry, but I can't do what you're asking." Through this exercise, the therapist recovers internal regulation and overcomes the feelings that were paralyzing him. In subsequent sessions, he is able to be firmer in interrupting IRT; fear of harming the patient and jeopardizing the relationship no longer dominates him. In the face of Marcello's reticence, the therapist is progressively firmer, even to the point of saying: "Marcello, if you continue to ruminate, that's fine with me, but I'll do something else in the meantime," and goes so far as to take out his cell phone and look at WhatsApp chats and social media. Thanks to this paradoxical intervention, Marcello finally realizes that he is falling prey to endless rumination and, more importantly, that he is not allowing the therapist to work. Only at this point does he take the interventions seriously and agree to make reducing interpersonal rumination a priority goal.

Without the deliberate practice work, the therapist would not have been able to take the necessary steps to interrupt Marcello's IRT. The therapy would probably have continued to stagnate or would have stopped without proving useful.

Invite patients to communicate their negative thoughts about therapy and the therapist

In this and the next section, we describe two interventions linked by an underlying theme: allowing the patient to express concerns about therapy or the therapist. The purposes are a) to bring relational problems to the surface and examine them together, reducing the possibility of their acting underground, undermining the alliance; b) to facilitate the identification of elements of the patient's schema, for example, the wish or the other's feared response, by catching them in the bud in the session, in the relationship with the therapist; and c) to act to defuse early relational ruptures that could lead to dropouts.

The first step is simple and consists of asking the patient to verbalize negative feelings or concerns about the therapist or therapy. Almost by default, in the first few sessions, we intervene like this,

> If you happen at any time to feel uncomfortable with me, feel free to tell me. It is very helpful, almost valuable. If I do or say something that you feel is unpleasant, irritating, hurtful, or troubling, tell me, really. Don't worry about hurting me. In fact, if you do, it helps me because if we worked while you were uncomfortable, I would be of no use to you. Instead, if you tell me what's wrong, it helps me understand what's going on, and at that point, I can correct myself, or we can figure out how to align with each other to work well.

We also formulate the same intervention at specific times, tailoring it to the patient's themes. The most frequent case is when the patient recounts episodes of high emotional intensity, and a pattern appears clear to the therapist. In this case, it is likely that the patient will sooner or later also read the therapist in light of the pattern. The therapist, therefore, intervenes preemptively like this:

> You are telling me how, when you needed attention, you mother was not there, too caught up in her own worries. You tell me that seeing yourself neglected is something that happens to you often in life, and you suffer because of it. I thought that if you see me absent, distracted, or disinterested at any time in our conversations, you would have no qualms about telling me instantly! The last thing you need is a therapist who puts you in the same condition that makes you feel bad. If it doesn't happen, I'm happy, but if it does happen, tell me! Maybe one day I'm tired, or you read something in my face that may make you think

I am far away, even though maybe I am not. In short, feel free to talk to me about it, and we can think it over together.

Inviting patients to explore the therapist's mind

This intervention is similar to the previous one but is specific to times when a breakup is in progress, and the patient has manifested it in behavior or words. Silvia, 30, suffering from covert narcissism, talks about difficulties with female colleagues in the law firm where she works; she is tense and controlled. The therapist, noticing the non-verbal signs of reluctance, asks her what is going on, and Silvia admits, with some embarrassment, that she is anxious: she believes the therapist thinks she is boring, whiny, and unpleasant.

At times like this, many colleagues, in an effort to repair the relationship, make mistakes. The typical example is appeasing the patient by declaring themselves benevolent and appearing welcoming. In reality, what drives them most often is anxiety to put the patient back at ease, driven by patterns of inadequacy and compulsive caregiving tendencies. The patient usually does not respond well to reassurance, but therapists do not realize the error and do not correct it. They persist and are motivated not only by personal reasons but also by theory. Indeed, they are convinced that they are providing a corrective emotional experience (Alexander & French, 1946), or that they are acting as a secure base (Bowlby, 1988) for repairing the patient's attachment patterns, or that they are functioning as a "good enough therapist." In the cognitive-behavioral field, therapists do not infrequently believe they are acting to correct the patient's irrational beliefs (Ellis, 2010). In the case of Silvia, who is concerned about being seen as insulting, the cognitive-behavioral-oriented therapist might intervene in this way: "But no, please, I think in fact you are doing a brave thing in expressing these feelings, and I don't feel bored or numb at all."

Let us be clear: in some circumscribed cases and in the early stages of therapy, it may be helpful simply to reassure the patient. But we do not have the goal of convincing her of our good intentions; it would be, on second thought, an intervention of rational refutation of the belief: "You are afraid I am bored, but I am interested." This is a type of intervention that does not work with PD: if patients have a schema-dependent idea, they will not change it just because therapists reassure them.

Instead, we invite the patient to explore the therapist's mind. We begin by asking her to anchor her hypotheses to precise markers:

Silvia, you are almost convinced I am bored. Actually, I'm not bored; in fact, I'm interested, but it's really not important. Instead, I'm curious, what markers do I give you that make you think I find you boring? Does it depend on something I said, my face, tone of voice, posture?

Then we explore the cognitive content she ascribes to us: "What attitude do you think I have toward you as you tell me that you are uncomfortable with your study colleagues? You tell me about the problems, and I think . . .?"

In this way, the patient is forced, in a sense, to move from attributing ideas to the therapist in a schema-dependent way to exploring what is happening at that moment. This intervention is beneficial for many reasons. In inviting the patient to explore her own mind, the therapist comes across as confident, open, and non-defensive, something that, on a non-verbal level, the patient can sense. Moreover, the patient, finding herself having to explore the signals the therapist manifests, is performing a live behavioral experiment, which often makes her discover that the therapist's attitude is not negative. If so, the therapist can use this discrepancy to move on to reason about the patient's patterns:

> That's interesting. You have noticed that I am not bored. You are telling me clearly. At the same time, though, the belief remains. Could it be that it's just your way of seeing others, as if you have become accustomed to taking it for granted that you are uninteresting? What do you think about that? If so, can you think of any episodes?

Usually, these interventions repair the rupture and reassure the patient far more efficiently than the usually futile attempts to convince her that we like her. If, on the other hand, the patient persists in reading negative signals in the therapist, and the therapist is reasonably certain that she is in a modulated state of mind, we are in the presence of a major, schema-dependent relational rupture, and so more extensive work will need to be done to repair it. The first step is metacommunication.

Metacommunication

This is a communication whose content is the ongoing relationship (McCarthy & Betz, 1978; Kiesler, 1996; Safran & Muran, 2000) and, if used properly, has the power to solve major relational problems.

Its object can be as follows:

1. *The patients' state of mind:* "It seems to me that while I am asking you X, you are feeling Y." Here, therapists voice what patients think and feel about the therapists. Therapists focus on the content of the moment and anchor it to specific behavioral indicators.
2. *A certain relational configuration of the therapeutic dyad:* "It is possible that you and I are behaving as if . . . ." Here, therapists invite patients to reflect together on what is happening to both of them in the session, how the actions of one affect the other and vice versa.
3. The *therapist's state of mind:* "I realize that now toward you, as you are saying . . . I feel . . ., I get to . . . ." Therapists here give voice to their own thoughts and emotions about what is happening in the heat of the interaction or what is happening in therapy on a recurring basis. It is, therefore, a self-disclosure whose content is the therapist's thoughts and emotions with respect to the patient.

The goals of metacommunication

The therapist metacommunicates not only to mend ruptures but, for example, to identify and validate the emergence of positive states: "Just now, when I was pointing out the progress you are making, I saw a smile from you that seemed to indicate to me that you were enjoying it. Is that so?" Or,

> Earlier, when you were talking to me about how painful it was to grow up with an abusive mother, I saw that you looked at me with . . . I don't know . . . hope? Like you were asking me if it was true that you were abused. I felt called in, grieving for you, and that you were asking me to be there for you, and I felt it was important. What do you think?

If we face major alliance ruptures, metacommunication is essential for repairing them. By definition, good metacommunication occurs only after therapists have achieved a self-regulated state and anchor their communications to the case formulation. If therapists express themselves only as a result of their own emotional activation, without an idea, at least an intuitive one, of how their own communication will impact patients' schemas, this will probably be doomed to failure and not solve the relational rupture or will exacerbate it. Thus, the goals of metacommunication can be summarized as follows: breaking an interpersonal antitherapeutic cycle, restoring cooperative motivation in both patient and therapist, renewing the working alliance to make the patient aware of his own relational functioning, that is, of the structures and processes that guide it, and making the patient aware of healthy parts and of the good bond with the therapist.

The structure of good metacommunication

Let us now look at the elements needed to make metacommunication effective.

BACKGROUND/PERMISSION

Metacommunication requires a dedicated space and often represents a "change of pace" in conversation. One puts life issues or symptoms on standby and shifts the focus to what is happening in the session. This change of pace cannot be abrupt, so let us start with a kind of premise. Therapists first shift the focus from the topic at hand and direct it toward the therapeutic relationship; then, when patients agree, therapists explain why they are talking about the relationship. They specify that they are going to say something subjective and will, therefore, care about getting feedback:

> Excuse me, but I would like to talk to you about something that has been going on inside me for a while . . . I was hesitating because I was afraid that I wouldn't be able to find the right way or that I would create some stress for you anyway. Would you like me to try?

ANCHORING THE INTERVENTION TO SPECIFIC MARKERS

We always metacommunicate from observable markers at a given time in the session. Why is it such a priority to anchor ourselves to visible markers? Because it allows us to minimize defensive attitudes. We want to reduce the risk that the patient perceives the therapist's intervention to be critical or carried out from a position of dominance. For this reason, we have to express ourselves based on what the patient manifests and what we feel at that moment. We specify, therefore, to what visible signals – posture, phrases, tone of voice, and behavior – we link our observations. In this way, the patient will be able to reflect on the material we have reflected on and, if necessary, disagree. Moreover, by talking about specific elements, it will be easier to show that we are not talking about his whole personality or how we experience him as a whole, but about something that belongs to him and with which we are resonating, about a specific relational arrangement that does not exhaust our relationship with him in its entirety. In doing so, the therapist reduces the risk that the patient will read her communications as stigmatizing or oracular. Often, in fact, if patients have this impression, they have a good reason.

First, the *when* should be indicated: "I was noticing just now . . ."; "It's been a while since . . ."; "Even at the beginning of the session, I got the impression that . . ."; "When I told you that . . . it seemed to me that you reacted . . . ."

The *behavioral/expressive marker* consists of *what* happened: "You're speaking in monosyllables"; "I know it's a subject that gets you heated. However, I saw that you tended to talk over me"; "You made an expression that struck me, like a grimace of irritation . . ."; "You lowered you head, shifted your gaze away from me . . ."; "Whatever I said to you, even if I repeated almost verbatim the words you had used a second before, you replied it wasn't so."

The behavioral/expressive marker may also relate to behaviors and attitudes of both parties: "I feel like we're playing tug-of-war"; "The more I cheer you on, the more you seem to put yourself down, and the more you put yourself down, the more I try to motivate you to fight back"; "We seem to be competing for who gets to talk."

MAKING ASSUMPTIONS (NOT INTERPRETATIONS!) ABOUT
THE PATIENT'S MENTAL STATE

Once it is defined *when* something happened in the relationship and *what* happened, the therapist makes hypotheses about the underlying reasons. It is critical for the therapist to make a prediction about how the patient will accept her hypothesis. Will it go to reinforce the pattern? It may create inevitable friction, but is there a healthy part of the relationship that will allow the patient to accept the observations and cooperate? Is it an intervention that will break the cycle?

Another element of metacommunication is thus to *formulate hypotheses about the mental state underlying the patient's behavior*. Remember that the therapist formulates them only after self-regulation. She must know that they are hypotheses;

that is, subjective and falsifiable ideas. It is important that the degree of inference be minimal, a little more elaborate than the observable data. One thus moves
into the therapeutic zone of proximal development, helping the patient understand
something just above what she would be able to comprehend spontaneously (Leiman & Stiles, 2001). Too high a degree of inference corresponds to "You, when
you behaved that way, were trying X because in my opinion . . . ." A minimal, and
therefore adequate, inference sounds like, "Seeing behavior X made me think that
you were feeling Y at that moment. Is that right?" If the patient accepts this first
observation, a slightly more complex inference can be made: "Could it be that you
were guided by fear of . . .?" Otherwise, this would be an interpretation, something
MIT avoids as much as possible since it often raises defenses, wears down the alliance, and contributes to passivizing and disempowering the patient.

Remember that the goal of this step is to interrupt the interpersonal cycle. Consequently, it is not crucial that the hypothesis is right but that it invites the patient to
think together about something that was automatically damaging the relationship.
Our action makes the mechanism that previously controlled the relationship an
object of reflection.

If the observation is about the therapeutic couple, the transition to psychological
cause-effect relationships sounds like this:

> I used to notice that the more I encourage you, the more you close down and lose
> confidence in the possibility of getting better. I, at that point, feel almost obliged
> to make you feel better and push you more. And the result is that you close down
> even more. Have you noticed that yourself?

When the patient recognizes that the therapist's observation is correct, or after
they have thought about it and found a shared reading, the therapist invites him or
her to think about what was driving both of them, although the patient at this point
often begins to think about it spontaneously. The therapist may observe,

> I think I was driven by feeling guilty if you were not getting better. Could it be
> that you, on the other hand, felt as if I underestimated your pain? Or, at any rate,
> that you were experiencing me in a way that not only didn't help you but made
> you feel worse?

DISCLOSING THE THERAPIST'S MENTAL STATE

Every metacommunication involves some degree of disclosure. Even when the
focus is on the patient's mental state, therapists nonetheless disclose something
about their own cognitive processes: "When I saw your eyes bulge, *I thought you
were* feeling some emotion and trying to hold it back."

With what attitude do therapists metacommunicate? The first prerequisite is that
the unveiling is done in a tone that is neither critical nor judgmental. It is, therefore, necessary to access painful emotions and thoughts, to recognize irritations or

criticism, and to unveil the former and not the latter, except in special cases that we will see in a moment. It is correct to say "When you don't give me space, you don't welcome any intervention I make; I feel useless, powerless," while it is wrong to say "If you keep not letting me speak, that's annoying."

In many cases, especially in advanced stages of therapy, it is instead appropriate to include reactive mental states in the communication, as, for example, when we aim to show the patient the effect their behaviors have on others. We explain that we are reacting to a painful state and we also explain what this painful state was while self-regulated. For example, completing the metacommunication from earlier:

> When just now you did not give me space, you did not welcome any of the interventions I made, I felt useless, powerless. At that point, I felt the need to break free from that state; I got irritated, and I felt like protesting; you must have noticed . . . . But then I wondered why you had to reject everything I said. At that point, frustration and rebellion slipped into the background. And I began to wonder what was going on. What do you think?

This is a useful type of metacommunication, especially when conflict is heated.

Therapists can disclose intense negative emotions only if they have at least temporarily regulated them and also have access to some form of pain, along with the curiosity to cooperatively explore what is happening, however unpleasant.

In advanced therapy, when the alliance is solid and the patterns have been reviewed together several times, the metacommunication can have a different, even blunt, ironic, or irreverent, tone: "Look, I swear if you start saying 'and no to what you said and no to this other one too,' I'll go on strike and not say a word for the next ten sessions! I really do, huh!"

Self-disclosure occurs after the therapist has formulated in his or her mind the idea about what impact the metacommunication will have in light of the patient's schemas. If the therapist says, "I acted because I felt that . . .," he is automatically making a mistake; there is no room for intuition without reflection in rigorous therapy. However, since these are emotionally heated interventions, under the pressure of a relational breakdown, the therapist may make mistakes. It is important that the therapist has formulated a hypothesis before intervening and is ready to correct it based on the reaction.

Therapist-centered metacommunications occur at various times during therapy and for different purposes. Even in the early stages, it is advisable to engage in self-disclosure if the patient's behavior makes the relationship difficult to endure, net of the role of the therapist's own schemas. The therapist, in such cases, can show the difficulties he or she feels in the face of certain behaviors to set limits or to begin to modulate the ongoing interpersonal cycle:

> I notice that you often speak to me in a critical, sometimes dismissive way. If you despise what I say, it is difficult for me to remain calm and help you because

I feel pressured to defend myself and react, and this does not benefit you or the therapy. Are you aware of this tendency? How come you do it?

At intermediate stages, self-disclosure helps to change the patient's idea of the therapist, and this is one of the ways to start changing patterns, as we shall see in the coming chapters. We help with an example of a correct disclosure.

The patient repeatedly criticizes the therapist. Two configurations exist in his schemas: either others criticize him, and he surrenders, or he criticizes others, who tear down or react with anger. The second configuration arises from a typical passive-into-active shift (Weiss, 1993). The patient always moves within the same script and only manages to change the role he plays in the drama. If the therapist metacommunicates, she gets out of the script:

I noticed in your words a critical, almost dismissive tone. There and then, I felt a certain humiliation; I felt like defending myself, almost counterattacking. But then I asked myself, 'But why is he talking to me like that?' Then, it occurred to me that perhaps you might have first feared my judgment. In such cases, it is common for one to enter the 'whoever hits first, hits twice' mode; you told me about it on several occasions with a certain pride. It's just a hypothesis, for goodness sake, but what do you think?

At advanced stages, disclosing the therapist's mental functioning can serve as true *modeling*. We show the patient a functional way of being in a relationship. This is modeling in action, quite different from giving advice from the heights of one's own supposed wisdom, pointing the patient to the correct path, as if he or she were a disciple coming to us to learn how to live.

We repeat that self-disclosure is for many patients a surprise, almost a revolution. They have never experienced, in fact, reference or care figures telling them, "You are authorized to explore my mind and also to tell me if anything of what I think causes you problems."

CLOSING: PROPOSAL FOR SHARING AND FEEDBACK

This is a fundamental element. The therapist does not have to be attached to what she thinks and feels, to the reasons why she metacommunicated, for example, or self-disclosed. What matters is the impact that our words have had: "Does what I said to you correspond to your experience, or is there something that doesn't fit? Do you have a different idea?" Any metacommunication must therefore close by asking the patient what she thinks and how she feels. The therapist has to be curious and open to answers that wrong-foot her. We try to help the patient discover that the therapist is genuinely interested in understanding the relational phenomenon going on between the two of them, that she is exploring and not reacting.

It can happen that the patient reads the metacommunication in a schema-dependent way, and, in this case, it will be necessary to continue working on the rupture. It is also possible that the patient catches realistic aspects of the disclosure that the therapist was unaware of! If so, the therapist will have to come to terms with aspects of self that the patient has recognized beyond his or her own willingness to communicate them.

As a result of the request for feedback, the patient will enter more easily into an attitude of cooperation and exploratory curiosity. He will understand that the therapist expresses hypotheses and not disclosed truths and will feel empowered to correct them, without feeling in a position of reverence and submission. The patient will also increase agency and find himself active in reflecting on the therapist's mind and the relationship.

Conversely, forgetting to ask for feedback would lead the patient to perceive the content of the metacommunication as an oracular, authoritarian interpretation. At this point, he either feels pressured to submit or rebels. Either way, the relational breakdown tends to escalate (von Below, 2020).

METACOMMUNICATION RESPONSE MARKERS

How do we know if this intervention has worked? There are several indicators (Austin, 2011; von Below, 2020). First, precise non-verbal markers: for example, astonishment emerges on the patient's face, indicating the ignition of exploratory motivation.

It is possible that the patient openly manifests an attitude of trust in the therapist and/or therapy and/or that she recognizes herself in the therapist's observations. Another positive marker is when the patient asks questions designed to look deeper into the relational problem: "So you are telling me that when I became so stubborn and touchy, it is because I felt devalued and believed it to be true?" Or when she expresses needs or seeks solutions to the relational problem, now seeing the therapist as understanding and supportive: "It's true, I often feel useless and shout for attention from the other person, making him irritated. Now what? How do I get out of this?"

It is common for the patient to bring in new material: "In fact, this is how I feel in other contexts as well. For example, at work with a colleague . . ." Finally, reliable evidence of the effectiveness of metacommunication is when the patient picks up the topic she was working on with the therapist before the break but reads it from a new perspective (Austin, 2011).

Metacommunication in action

Let us now look at metacommunication in the heat of the session, taking up some of the examples described earlier.

Repairing alliance ruptures

Rose is 41 years old and suffers from narcissistic PD, depression, and fibromyalgia. In the fourth session, she devalues the therapist's interventions for the umpteenth time while minimizing her own pain. The therapist first self-regulates and then focuses on the elements to metacommunicate, focusing on the patient's mental state.

Therapist: "Rose, excuse me, but I was noticing something that I think is important for the purposes of therapy. You recount several interesting episodes. However, when I try to explore them, I regularly notice a difficulty. When I ask you what you felt or thought in such and such a situation, you downplay the experience, 'Well, but that's normal, isn't it? What do you want me to have felt?' And then you go off to say that it depends on the rudeness of modern society. I just don't understand what chords the event touched and why you're telling me about it. I was wondering, how come you belittle what you say and my interventions? Maybe you don't give importance to what you feel, either? Or does my insistence on understanding how you feel bother you? What do you think?"

Rose: "But a lot of things like that happen to me. I didn't even know what was going through my head at that time. I try not to give it any importance; I go over . . ."

T: "Okay, and with respect to annoyance with me?"

R: "Well, yes, I find these things silly, insignificant . . ."

T: "So my questions are also silly, right?"

R: "Yes, they are about useless thing. The important things are how mom rejected me and manipulated me, the abortion, those yes . . ."

T: "True. But you talk to me about those everyday things when you see yourself neglected or cheated. I understand that you don't give them importance, but at this point, it escapes me why you talk to me about them."

R: [*Silence*]: "Like my mother . . . Whatever I did was not important, it was totally other things that were important . . . I was never worth it . . . I mean, am I doing with myself what my mother always did with me?"

T: "Don't give importance to what you feel? Yes, I think so."

Relational indicators, verbal and non-verbal, signal a radical change in the stance she takes in therapy: after metacommunication, metacognition has visibly improved. Rose has stopped speaking in abstract and moralizing terms, she recognizes emotions, and grasps connections with her life history. The therapist senses that the tension has ceased. Metacommunication has triggered virtuous interpersonal processes, which makes the continuation of the session cooperative.

Restoring agreement on goals

Let us return to Donatella, the patient with dependent PD who was coping with the end of a relationship. She was passive, expecting the therapist to solve her problems for her. The therapist pointed this out to her with a metacommunication centered on both the patient's behaviors and her own mental state.

T: "Donatella, excuse me, I'm thinking something. When I tell you that there is a solution, a possibility, I notice that you slowly change your attitude. First, you get irritated, protest, opposing all my proposals with 'yes, but . . .'. Then you get discouraged, hunch your shoulders, and look at your hands; you look almost depressed. I don't know if you've noticed. Something happens to you at these moments, and I would like to understand it better. Now, I don't know if it will help us, but maybe what I feel will help us. At these moments, I feel helpless and useless, and I have a tendency to break down. Then, I also felt a tinge of anger because it seemed unfair. For a moment, I even felt like giving up: 'I can't do it, it's all useless, she won't get out of it'. But then I thought about it and told myself that first I had to understand how you were feeling at these moments. I mean, I think I'm encouraging you, but you, at that moment . . .? I thought, 'It may be that Donatella is not putting a wall up against me, but she really believes that she has no hope. What do you think? Correct me if this is not the case."

D: "Yes, exactly! But that's what my mother always did: when I would tell her I wanted to do something, I had a desire, a passion, she would say: 'But where are you trying to get to? . . . look, you're not able . . .' At the time of the school trip, my mother told me that it was not stuff for me. I didn't listen to her, I went and what happened? I broke my leg! There, you see, she was right! I can't do it, I'm not able to take care of myself like other people do. I hate it, you know! I always thought I wasn't like my mother, and instead . . . inside, I do the same. How can I get out of it?"

At this point, cooperative motivation is restored and the therapist reformulates the contract. If Donatella wants to break the conditioning that paralyzes her, agreement on the purpose of therapy is necessary, which is not to be rescued and understood to the bitter end, but to pursue autonomous exploration and action in the real world. This is exactly the healthy purpose that Donatella is avoiding.

Through the exploration and action of restoring a rupture in the alliance, the therapeutic couple was able to reestablish agreement on purpose, and this allowed them to move on to the stage of promoting change, hitherto obstructed by Donatella.

Stop devaluation and aggression

In some situations, metacommunication must be firm and direct. These are the cases when patients are dismissive, sarcastic, or defiant. Or they present with symptoms such as self-harm or drug addiction but state that they have no intention of getting a handle on them. In these cases, it makes no sense to assume a cooperative tone because there must be two people for cooperation to occur. At the same time, it is impossible to reflect together with those who despise, devalue, or blackmail us. The therapist has a full right to remain within the rank motivational system because the patient would put him in a submissive role. It is necessary for the therapist to modulate the internal state, avoiding either accepting submission or becoming, in turn, dominant or tyrannical. Instead, it is useful for him to seek a confrontational, forthright, open position and point out to the patient the futility of the latter's position, the harm it generates, and the total absence of a therapeutic contract, making therapy thus useless.

Brad, suffering from narcissistic PD, is stalled in his university studies and does not know why. He speaks abstractly as if the problem does not concern him. The therapist senses that this is avoidance and asks him how he would feel if he forced himself to study. Brad comments sarcastically, "Well, of course, you have to have studied a lot to ask questions like that." This is just the beginning. When the therapist asks questions to understand Brad's internal state or psychological cause-and-effect linkages, the latter responds with an irony that borders on derision. After a few sessions, the therapist feels angry and frustrated. She regulates her state through inner discipline operations and discloses a sense of powerlessness and of not being respected. The patient further devalues her, "So what, now you get upset about something like that . . . I just told the truth. Of course, doctor, you really are oversensitive."

The therapist finds herself trapped in a position of inferiority and low value. She seeks help from the supervisor, who helps her realize that this is the same relationship she had with her aggressive and overbearing mother. Through this realization, she plans to do a deliberate practice exercise. Before the session, she recalls in her imagination the face of her critical mother and adopts a solid body posture, planted on the ground, addressing kind words to herself. She then begins the session in a regulated state, ready not to succumb.

Brad talks about a conflict with his partner. The therapist is tense before intervening, expecting the patient's sarcasm, but does not give up. Brad, as expected, blurts out, "Whatever, but what's the point of this whole thing? What's the point of wasting time on this stuff? Excuse me, but have you really studied to say these obvious things? Or do you psychologists get your degrees by correspondence?" The therapist understands that accepting contempt means placing herself in Brad's agonistic pattern and that remaining submissive would create a self-feeding interpersonal cycle. Brad despises, the other submits, and he despises even more.

The therapist maintains a firm stance and anchors herself to solid self-esteem, neither submitting nor prevaricating: "Excuse me, Brad, let's start from an important point. You cannot treat me with contempt. It is a matter of respect, and it must be mutual." Brad tries to talk over her, but the therapist interrupts him,

No, let me talk. This tone is of no use to me, nor to you. You brought me a problem, and I've been doing my job. If it was nonsense, we could just not talk about it, but if you talk about it, you leave me the opportunity to intervene. Then, I can also talk nonsense, but not always. It's also okay for you to criticize me; for goodness sake, that's fine, but you do it systematically, and this tone is not good in a working relationship. I need to understand why it comes so naturally to you to devalue. Moreover, I don't understand why, if everything I say is nonsense, you keep coming. What's going on?

Warning: this is a thoughtful intervention, not an impulsive one. Not confronting Brad with this firmness would have maintained a pattern based on crystallized roles of dominance and submission that prevented the transition to any healing operation. The therapist knows that waiting in silence for Brad to be lenient or hoping to do the right thing and be approved would have been futile, just as with her mother. The goal of her intervention was not to overrule the patient but to pass the passive-into-active relational test: Brad despised the other, whereas, in the past, he had been mocked and humiliated. The therapist, metacommunicating assertively, breaks the pattern, and Brad changes his attitude. He admits that he has been defiant and that he is used to this, even with his girlfriend. Now, a gap has opened that is possible to explore. Brad understands that his aggression is defensive: "Mock first because if not the other person will humiliate you." This is the beginning of change.

PART II

The therapeutic contract

In PD therapy, it is crucial to have a clear and explicit therapeutic contract. It is necessary, for example, to counteract self-harming acts in borderline PD (Linehan, 1993) or to counteract passivity and social withdrawal in various PDs from borderline to narcissistic (Caligor et al., 2019; Dimaggio, 2022; Links et al., 2015; Magistrale et al., 2024).

For therapy to be effective and the relationship to be stable, it is necessary for contract negotiation to be continuous. That's right: continuous. This is one of the cornerstones of treatment, especially in PD. What prompts us to state it so clearly? Too often, in supervision, even experienced colleagues tell us about patients who do not progress, in whom symptoms and relational problems persist and seem unassailable. They try, with zeal and enthusiasm, to use experiential techniques. But the patients do nothing; they do not move a step. The colleagues try to get them active, break the automatisms dictated by patterns, and look for more incisive and creative ways to apply the techniques after using them without benefit. They insist on behavioral tasks that, yes, are necessary, but patients show no intention of putting them into practice or declare themselves willing but do not move a finger during the session. Nothing works.

Frustration draws therapists into dysfunctional interpersonal cycles. More reticence and passivity on the part of the patient induces more alertness in the therapist, who insists on trying change, which causes the patient to feel judged and misunderstood and thus close down and protest, making the therapist more frustrated and irritated. A spiral that results in stalling and, at times, drop out.

Why do colleagues repeat mistakes, with the only result being that they leave the session tense, nervous, and loaded with every negative idea possible about themselves and the patient? The solution is before their eyes. Have they not asked themselves: "But does the patient share with me the same purpose and the same path to achieve that purpose?" And, if they have asked, they have forgotten one of the basic principles of cognitive therapies: that the answer must come from the patient. Not from one's own internal dialogue.

If therapists do not pay almost manic attention to the explicit sharing of goals and tasks with some patients, especially with PD, it is inevitable that they will lose a realistic sense of efficacy: they will swing dramatically between the poles of omnipotence and impotence. Especially the latter, in fact. They will either turn on their heels or become demoralized; either way, they will spin out of control and lose their therapeutic bearings.

At all times, the therapist must identify what direction would lead to the patient's good. But even more, he must ask himself, "Does the patient understand this? Does he agree with it? Is he going to implement the necessary actions?" At this point, he must ask the patient these questions: "How do you imagine therapy will help you? Are you going to do anything to get better? Do you want to become a therapist between sessions?"

But why do patients not enter therapy with goals they really want to achieve? After all, they are suffering, and it would be natural for them to try to ease the pain. So, if they have a reasonable purpose, why do they not take action to achieve it?

Why do patients not adopt an active position?

The reasons why patients fail to determine therapy goals or engage in tasks are (Dimaggio & Valentino, 2024):

(a) *Impaired metacognitive monitoring.* Deciding a direction requires awareness of the internal world: knowing what causes suffering and why, and knowing one's desires (von Below, 2020). If patients recount pain vaguely, without naming emotions accurately, and without understanding the cause-and-effect links between thoughts, emotions, and behaviors, it will be difficult to understand what therapy should aim for. If they do not know their desires, the problem is the same: where do we take them if they do not know where to go? In these cases, the therapist must stop pushing toward health and work on metacognitive monitoring. Only when the aims have emerged can he work to achieve them.

(b) *Disagreement on goals.* Sometimes, the problem lies in the goals of therapy. Therapists believe that, to overcome relational problems, it is essential to go in a certain direction. Patients, however, find such goals senseless or contrary to their values. Those suffering from narcissistic PD, for example, consider the goal of devoting time and energy to activities that will not lead them to the lost Olympus to be meaningless. To many, the idea of taking time away from suffering partners or family members seems immoral despite the fact that compulsive caregiving clearly causes their suffering. Those who adhere strictly to religious beliefs may not consider options such as stopping sacrificing or separating viable. In these cases, the contract is essential. Therapists must validate and respect patients' goals and, at the same time, bluntly show that pursuing them has negative consequences for their psychological health. It will then be necessary to renegotiate the contract and define goals that patients feel are their own and that therapists consider reasonable and beneficial, with the understanding that the effectiveness of the treatment will be limited to the areas that are actively worked on.

(c) *Maladaptive patterns: the image of the therapist.* Therapy works when patients have a view of the therapists that is, at least in part, positive. In more severe PDs, trust and esteem are often jeopardized. Patients may question the therapist's good faith and professional abilities, as well as his or her sincere interest. Sometimes, unfortunately, they may be right in reality, but here we are referring to patients whose patterns foresee *tout court* that the other person deceives, manipulates, and is incompetent, disinterested, or cynical. In all such cases, the therapist must refrain from setting any therapeutic goal. That would be risky for him because it would give the patient the opportunity to devalue him, despise him, or protest the ineffectiveness of a therapy that he actually hinders. The therapist must limit himself to working on the therapeutic relationship, and only when at least partly positive patterns emerge can he seek shared goals. Since patterns are pervasive in these cases, it is important that the therapist not view such arrangements as stable. It is wiser for him to see them for what they are, houses built on sand, which will easily collapse at the first storm. At this point, he patiently goes back to working on the relationship and looking for room to return to the same purposes or to define new ones.

(d) *Maladaptive patterns: self-image.* In previous cases, the patients' attention was focused on the other, the therapist. Here, the focus is on the self-image. For therapy to work, patients need to have stored in their repertoire of memories and schemas of action at least some positive ideas of self. Remember that a schema is almost always supported by a negative image that obscures, most of the time, the positive image (Chapter 2). However, the latter exists, is accessible, and at various times surfaces and controls the action. There are patients in whom the negative image is so intense and dominant that it leaves little room for benevolent views/images. Or the latter are really lacking, sometimes absent altogether. In these cases, the patient is moved by pain, but he is driven by crystallized images of himself as incurable, unlovable, radically inferior, and powerless. On this basis, he can only construct the therapist as useless, distant, judgmental, or powerless in turn. The core problem, however, is precisely the negative self-image. In this situation, there is no point in thinking about the contract. The therapist can only work to try to bring out a minimum of positive self-image to serve as a starting block to make at least a few steps and counteract the suffering. Until a positive image emerges, the therapist can only be a witness to the pain for the time of the session, at most mildly soothing, and must not promise anything else.

(e) *Focus on others as the sole source of the problem and lack of agency over the internal world.* A very frequent problem is that for patients the sole cause of their pain is others (Dimaggio & Valentino, 2024; Magistrale et al., 2024). They do not take into consideration that suffering and problems depend in part on reality, certainly, but this is not what brought them to therapy. Their turning to the therapist is thus just an accusation of the other or a desperate plea for the other to bring about change so that they can finally be well, free themselves, and be autonomous. It is the "the other does to me" and "if only the other," and the only seemingly more evolved version, "the other makes me feel" modes that invariably accompany repetitive interpersonal thinking. Underlying them is the perception of the self as passive, powerless, and unable to influence the world. Patients in this setup come to the therapist with the idea or expectation that he or she will change them but without offering him or her any leverage to effect transformation. Many therapists become paralyzed when confronted with the question, typical of those with this attitude, "Doctor, you have to tell me you are the expert." The therapist must know that the answer is very simple: "No, therapy doesn't work that way." Of course, said in a calm and gentle but firm manner. He has to explain that psychotherapy is not like other professions where we ask the expert for the solution, and he provides it. And actually, even in situations where the client-professional relationship is more defined, collaboration is necessary. Think of someone who asks a financial lawyer for help but does not tell him what he is aiming for or what amount he wants to receive, and above all, does not bring him the papers. Think of a patient who goes to the doctor for an infection but does not want to take antibiotics. In such cases, the therapist will first have to explain that therapy requires that the focus be on changing the internal world. And that the goal is clear, wanted by both of you, and that the path is concrete and decided by both of you. The therapist proposes and assesses whether the paths envisioned are viable, whether they lead in the desired direction, and what risks and obstacles they conceal. However, therapy begins when the patient decides to go down this road.

Let us now see how to define and continuously update the therapeutic contract.

Define the purposes

The therapist must understand what the *patient* wants to achieve. The purpose of therapy must never be left implicit! From the first moment of the first session, and then on a regular basis, the therapist must ask, "Did you come to me because you need to be helped to . . .?" A good question ends with a series of dots. And frequently, in session after session, the therapist will still ask the same question, either when it seems that goals change or if the patient is talking without a goal in mind, perhaps brooding.

In the first case, the therapist begins by summarizing the points agreed upon up to that point. She then introduces the new topic:

Now you're talking to me about X . . . do you want this to become the topic we focus on? If so, let's think again about the goals we would like to achieve together and what we can do to achieve them.

In the second case, when the patient speaks ruminatively, as we saw in the first part of the chapter, the therapist, with timeliness, emphasizes the theme of the discourse: "You are again telling me that your wife is jealous, obsessive, doubting you, and asking you a thousand questions." Then she notes this is not a new topic and formulates the decisive question that the therapist must know by heart: "But it is something you have told me many times before; it is information that you have, and I have; we both remember it. So, are you telling me about it today in order to . . .?"

Here again, the decisive part is the suspension dots. It involves inviting the patient to move from purposeless telling, except from continuing to ruminate, to becoming active and engaging with the therapist in shared work aimed at an explicit goal. Therapy finds direction only after the patient shows signs of wanting to become active toward a goal.

Clarify the emotional costs that change requires

The therapist must always keep in mind that one of the reasons patients remain imprisoned in their psychopathology is to protect themselves from psychic pain. Healing means accepting and experiencing a share of suffering without letting it overwhelm you while pursuing healthy goals. Overcoming emotional dependence and leaving a partner who, in a manifest way, is a source of dissatisfaction means exposing oneself to loneliness and the idea of not coping. Emerging from isolation requires facing the risk of critical judgment, of looking bad, of shame. To become autonomous, we must overcome feelings of guilt at the idea that the other is suffering – "I can't get away from my mother, she would be too hurt" – or the fear of retaliation – "If I go out with friends, she will be angry, she will give me a load of accusations and protests." The patient may not necessarily want to pay these costs.

We, therefore, need to ask the patient what he is willing to do to overcome problems and symptoms, break free from dysfunctional relationships, and gain freedom of action and choice.

Sharing a commitment to take action toward health

What are the steps to follow? The first step is to agree explicitly and in detail on the goal; it is the *goal* component of *the alliance* (Bordin, 1979): what goal is both desired by the patient and realistic in the eyes of the therapist?

The second step is the joint definition of the tasks necessary to achieve the goal, the *task* component of *the alliance*. Here it is a matter of showing the patient that there is a means-end relationship. Achieving health does not happen only through a change in cognitive perspective, a new arrangement in the therapeutic relationship. It requires acting in daily life in a way that brings one closer to the goal.

Therapists must make sure that patients' attention is focused on the path ahead. When they are certain, through explicit consent and congruent non-verbal signals, they will draw on the map, together with patients, the road to health. By explaining that along the way a quota of pain will emerge, but that immediately beyond it will appear the possibility of fulfilling one's desires, and one will find more health and greater freedom. If patients stop in the face of pain, this will remain, for longer or shorter.

The third step is to show the benefits and costs of healthy actions. Therapists must be optimistic, confident, and realistic at the same time:

> You want autonomy and to follow your own choices. To do so, it will be inevitable to say no to others' demands. It is impossible, as it were, to have it both ways. Saying no will be healthy; it will allow you to achieve something you care deeply about. But it is inevitable that it will come at a cost: disappointing your father and making your mother suffer, and this will make you feel bad and see yourself as a bad, ungrateful son. Unfortunately, it is inevitable; these are ideas and feelings that anyone would have. In part, they are normal, indicating that you feel affection for your dear ones. But if you decide to protect yourself from these emotions and the idea of being bad, you won't become autonomous. You will remain stuck waiting for permission that does not come, will continue to complain about your parents' attitude, to protest, to claim freedom of action that you first do not give yourself. It is a matter of choosing to pay that transitional price. Then, of course, when those painful ideas and feelings emerge, I will be there; we will work to make them harmless and put them aside. But a period of pain will be inevitable. What do you think? Do you feel up to taking that step?

This same principle applies to all therapeutic goals and to every area of suffering. It, therefore, applies to symptom treatment: "To get out of depression, it is necessary not to ruminate, and I need you to have the intention not to ruminate"; "To reduce anxiety, it is necessary that we engage in reducing avoidance. Do you want to try that?" It applies to work functioning:

> I understand that you are skeptical of the offers and possibilities in front of you. However, how can I help you find a job that will satisfy you if you don't try? Do you feel up to showing up for a job interview?

It applies, finally, to relationship problems:

> You can't find a partner who leaves you satisfied. I realize that it is as if you are looking for the perfect partner. This leads you to consider all the girls with whom a relationship might blossom inadequate, and lately, you have been isolating himself. I cannot promise that you will find a relationship that will make her happy. But by staying at home or rejecting all of them immediately, we certainly don't stand a chance. What about if you try and give yourself a chance, and when the next relationship starts, you try and resist the urge to end it right away?

The therapeutic contract, therefore, is an irreplaceable tool for overcoming deadlocks and helping the patient not to lose confidence or enter states of frustration, guilt, shame, anxiety, or helplessness. Above all, it is decisive in promoting agency.

Letizia, 50, suffers from dependent PD and major depression. She begins each session like this: "Everything as usual, nothing new," as her face, voice, and posture disclose sadness, devitalization, and passivity. As always, over the weekend, she stayed at home ruminating, fueling negative emotions and a lonely and inadequate self-image. In previous sessions, she has learned, through attentional techniques (we will see these in chapter viii), that it is within her power not to ruminate and to choose alternative content to pay attention to. She knows that she ruminates because she is guided by a specific purpose: to reassure herself that she has done everything possible so that her father and mother do not separate permanently, breaking up the family she comes from. She knows that not ruminating would make her feel better and, more importantly, allow her to invest in the profession she is laboriously pursuing hundreds of miles from her hometown. She also knows that to stop ruminating when thoughts regarding family surface makes her feel guilty; not thinking about her parents means neglecting them. But again, the weekend brings back the repetitive thought processes that fuel depression and freeze her plans. In short, she has ruminated all weekend and did not even attempt to curb IRT. Is it helpful for the therapist to use one technique for the umpteenth time or adopt others? No. Is it useful for him to change the subject? It would not work. It is necessary to rephrase the contract:

> Excuse me, Letizia, how do we get out of depression if you don't decide to stop ruminating? How do you think you are better off if you don't give up the purpose of monitoring what might happen to your parents, accepting that you feel guilty because you dare to think of something else, even something good?

Some might object: "But you, by doing so, are asking the patient to do what she cannot do; you are transferring the responsibility for her own discomfort onto her." This is not so; the crux is different. Letizia already understands the nature of her problems and has developed the skills necessary to get better. The techniques have been effective, but the patterns are less pervasive in many areas. Now, however, residual change is in her hands, but it comes at a cost: feeling transiently guilty. The therapist is not asking her to use tools unfamiliar to her, but to declare whether she is going to use them and deal with the guilt! The therapist cannot relieve her from paying this toll, and if he tries to protect her, he is wrong; he is promoting chronicity.

The therapist is not conveying to her the idea that it is normal and human to disregard the family she comes from. On the contrary, he validates it: that she feels guilt is natural; it is a sign of intact affectivity. The problem is that giving in to guilt supports action paralysis, which leads to the devitalization and depression she would like to get rid of.

The therapist must leverage the patient's agency and ask her if she is going to take steps toward health or continue to act out of guilt. The therapist should pay attention: now Letizia is no longer acting out automatisms. She is making a conscious decision to sacrifice herself not to feel guilty. It is a deliberate choice. Fortunately, Letizia chooses the path of health and accepts pursuing autonomous goals while feeling guilty. As a result, she soon emerges from depression.

A key principle of MIT sounds like this: the goal of therapy is not to change the patient but to help the patient build a mental model of the mechanisms underlying his or her suffering. If the patient has this model of self in mind, now the therapist must check whether the former has the conscious intention to use it as a map for action and change.

The idea that therapeutic change is all in the corrective emotional experience (Alexander & French, 1946) seems naive to us. Even if the therapeutic relationship, after initial problems, becomes good, repairing developmental pains, the patient does not heal except in rare and fortunate cases.

Disrupting schema-dependent actions in daily life happens only through the intention to act differently. This requires commitment, training, and repetition. An explicit therapeutic contract is needed to verify that the patient intends to apply himself continuously to get better.

Passively recounting pain to an immobile witness or engaging in soothing it?

Another frequent case is when patients recount, in session after session, objectively painful events, such as separations, bereavements, and betrayals undergone. After validating and normalizing the suffering, the question the therapist has to ask sounds something like this: "I understand your bitterness; these are universally painful experiences, and it is good that you shared it with me. I wonder, though: are you telling me about it yet again today because this is useful for . . .?"

As we have seen, it is a question that the therapist continually asks when the patient tells him facts he has already told him and makes him aware of events he already knows. This question also aims to formulate the contract.

The therapist emphasizes to the patient that the latter is holding him in the position of a static and powerless witness. And that this position leaves the patient in passivity. He then asks him if he is going to access a problem-solving mode, focused no longer on past events but on what can be done to change things after the session, during the following week.

It is an intervention that we already mentioned a little while ago, but it is so important that we repeat it:

I hear the pain and I see it, and I am close to it. I'm just wondering – you're telling me something that we already know, it's information that we shared, right? Are we repeating it because telling it is still useful for . . .?

After these suspension dots, therapists must wait because the continuation of therapy is now in the hands of the patients, who may also decide to use therapy as an outlet space, where they seek only a benevolent listening ear. Patients may decide to continue ruminating, and therapists can certainly accept that. However, patients will have to do so consciously and intentionally, aware of the consequences. That is, the persistence of subjective suffering and relational problems! One may even come to share the purpose of non-action: "I don't want to do anything about it; I simply want to tell you that I am in pain, and it is important to me, doctor, that you listen to me." We repeat that this is not wrong; the difference being that, again, it is a joint and explicit purpose: therapist and patient know what they are doing and why, and that, under these conditions, the therapist does not promise healing.

The psychoeducational component of the therapeutic contract

A somewhat psychoeducational and motivational component is present in the contract. For example, in narcissism, the rank system dominates, so it is common for the patient to be exalted by his or her own successes and dejected by failures. What is often lacking is acceptance of the link between effort/commitment and success in the task. The narcissistic patient cannot be expected to know this on his or her own or to arrive at it through an epiphany arising from looking at the furniture in the therapy room. It is something that must be explained, accompanied by universal or personal examples. Nothing is achieved except through perseverance and tolerance of frustration, not even therapeutic change. It must be said explicitly, and then the therapist comes back to ask, "Are you up to it?" (Dimaggio, 2022; Dimaggio & Valentino, 2024).

In relational dependency, however, the attachment system dominates at the expense of exploration. Patients perceive vitality and a sense of direction only in the presence of their partner, while in his or her absence, they experience emptiness and shutdown. It should be explained to these patients that it is difficult to have a fulfilling, solid, mutually respectful relationship if one is unable to independently pursue goals, desires, and interests. Again, we state this and then immediately ask, "Do you feel able to act on this goal? knowing that this initially might make you feel lonely, purposeless, disoriented?"

The internal structure of the therapist

Negotiating the contract is, based on what we observe in supervision, extremely difficult for the majority of therapists. A large majority. What frame of mind should we assume when we formulate the contract? In the meantime, it is necessary to avoid competing and to care; we must not burden ourselves with omnipotent responsibility.

Many therapists are convinced about cooperating: they explain the problem to patients, explain to them what to do, and try to motivate them to act and perform behavioral exercises during the week. In fact, they are in the rank system, guided by a kind of benevolent paternalism: "Listen to what I tell you, it's good for you, believe me." Or, they act like a loving but actually controlling mother: "Careful, on that road, you're going to get hurt; you're going to stop first, aren't you?" The problem is that when the patient does not move, these therapists go into crisis, swing between frustration and guilt, and get irritated. We repeat: it is not the cooperative system. It is rank!

The cooperative system requires drawing together the boundary of the game and its rules (in other words, therapeutic goals and necessary actions) and then asking, "Do you feel like playing? That is, do you feel like doing what is necessary?" True cooperation requires the therapist to wait for the answer and especially to contemplate that that answer may be 'no'. At this point, they have to reformulate the contract and explain that saying no is all very well, but therapists cannot promise progress and relief from pain.

Another problematic therapist attitude concerns the sense of paralysis. In the face of the patient's suffering and immobility, they feel powerless. And to this helplessness, they react by activating themselves, even though the patient has given no sign or intention of making a move. This helplessness should instead be accepted with serenity.

We call it *leaning forward helplessness*. It is an attitude that requires being present and, as much as possible, warmth. It means showing the patient that we are with him whatever. We declare that we do not know how to act; we show ourselves waiting for the patient's intention to change. At the same time, we are leaning precisely toward the patient:

> I am with you; I am with you even if you decide to persist in actions that give you pain. I don't promise you well-being, but I'm here; I just ask you if that's what you want, my presence when you suffer, or are you asking me to help you change?

It is not easy to take this position. At such moments, therapists come to terms with emotions that drive them towards action. They experience rank-related anger when patients are disappointed and devalue them: "I thought psychotherapy would be of some use, but I realize it's just words." Or they experience frustration and anger when patients continue to pursue maladaptive goals: "Yes, we agreed I would try to get out of the house, but then I stayed home with Mom." They may experience shame when, in the face of patients' immobility, they consider themselves ineffective and unprepared.

It is common for them to be anxious about failing, about losing their reputation if patients get worse or leave therapy, even to the point of fearing professional ruin: "Colleagues will think I'm poor and won't send me any more patients." It is easy for therapists to feel guilty at the idea that, because of their inability, patients will continue to suffer or hurt those around them.

The contract can fall apart in various ways when addressing problem behaviors and severe symptoms such as, for example, eating disorders, substance abuse, behavioral addictions, and aggression. However, the spirit remains the same: explicitly define the goals and the tools needed to achieve them. This will make it easier:

(a) to build and maintain the working alliance and repair it if ruptures occur;

b) to increase treatment adherence and commitment to treatment goals;

c) to prevent the therapist's contribution to interpersonal cycles and, if they are activated nevertheless, recognize and interrupt them;

d) to empower agency by verifying that the patient has made a conscious decision to discontinue the use of coping: "Would you like to try to resist when the urge to . . .?"

e) bring out the healthy parts no longer overwhelmed by passivity, resignation, or protest.

Chapter 4

Decision-making and relational procedures

Shared formulation of functioning

The shared formulation

One of the elements on which psychotherapy, in general, and for PD, in particular, should be based is a correct case formulation (Critchfield et al., 2022; Gazzillo et al., 2022; Kramer, 2019). In MIT, we add: the pillar of clinical action is a formulation that is both correct and *shared*. In other words, a formulation that is right but localized only in the therapist's mind is useless. The reason is that the patient, to change personality structures, must act deliberately and consciously.

Patients can only engage in the necessary activities if they have a clear, explicit model of how their own mental functioning triggers suffering and dysfunctional behavior. A model that includes pathological and healthy aspects. With such a model, they can decide to operate to interrupt the pathology-maintaining circuits and move in the direction of well-being.

MIT (Dimaggio et al., 2015, 2020) therapeutic work revolves around the idea that first the formulation is shared and only on this basis is change made. There are two macro-areas: *shared formulation of functioning* and *promotion of change*.

In this volume, we show how the steps of the procedures are a) accompanied possibly by the use of experiential techniques; b) performed under the continuous monitoring of the therapeutic relationship and its ruptures, which, if they occur, the therapist acts promptly to repair (Muran & Eubanks, 2020; Safran & Muran, 2000).

We describe how to interweave decision-making procedures with experiential techniques. Therapists:

- execute each action from an accurate, detailed case formulation shared with patients and updated continuously;
- propose an experiential technique after assessing the state of the alliance;
- continually make sure that patients have understood the purpose of the technique and share it;
- assess whether patients have consciously decided to engage in the experiential practice or task and whether they state this explicitly;
- attempt to predict whether the technique will push patients toward health or, conversely, whether it might confirm dysfunctional ideas about relationships;

DOI: 10.4324/9781003570967-4

- monitor the alliance from the time they propose the technique, during its implementation and immediately afterward;
- as soon as they notice signs of relationship breakdown, they first interrupt other actions, then bring it to patients' attention, and begin the work aimed at repairing it.

Each step in the procedure is accompanied by an assessment of the interaction between the technique the therapist is proposing or performing and the therapeutic relationship. As already shown and as we will repeat again and again throughout this volume, apart from where the technique does not have a significant impact on the alliance (it happens!), there are five possible patterns:

1. The same proposal or initiation of execution generates a major rupture that should be repaired while the use of the technique should be suspended;
2. Patients initially accept the technique and prepare to practice or initiate it, but while preparing or during its execution, experience negative effects that generate a rupture in the relationship. Again, therapists stop the exercise and work on the therapeutic relationship until the rupture is repaired and the technique can be continued;
3. The proposal of the technique or its execution generates transient negative emotions and thoughts, so that a relational micro-rupture is created, but this does not require stopping the experiential work. At the end of the practice, the relationship is consolidated or strengthened;
4. The experiential technique reinforces the therapeutic relationship either from the proposal itself or during its execution;
5. The experiential technique generates improvement in symptoms or behaviors as early as the end of its execution or during the weeks following the session. Patients' trust in the therapist increases, and the therapeutic relationship is strengthened.

What does shared formulation mean?

That case formulation is the operation on which treatment should be based is an idea held by many (Critchfield et al., 2022; Kramer, 2019) and divides therapies based on careful reflection on the individual patient's functioning from protocolized therapies. It goes without saying that MIT ranks among the former: it is a manualized and empirically supported but not protocolized therapy.

Instead, it is rarer that therapists pay attention to the keyword: *shared.* The vast majority of colleagues spend mental energy and time formulating the case in the confines of their own minds. They are guided by the implicit idea that the onerous task of figuring out how the patient works and guiding him or her toward health is up to them. They take on their shoulders the burden of understanding the patient's functioning, often without having obtained the necessary information or without having simply noted that that information is currently lacking. Based on this intellectual work, which is often exhausting, they try to explain to the patient what they themselves struggle to understand.

It does not work this way.

The logic of the shared formulation is as follows:

a) one must construct a model of the patient's mind that accurately accounts for the subjective experience and psychological reasons for suffering and dysfunctional behavior;
b) one must first verify that patients recognize such a model as plausible; that is, that they see themselves reflected and recognize the elements of the formulation as their own. The next step is to verify that patients feel that the model is correct on a subjective level. This is not an operation in which therapists can rely on intuition. In fact, they must avoid relying on their own judgment. Instead, they must ask clear and focused questions. Only if patients respond with a clear, convinced yes, accompanied by congruent non-verbal signals, can the clinician consider the formulation truly agreed upon;
c) the model must guide treatment planning and easily connect to the actions needed to move toward wellness, both in patients' and therapists' minds. In other words, the shared formulation is not meant to lead patients to say "Okay, I see that I work this way," but "I see that I work this way, I can do something to change, and I'm going to try."

The first operation in the shared formulation is to attempt to identify with patients, moment by moment, the elements of internal experience: thoughts, emotions, somatic correlates, and fluctuations in arousal. *Together* means that if therapists deduce from verbal and non-verbal cues that patients experience guilt, they ask them, "From your story, facial expression and voice, I seem to infer that you have given up going to the party through feeling guilty about leaving your mother alone, is that correct?"

In metacognitive terms, this is an intervention that promotes the monitoring of thoughts and emotions, guilt, and attempts to get patients to establish a simple cause-and-effect link:

I wanted to go to the party, but I thought that, if I did, my mother would be sick. At that point, I saw myself hurting her and thought I would be a bad son. I felt guilty and gave up.

If such an intervention is successful, it is not because the therapist formulated it intelligently. Mind you, it may indeed be so; the therapist's psychological intuition and deductive skills may have led him or her to hit the mark. However, MIT does not consider this the definitive formulation.

The formulation is successful when, to the question "Is my observation correct? Does it correspond to your subjective experience?" patients answer with a firm, fully conscious "yes," accompanied by congruent non-verbal markers. In the event that therapists fail to check whether patients have made the formulation their own, they are, from that moment on, acting on the basis of a map of the patients' mind that is theirs alone. They are, consequently, preparing themselves for a series of frustrations when they discover that patients do not make the desired progress.

The formulation, therefore, must be shared at every step and always consistent with the patient's metacognitive abilities, from the lowest to the highest.

If the intervention is "You seem angry," and the patient responds, "I don't know, I'm tense," it means that already at this basic level the formulation is not shared. Consequently, the only sensible work, apart from symptomatic or regulatory work if necessary, is to increase emotional monitoring (Bateman & Fonagy, 2004).

At a higher level, let us imagine that clinicians try to determine what triggered a fluctuation between mental states, a first attempt at integration,

> You were excited about the journey you were about to embark on; you told me enthusiastically about it last session. Now, you are less motivated; it almost seems as if you care less. Could it be because of the problems with your husband or the fact that he criticized you? Let's say that the criticism you received is as if it has, I don't know, taken you apart? Almost as if you were no longer convinced of your own desire.

If the patient replies, "Yeah, maybe, I don't know, I'm kind of over it, that's it," the hypothesis has fallen on deaf ears. It was probably correct but not usable. The next step is not to push the patient toward wish fulfillment but to learn about aspects of internal functioning that are obscure at this time. How come she cannot describe her mental state? Are there other contents of the experience other than those hypothesized? Is a relational rupture in progress?

Only when the patient comes, for example, to say "Yes, I realize that when I am criticized, I get turned off, and what used to seem important to me becomes insignificant, to the point where I no longer know whether I like it or not," will the map of her inner world really be shared. This is a reliable guide for traveling to health.

The most problematic passage for clinicians, the one in which the word *shared* escapes attention, is when they attempt to summarize various episodes by organizing them according to the schema structure. It is an intellectually demanding effort, and often, in the end, the patient agrees with the description. At this point, therapists are convinced that patients are aware that they are being guided by a schema. In other words, therapists believe that patients are differentiating, gaining critical distance from their own ideas about themselves and others to the point that they consider them not true but schema-dependent. This is almost always not the case.

Warning: the real differentiation is as follows. At first, patients think "I wish to be appreciated, but, if I show my real abilities, the other person despises me and is right because I am incapable." Later, thanks to therapeutic work, they are able to say

> I realize that whenever I seek the other person's approval, I pay attention to every sign of criticism, and I believe it is because I have this idea of being incapable that doesn't go away, it's hard to get rid of it.

As can be seen, patients partly still believe the schema-related ideas, but they have gained a perspective from which they realize that they are not necessarily true. They would sincerely like to consolidate the new, more benevolent reading, but they find it difficult. With this awareness, change operations are possible.

Clinicians, on the other hand, very often mistake this thought for schema awareness: "I wish to be appreciated, but when I show my real abilities, the other person despises me, I feel ashamed, at which point I isolate myself and stop pursuing my goals." Patients describe themselves in a well-organized way and using the schema structure, but therapists mistakenly convince themselves that the former also know that they are describing a schema and not reality.

It is not true differentiation. It is just a high level of metacognitive monitoring, coupled with some capacity for integration. Patients, in fact, continue to adhere to their own ideas, know their own way of reacting to relational events, but take the other person's criticism at face value and remain anchored in the belief that they feel ashamed because they really are defective and inferior. They do not, therefore, assume an alternative perspective.

If the therapist does not realize that such a patient is still guided by the schema, that he still believes that his own negative ideas about himself and others are true, he will be making a mistake. The therapist is convinced that the formulation is shared and is deluding himself.

We show two examples below. In the first, the therapist is convinced that the patient has realized that she is schema-driven, proposes change operations to her, and fails because the patient took the schema-dependent ideas as true. The therapeutic contract (Chapter 3) was thus missing. The second is, on the other hand, an example of real differentiation, and so the intervention succeeds.

Julia, a journalist, is 31 years old and has entered treatment for binge eating and dependent PD. She is consumed by perfectionism and a sense of abandonment. The root is in the memories of her depressed mother, whose eyes only sparkled when Julia told of getting A's in school. Her father was harsh and strict, which also contributed to her perfectionism. Moreover, the father would wake up in the middle of the night crying after separating from his wife, waking his daughter, and desperately begging her to talk to her mother and ask her to get back together. Julia would remain dismayed and frightened, with the idea that no one cared for her and that she was alone. The central wish thus appears to be related to the attachment system, but Julia is prey to rank-related rumination, and only gaining approval matters to her. Moreover, because of her perfectionism, exploration is paralyzed, and the therapist attempts to promote it. He is guided by the idea of promoting exploration, helping Julia to give space to her creative part and leaving aside the wrong and disgusting idea of herself when she is not perfect.

Julia has an idea for a book she would like to write; she cares about it, and she feels it is hers. She recounts one of the many moments when she faces the blank page. She starts writing and, after a while, tears up the sheets; every smudge is intolerable, and "It sucks." At the slightest mistake, she despises herself. Starting again is so exhausting that she stops writing, and therapy is blocked.

The therapist is convinced, therefore, about supporting the exploratory system and intellectual creativity. At various times, the part of Julia that believes in the idea of the book surfaces, accompanied by very positive feelings. It is a healthy self-representation that, however, quickly slips into the shadows since, in the face of vital momentum, Julia does not encounter another who encourages and supports her. Instead, in her mind, she encounters a mocking gaze in the mold of developmental memories related to her harsh and stern father and her depressed mother, who could not give her attention and locked in her suffering.

In the story with her first boyfriend, new memories are formed that consolidate representations of self with the other: "We were on the boardwalk and he was looking at girls and saying, 'Holy Mother, what I would get up to with that one!" This leads her to focus her sense of imperfection on physical appearance and then to extend it to other areas.

By now, Julia has internalized this look in the form of fierce self-criticism. The contemptuous eye deactivates exploration and triggers rank. With respect to this motivation, Julia barely accesses the idea of worth, remaining flooded with sadness, despondency, and shame, which indicates how the nuclear self-image is "wrong/defective." When such an image emerges, Julia resorts to obsessive and exhausting perfectionism coping, devoting herself to endless corrections. Even the *perfected self,* however, keeps encountering a dismissive other, and this consumes her energy, and Julia gives up. The sense of failure and helplessness is at its peak; the primary wish of exploration and the secondary wish of rank remain frustrated.

The therapist assesses that Julia, having awareness of what she is feeling and thinking and what activates her, and having associated congruent memories, realizes that she is pattern-driven. He points out to her how, when she gets stuck in front of a Word document, she is convinced that she is defective and oscillates between renunciation and ruthless perfectionism. Julia sees herself in the description: "Yes, that's me, that's right."

The therapist explains to her that to overcome this negative idea, "it would be helpful for you to expose yourself to sustainable doses of imperfection, trying not to give up and anchor yourself in your vital aspects." Once again, Julia agrees.

At this point, he offers her a guided imagery and rescripting exercise. He anchors her to memories in which she is curious and creative, then leads her to recall a moment when she notices an error in her writing. Julia's reaction is startling; she dissociates: "My legs have become gigantic, my shoulders are tight, my head is tiny, my stomach gigantic." She sees herself as flawed, wrong, and deformed: these are the body images she had at the beginning of therapy that were connected to binge eating, and now they resurface. The therapist uses regulatory tools, but they do not work.

What happened? The therapist finds out by only now completing the cognitive inquiry that would have been necessary before beginning imagery.

T: "Julia, I would like to understand, but you, the idea of being defective, how much do you believe in it?"

J: "Completely."

Only in a few good moments in the session does she believe that she is of worth and entitled to create, but negative beliefs dominate. It was not, therefore, the imagery that had a transient iatrogenic effect but the fact that it was performed without the formulation of the schema really being shared. Julia entered imagery thinking, "I am disgusting," an idea with an untenable reality value. From this point on, the therapist carefully monitors the degree of belief in the negative idea, and it will take months for Julia to begin to understand that it was a schema and to have faith in the idea of being of worth. Only then will imagery exercises prove useful.

Above all, Julia comes to realize that perfectionism was the only way to ensure proximity with her parents, who were in effect unavailable and so caught up in their pains. At this point, therapy shifts to the frustrated nuclear wish, attachment, connected to the image of being destined for loneliness, as in childhood.

Let us now look at a case in which the therapist correctly assesses how much the patient shared the pattern before involving her in experiential work. Veronica is 50 years old and suffers from narcissistic PD and emotional dependence. She fears her husband will abandon her and reports an episode in which he does not respond to a text message. She thinks, "I suck," but immediately becomes resentful and angry.

In contrast to the previous case, the therapist, before attempting rewriting, makes sure that the patient knows at this exact moment that she is being guided by a pattern.

T: "When your husband didn't text you back, you got sad; you thought you sucked, and you were ashamed, right? We've talked about this several times, and we know it's part of your story, but I still ask you: right now, what do you think about the self that doesn't get a response? Does it really suck? Right now, the impression is that, on the one hand, you are rebelling; that abandonment hurts you because you see it as unfair. But more importantly, on the other hand, it seems to me that you agree with your husband; you do think you deserve abandonment. What do you think?"

V: [*reacting with pride*]: "No, it's not fair; it makes me angry that he treats me like this."

T: "Well, so you now don't feel that you deserve abandonment, right? We can say that a part of you, on an almost physical level, feels that abandonment is her destiny, but now, in talking about it, you know that it's not really like that, that it's a pattern of yours that gets reactivated. Right?"

V: "Yes, I realize that. It's just that, when he ignores me, very primitive stuff moves around. I feel like an abandoned kitten left out in the cold."

T: "The image is strong! Look, just in case, Veronica, does a part of you feel that you are really that kitten? I mean that you have been abandoned, and, basically, it's okay because you deserve it."

V: "I feel it so much. But, no, I realize it's not really like that, it's just that the feeling is so intense."

T: "Sure. Would you like to work on that with exercises? So as to help you get rid of the idea that you deserve that sense of abandonment that often grips you?"

Veronica accepts, convinced. The therapist has her imagine being that kitten and adopting a slumped posture to the point of almost physically feeling herself. When the arousal has increased, and the feeling of being a "kitten left alone that no one cares about" is vivid and accompanied by intense sadness, the therapist invites her to stand up slowly and report how cognitions and feelings change moment by moment. Veronica comes out of the "lost kitten" character and, as she stands up, she regains a sense of worth, dignity, and relational security.

How was this experiential practice successful? Because it was based on a correct formulation! The therapist asked specific questions aimed at understanding the patient's nuclear cognitions about herself: "What do you think about your idea of . . .?" This revealed that Veronica had reached the level of differentiation necessary to attempt the first exercises aimed at change. The two tested together how much Veronica did or did not believe in her ideas about herself and the fate of her wishes. Resting on solid ground, the experiential work was effective.

Reconstructing patterns and recognizing them as such

The decision-making procedures are carried out in the following order: 1) we first describe the steps for moving progressively with patients from understanding their functioning to attempts at change; 2) we show how experiential techniques contribute to the successful achievement of each step; and 3) we show how the therapeutic relationship interacts with the techniques in the aspects of treatment described in each section. We will then refer back to the general modes of relational work described in Chapter 3, with a specific focus on the techniques-relationship interface.

PART I

Narrative episodes, awareness of internal states, and cognitive-affective-somatic processes: access to healthy parts (Figure 4.1, Box 1–5)

An underlying principle of MIT is that it starts with trying to understand what the patient is thinking and feeling (Semerari et al., 2003). This step focuses on collecting narrative episodes and exploring thoughts, emotions, and somatic states, as well as their cause-and-effect links. We describe how experiential techniques and therapeutic relationships are intertwined with the following steps.

1. Search for narrative episodes.
2. Recognition of mental states.
3. Early access to healthy parts.
4. Dynamic assessment.
5. Reconstruction of psychological cause-and-effect links.

Collecting specific autobiographical memories Box 1

Identifying the elements of subjective experience Box 2

Early access to healthy self aspects Box 3

Reconstructing psychological cause-effect links Box 4

Dynamic assessment: Behavioural homework and experiential techinques to improve monitoring Box 5

Structured summary of the episode Box 6

Evoking associated autobiographical memories, past or collected in the weeks after the session Box 7

Further exploration of inner states into associated episodes through experiential techniques Box 8

Identifying behavioural coping and repetitive thinking

Low metacognition strategies to deal with symptoms and problematic behaviors Box 13 a

Reconstructing regularities among episodes Box 9

Hypothesize that regularities correspond to underlying interpersonal schemas Box 10

Identifying which coping strategies are triggered by the response of the self to the others

Strategies to tackle coping and maladaptive behaviors when metacognition is low to medium Box 13 b

Explicity identify the core self-image and make sure patient considers it an idea and not a fact Box 11

Recognizing the shifts between healthy and maladaptive ideas about self and others Box 12

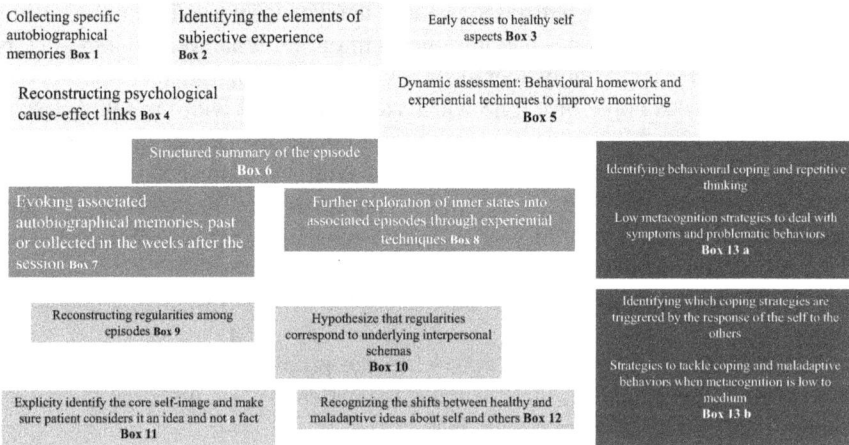

Figure 4.1 Shared formulation of functioning

The goal of these initial operations is to form a detailed, shared knowledge of the patient's internal world. In MIT, it is necessary to refer as little as possible to abstract, semantic reasoning and generalized narratives. Patients speak in terms of "That's the way I am, I have understood about me that . . . People tend to . . ."

When they then attempt to describe internal states, either while speaking abstractly or while describing specific episodes, they refer to internal experience vaguely: "I am tense, nervous, agitated, I feel discomfort, fatigue." This indicates poor monitoring of internal states. Initial operations, therefore, turn to learning about the cognitive-affective-somatic processes underlying relational problems and symptoms.

Therapists can look for them in four source areas of information about the inner world: what we metaphorically call the *four lakes*. The *first lake* is the most natural, autobiographical narrative episode. The *second lake is the* reading of non-verbal behavior. The *third lake* is a reflection on the therapeutic relationship. The *fourth lake* is the use of experiential techniques aimed at recognizing internal states, that is, dynamic assessment.

When patients do not recount episodes spontaneously but speak in an abstract, generic, intellectualized way, the therapist first engages in a conversation similar to afternoon tea talk. As it flows, she fosters an atmosphere of sharing and begins to identify cognitive-affective content. Commonly, patients begin the session with doubts such as "Why do I always choose the wrong partner?"; "Why doesn't my partner understand that I'm just worried about my parents and need to be with them?"; "I have to get it right, that's normal. If not, there are consequences. Excuse me, doctor, would you do things like hell in your job?" Therapists validate, empathize, and notice the universality of the processes described. If a patient talks about his or her work, he or she gets curious about the details and, to evoke the healthy parts, may ask what activates and intrigues him or her. Whatever the introductory theme, at the first opportunity, therapists ask for specific narrative episodes: "Can you give me an example of a time when you had to deal with the selfishness of people close to you?" Then, look for the content of the experience in the first lake.

A good narrative episode must be located with some precision in space and time. It can be accepted that the patient does not remember the exact day and often places an episode in a span of years: "I don't remember, between 9 and 11 years old, I think." These are valid answers; what matters is that the therapist reconstructs a precise scene, accompanying the patient into the details of where the interaction took place.

The episode must be about a time when the problem happens in the context of another doing something that frustrates the patient's wish, not a time when the patient expects a negative response. In the latter case, it is not an autobiographical episode. It is a recollection of a moment when the pattern was activated independently of the relationship, and, probably, the patient was already ruminating! So, if patients fear criticism, they must recount an episode in which someone criticized them. If they fear abandonment, the episode must include someone who left them alone in a time of need.

When the narrative is sufficiently detailed, therapists ask questions about thoughts and emotions and their evolution over the course of the episode. The questions are used to understand what the patient thought and felt at the moment, if he or she gives signs of activation, and what he or she thinks and feels now. It is crucial that the questions do not activate abstract reasoning, so one does not ask "Why did you act that way?" but asks, "At the moment when your colleague criticized you, what did you think, and what emotions did you experience? What prompted you at that moment to . . .?"

The investigation continues to learn about the evolution of the stream of consciousness: "When your colleague told you that she didn't give a damn about your situation, what did you think and feel? What prompted you at that moment to slam the door and leave?"

The second lake is the observation of non-verbal behavior. MIT is attentive to changes in facial expressions, tone of voice, posture, and behaviors such as arriving late, texting insistently, complacency, and so on. Our suggestion is if the therapist notices a significant non-verbal signal, make it explicit right away and do not delay for fear of hurting the patient! Point it out aloud and ask for feedback. Many therapists are afraid of hurting the patient with these actions, which are instead necessary.

If the patient says she is sad but her face expresses anger, the therapist observes, "You said you are demotivated but, I don't know, from your tone of voice, from your expression, it seems to me there is irritation in you, maybe anger, am I wrong?" Or, "You tell me it's not a problem for you to travel even though your mother is hurt, but you lowered your eyes and head, your voice hesitated. Could it be that you actually feel guilty?" It is a *contingent marking* exercise (Fonagy et al., 2018), that is, "I notice that you have this, and I tell you that you have this," is the communicative style that naturally fosters the growth of mentalistic ability in the child.

Fishing, metaphorically, in the third lake requires monitoring the relationship itself. Therapists pay attention to how patients find themselves in the relationship: Do they show signs of withdrawal? Do they shut down? Do they show dissatisfaction and refuse behavioral exercises, or do they accept them but then not even think about them at home? Do they sound resigned or critical? In parallel, therapists must watch over their own internal world: how do they position themselves vis-à-vis the patient? In a concerned and caring way? Do they act hesitantly for fear that patients will suffer or criticize them? Do they fear doing harm? Or do they fear that their actions will be misjudged by colleagues if the patient does not improve or discontinues treatment? Do they feel sympathy, dislike, disdain, sexual attraction, or are they frightened of the sexual attraction the patient displays even if not explicitly?

Therapists must get to know themselves so that they realize whether what they think and feel vis-à-vis the patient is patient-specific and whether, at that moment, they feel sufficiently regulated. If they are calm enough, this means their thoughts and emotions are true countertransference, that is, reactions to how the patient is. In this case, we are really in the third lake: the therapeutic relationship is a source of good information for understanding the patient's interpersonal patterns.

However, it is necessary for therapists to be aware of their own role because, often, it is not countertransference but the activation of their own schemas, which require recognition and modulation. In summary, once therapists, alone or with the help of supervision (chapter III), are free from the influence of their own schemas and are not contributing to the dysfunctional interpersonal cycle in session (Muran & Eubanks, 2020; Safran & Muran, 2000), the relationship provides valuable information about the patient's interpersonal schemas.

The fourth lake is located at the heart of experiential work. Paradoxically, it is an artificial lake, yet capable of providing pure, fresh, and reliable psychological material. It is about using experiential work to increase access to internal states. The fourth lake corresponds to *dynamic assessment* (Dimaggio et al., 2020). The therapist uses behavioral experiments, guided imagination, body work, two-chair play, and role-play for the sole purpose of uncovering thoughts and emotions at that moment.

All these practices have one thing in common: they increase arousal. They do this by counteracting automatisms, often hindering coping activation. The therapist brings the patient into a narrative episode through imagery by asking him or her to scan the faces and behaviors of the characters and, at the same time, to monitor the flow of thoughts and emotions: "You're looking at your boyfriend's face; what are you feeling right now?"; "Your mother is furious; you know she's about to scold you. What's happening to you at this exact moment?"; "Your parents aren't fighting yet. You're in the room and playing. Describe what it's like to touch the doll; how do you feel?"

In this way, patients discover details of experience they did not know before. Behavioral experiments with attempted abstention from coping are most useful at this stage. It is valuable, in particular, to ask for abstention from coping that is activated as a result of the self's response to the other's response: "When you see yourself being criticized, can you pause for *a moment before* giving up or reacting angrily and see what happens inside you in those moments?"

These are behavioral experiments whose sole purpose is to increase self-reflexivity: "Try not texting to ask your ex what he's doing, and note down what's going on inside"; "Next time you have the urge to cut yourself, try resisting it and record your thoughts and emotions";

> You would study until ten o'clock at night even if you were exhausted. Shall we try to cut off fifteen minutes earlier? It doesn't matter if you succeed; we just need you to try and pay attention to your inner world;
>
> When your friend asks you to go to her because she needs you to listen to her, you don't feel like it because you would like to do something else but you end up doing what you're asked. And we don't know why. When it happens again, try to resist and then you will tell me in the next session what you think and feel and what happens at the moment you are trying to say that you cannot be there for her.

These forms of refraining from coping can have both a negative and positive impact on the relationship, as shown in the classification of technique-relationship interaction patterns. On the one hand, patients perceive the usefulness of not enacting coping, become curious, and begin to realize that doing therapy means gaining power over their own mind and gaining confidence. On the other, guided by social rank, they may worry about failing and thus disappointing the therapist. Or the exercise immediately activates a pattern so that, for example, at the mere idea of saying no to her friend, the patient feels guilty and, consequently, fears that she will not do the exercise and that the therapist will judge her. In the latter case, in fact, the exercise has already had its effect; the patient is observing *live* that she is guided by an automatism, an information that the therapist can now include in the shared formulation. That is, the patient understands that the problem is not the disappointment of the real friend but her expectations that, if she is autonomous, the other will suffer, and, if she is not good, the other (the therapist) will judge her.

As regards relational breakup, the same rule always applies: the therapist asks the patient if she sees him as judgmental and if she has contributed in any way to this, and proceeds to repair the breakup.

In searching for internal states, it is crucial to pay attention to the emergence of healthy parts (Figure 4.1, Box 3). Schema formulation (Chapter I) requires the presence of positive nuclear images of self with related positive emotions. To notice them, the clinician must be attentive and responsive. In fact, at the beginning of therapy, the healthy parts surface fleetingly, often unexpectedly, and the therapist easily overlooks them. The patient shows satisfaction with his work, which is evident in his face and voice. Or, in an episode, he is in touch with emotional pain and asks for congruent help despite the other person's denying it. Again, he describes a moment of leisure or curiosity.

Therapists must immediately notice such experiences and mark them, giving them a voice so that they remain in the shared working memory long enough to be remembered. Experiential techniques during dynamic assessment are invaluable in evoking the healthy parts. When patients refrain from coping or change posture from a negative state until they feel changes, they are more likely to discover that they have benevolent ideas about themselves or that they are capable of reducing pain.

The shared knowledge of the patient's internal world through observation of the four lakes tends to increase significantly and provides the information for the next step, which is the reconstruction of cause-and-effect links.

But meanwhile, what can happen at the relational level in these transitions?

The therapeutic relationship when searching for inner states with the use of techniques

We are in the midst of dynamic assessment. Relational ruptures are possible since the therapist immediately asks for active involvement in the therapeutic work.

Key among the techniques we use at this stage are behavioral experiments with attempted abstention from coping. Patients have described some aspects of their experience, but either bring a few narrative episodes or not, but, even if they do, they do not describe the elements of their inner world, obscured by the speed with which they switch to coping. Typical exercises always follow the logic, *stop a moment before you fall, that is, immediately before using maladaptive coping, just long enough to understand what is happening inside you.*

We can ask patients to avoid texting a partner by whom they feel abandoned; to refrain from binge eating or self-injurious behavior; to reduce perfectionistic behavior; to expose themselves socially, and so on.

To access internal states, guided imagery without rescripting is useful. This involves letting a narrative episode, often a recent one, flow through the mind, scanning the stream of consciousness moment by moment. Regarding the use of the body, it is possible to use tracking (Ogden & Fisher, 2015), that is, paying attention to bodily cues as the speech flows: "What do you physically feel now that you are telling me about that tense moment in college? In what parts of the body do you feel the sensations?"

Sometimes, the inner world remains opaque due to emotional dysregulation or dissociation. In these cases, breathing or somatic practices help to overcome them. At this point, reading ability is likely to improve quickly, and patients describe thoughts and emotions.

Some patients, then, are poor at relating between variables; that is, they describe an emotion or its physical correlate but without awareness of the trigger: "I woke up nervous"; "I feel anxiety today, and I don't understand why, I have this kind of breathlessness." In these cases, we can ask the patient to lie on a couch or bed with her knees bent and the soles of her feet planted on the floor. Then, we ask her to pay attention to her breathing and to the areas of the body where she locates the emotion (*grounding lying down*) and to remain in this position for several minutes, trying to notice if mental images or interpersonal episodes, that could be the triggers of the hitherto unexplained emotion, appear in her mind.

What impact do these techniques have on the relationship?

The patient may reject behavioral homework or forget it systematically. Some remain tenaciously attached to a position of passivity, either with resignation ("if only the other . . .") or protest ("the other makes me . . ."). They spend sessions in depressive or angry rumination trying to understand why they have been treated unfairly and, meanwhile, oscillate between putting themselves down and complaining.

The therapist asks a patient with dependent PD for a behavioral experiment: "Instead of writing long angry messages to your lover asking you to sleep together again, try not responding and see what happens to you." The patient replies that the therapist doesn't understand her, that she is in love, and so, "What would you do in my place? Wouldn't you feel bad about it?" She then says he should not behave like that and . . . ruminates again!

It often happens that techniques have a positive relational impact right away: this is interaction pattern 4. Patients get curious and see that the therapist is active and does not stop in the face of difficulties. They appreciate the therapist's tendency to curiosity and not-knowing during dynamic assessment and notice his open-mindedness and eagerness to get to know them without anchoring on theories. Finally, patients understand that they possess agency, can discover more about themselves and modify their internal world. This is the direct positive impact.

Then, there is the indirect positive impact (pattern 5): patients discover that the technique is useful or beneficial. It helps them improve their awareness of the internal world, and they begin to discover that behavioral automatisms are not inevitable. They do not know how to stop them, of course, but they discover that there is room for intervention. They thus understand that they have the power to improve and, as a result, have more confidence in the therapeutic process.

The impact on the relationship of early access to healthy parts

Therapists try to evoke healthy parts from the very first sessions. What do they look like, what are the positive cognitions? These are moments of satisfaction, competence, good self-esteem, the ability to reduce pain through therapeutic exercises, to disclose one's own vulnerability and ask for help. At other times, patients enter states of curiosity, irony, and playfulness.

Noticing and verbalizing the healthy and creative aspects usually has an immediately positive relational impact, again pattern 4. Sometimes, however, the pattern is followed by micro-ruptures. The therapist insists on the positive part that has just emerged, and the patient quickly moves on to seeing her suffering ignored. She thinks the therapist is being superficial, underestimating the seriousness of the problem, or even teasing her by offering her false hope. These are not worrying reactions, but it is necessary to notice them and work on repairing the rupture.

PART II

Associated memories and beginning work on symptoms, coping and regulation (Figure 4.1, Boxes 6–9, 13a)

In this section, we focus on how experiential techniques and therapeutic relationships are intertwined during the following operations.

6. Structured summary of events.
7. Evoking associated autobiographical memories, both past and emerging, in the week after each session.
8. Further expanding knowledge of the internal states in such memories with experiential techniques.

Added to these is the work on coping, viz,

13a. Using mastery strategies to reduce symptoms and coping, bearing in mind still-limited metacognition.

Once the elements of the internal world have surfaced, therapists perform the first real formulation operation, which is the structured summary of events (Figure 4.1, Box 6). This is a purely cognitive operation; the techniques have only helped to provide the content on which it is based.

It involves summarizing what emerged in the first episodes recounted and rearranging the material according to the structure of the interpersonal schema. Therapists must pay attention to the following elements: a) the formulation must start from the wish; b) the therapist must include the healthy parts? or, if absent, point out to the patient how this element is missing; c) a correct summary points out the metacognitively obscure areas, where the therapist notes that in sections of the episode he or she could not tell what the patient thought and felt or why he or she acted in a certain way. The structured summary thus also serves to improve knowledge of the internal world.

Let us see a proper summary where self-reflexivity is partly lacking and the therapist points out what is not clear to her:

As you talked to me about your partner, it seemed to me that you were driven by the need to be liked. Which is normal, it's the most human thing in the world. For a moment, I had the feeling, from the words you used and your face, that,

I don't know, you were more self-confident, that a part of you maybe thinks you're worth something. Do you? But beyond that, what next? If you seek approval, your partner appears harsh, distant, and critical. At that point, it is not very clear to me what happens to you. I understand that you withdraw and shut down. At times, you get angry and protest, and you find his harshness unfair. But it is unclear to me what you think and what emotions you experience when you face criticism and disinterest from your partner. In short, what happens inside you a moment before you withdraw and shut down. Particularly, the day you wanted to go out, he replied that he was down in the dumps, and you got irritated and went to your room. What did you think at that moment?

It is important that in the summary the therapist emphasizes what he or she does not know because of impaired metacognition. Skilled therapists talk to the patient only about what is manifest to both of them and, if there are knowledge gaps, they point them out to the patient, "Here I lack information; shall we think about it together?"

When self-reflexivity is good and information is adequate, the correct summary sounds like this:

T: "As you were telling me about your partner, it seemed to me that you were driven by the need to be liked. Which is normal, it's the most human thing in the world. And for a moment, you said that, basically, it feels right to you that you have something that deserves to be appreciated. However, what happens? If you ask for approval from your partner and he comes across as harsh, distant, and critical, your self-esteem collapses and gives way to believing yourself inadequate. At that moment, you get sad and sometimes ashamed. At other times, however, you become angry, and protest. For example, when you told him that you wanted to plan the weekend and he replied that he was down in the dumps, you thought that it wasn't true, that you deserved attention and he was lying to you, because he just thinks of his own interest and doesn't consider you, which makes you angry."

Step 7 begins immediately after the summary, after gaps in metacognition have been filled with the proper psychological information of course. It consists of asking for associated episodes to find regularities in functioning that will lead to reconstructing the pattern.

In MIT, therapists do not ask for the associated episodes with the *affect bridge* technique. Instead, they start with the structured summary of episodes just described. They ask the patient, after repeating the summary a second time, "And so can you think of an episode, perhaps far back in time, from your childhood, adolescence, that has a similar storyline? A story in which you longed . . . ." Or, "A story where you wanted . . . and then that desire went unfulfilled because the other . . . where did you learn that things turn out that way?"

If patients do not recall relevant historical episodes, at that point they will be asked to observe the episodes that surface week after week and note their nuances. Once episodes have surfaced, either past ones or those surfacing in subsequent weeks, it is possible that the psychological information they convey is insufficient.

We are now at step 8, where we use experiential techniques to enhance meta-cognition in the associated episodes. We can ask patients to relive them in imagery and simulate them in session through role-play or chairwork. If we have asked for attention to what happens in the following weeks, we now ask patients to add an attempt to refrain from coping, a practice that increases arousal and makes internal states more accessible.

Symptomatic and regulatory interventions? (Figure 4.1, Box 13a)

At the beginning of therapy, patients often seek help for symptomatic and behavioral problems: obsessions, anxiety disorders, post-traumatic disorders, eating disorders, self-harm, and aggression are just a few examples.

While trying to understand patients' functioning, the therapist agrees with them to use some techniques (Figure 4.1, Box 13a), and in some cases protocols that can be applied even without understanding the underlying PD-related mechanisms.

To use such techniques, when metacognition is still low, it is enough for the patient to ask for help in coping and agree to do something to get initial relief. At this point, we propose simple strategies and regulatory tools.

Classic examples include behavioral activation for depression (Lewinsohn, 1974), exposure for various types of anxiety disorders, exposure and response prevention for obsessive-compulsive symptoms, and food diary compilation and attempts to regularize calorie intake in eating disorders both to cope with problematic eating and to improve metacognition (Fairburn et al., 2003; Fioravanti et al., 2023).

In cases of emotional dysregulation or self-injury, we suggest classic regulatory strategies such as mindfulness, calling friends or texting the therapist before acting out self-harming behaviors and placing ice cubes on one's wrists to calm oneself (Linehan, 1993). For aggressive acts, we suggest paying attention to early signs of mounting anger and moving away from the person against whom one might lash out, or mindful breathing until anger subsides (Pasetto et al., 2021).

Among in-session experiential practices to reduce symptoms and coping, we often use specific attentional techniques to interrupt IRT (Chapter 2, 7; Ottavi et al., 2019) or work through the body to regulate emotions (Centonze et al., 2021; Dimaggio et al., 2020). When used in agreement? with the patient, these practices are safe and have numerous advantages: (a) the therapist monitors live both their effectiveness and their impact on the working alliance; (b) patient and therapist focus on the dysfunctional cognitive processes underlying symptoms, helping the patient understand that the problem is internal in nature and that it is possible to reduce pain by working on the internal world itself; (c) they increase metacognition, especially self-reflexivity, which is likely to be lacking at these early stages; (d) they enhance agency over mental states, for example, the ability to regulate emotion by for example discovering that one mental state seems unbearable when sitting down bending towards the floor, and appears tolerable when standing up and puffing out one's chest; and (e) they reduce metacognitive beliefs such as "I can't control my mind when I ruminate."

Remember that we are dealing with symptoms and coping at the beginning of therapy or at any rate when metacognition is low. Usually, under these conditions, neither attention-regulation techniques, nor behavioral prescriptions, nor embodied regulation completely solve the problem. It is a matter of offering the patient tools to regulate suffering and reduce it, showing from the outset that therapy means working together. Symptom work will return at various points in the treatment, and each time will require a renewal of the contract (see Chapter 5). Moreover, when metacognition improves, techniques aimed at symptom reduction will be more complex and will benefit from the increased understanding of the mental states the patient has achieved (chapter 13). In any case, using such techniques at the beginning of therapy reinforces the working alliance, providing patients with practical tools that allow them to be less at the mercy of symptoms.

If patients do not intend to implement strategies, it means that there is a major relational rupture, which does not depend on the technique. We must, therefore, stop any action and discuss the contract (chapter 3).

The focus on the therapeutic relationship should be greatest in steps 13a and 13b, where the therapist proposes techniques to be used with concrete goals in agreement with the patient. It is not dynamic assessment, that is using techniques to learn more about the internal world. We already now want to reduce symptoms, suffering, and dysfunctional behaviors, using tools consistent with patients' poor metacognition.

Therapists can and should try to reduce symptoms and regulate painful emotions, especially with patients asking for therapy for that reason, and the exposure-experiential part is indispensable. We recall, however, that we focus on patients predominantly with PD, that is, people who struggle to form a benevolent representation of the therapist, take agency over their problems, and cooperate. As a result, it is easy for the therapist to use practices that are, in theory, appropriate but will have limited effectiveness or that the patient will not implement between sessions.

On the patient's part, ruptures depend mainly on schemas. When the therapist tries to do something, the patient perceives him as dominant, dangerous, disinterested, mechanical and disabling – "He wants to get rid of me as soon as possible" – and so on. Patterns 1 and 2 of technique-relationship interaction are thus frequently encountered: the patient either rejects the technique, initiates it and quickly discontinues it, or enacts it but keeps a protective distance from her own emotions.

Other reasons for breaking the working alliance at this point are (a) the task of abstaining from coping is assigned without the clinician carefully verifying that the patient really accepts it, so that the patient says he will try but, in fact, left to himself, continues to drink, avoid, sacrifice or care for the other because he thinks it is right; (b) the patient sincerely tries to perform the task but fails and forgets that the goal is just to try and observe himself, so he goes into the next session convinced that he has disappointed the therapist and thus the pattern is activated, but only after he has tried.

In the first case, the contract needs to be redefined; in the second, reflect on why the patient fears that she has let the therapist down, until she recognizes that the therapist has no expectations about her performance.

Ruptures may depend on the therapist. While the patient is experiencing symptoms or acting out harmful behaviors, the therapist feels the weight of her mission to heal, but progress is not being made. At this point, it is typical for him to experience negative thoughts and emotions: "What am I doing wrong?"; "I am inadequate"; "Colleagues will think badly of me"; "I am hurting this person" "A better therapist would have already achieved better results." He may take a negative attitude toward the patient: "He doesn't cooperate," "He doesn't make an effort," "He is unhelpful," "He doesn't respect me," "He makes fun of me."

In either case, he will be in an anti-therapeutic position that activates negative interpersonal cycles. If he is self-critical, he may become hesitant or insistent, in the former case, out of fear of doing harm, and in the latter, to make some progress at all costs. It is automatic that the patient will react to both attitudes negatively by confirming her own patterns. If, on the other hand, he is critical of the patient, it goes without saying that the relationship deteriorates.

How do we move through this bottleneck? The solution is simpler than it appears. It involves proposing the techniques and immediately focusing on the patient's verbal and non-verbal responses. Does the patient accept the task willingly, explicitly and with congruent expressive signals? Does she perform the exercises at home? Or does she display facial expressions, postures and behaviors that indicate a breakdown? In all these cases, the therapist immediately stops giving herself the task of being effective and focuses on the relationship. In a word, she metacommunicates,

Is something not working? Do you feel the exercise is unnecessary or premature, or makes you anxious? How are you experiencing my presence right now? Do you feel close to me? Do you feel understood? Or am I making you uncomfortable, making you feel misunderstood, pressured, criticized?

Based on what emerges from the dialogue, the therapist will proceed to attempt to repair a possible rupture, as shown in chapter 3. Only if the rupture is repaired will she return to using techniques.

The problem is greater when patients explicitly refuse to use the techniques or accept them on the surface but do not apply them, so that technique-relationship interaction patterns 1 and 2 occur. The procedure now forces us to move immediately to reformulating the contract. The therapist first monitors the way she addresses the patient; she pays attention to not being annoyed, judgmental, or alarmed. It is important that her words do not sound like a therapeutic ultimatum. Instead, adopt from the outset the position of *leaning forward helplessness*:

> Look, I'm there, I understand your pain, and I want to help you. Only if we don't put something in place to deal with the symptoms and the problems will it be difficult for me to be of help to you. What can we do together?

Moving on to reformulating the contract is a position that does not allow other activities. The therapist asks the patient whether he shares the goal, whether he has understood that, to reduce suffering, it is necessary for him to contribute his share of the work, and whether he is willing to do so. And in the meantime? She waits for the patient's response. If this does not come, there is little point in starting to propose alternatives again. We take it for granted that we have arrived at this point after having tried a range of tools aimed at regulating emotions and reducing symptoms, and none have worked.

It is a delicate moment because the therapist needs a high self-regulatory capacity. But it is a position that must be held; we repeat this here and will return to it later. Only when the patient declares out loud and with conviction, "Okay, I get it, I'll do something," does the therapist become active again.

PART III

Reconstruction of functioning and recognition of schemas as such (Boxes 9–12, 13b)

This section is the real treatment turning point. Correctly performing the steps we describe is often the key to success. Conversely, it is easy for treatment to get stuck at this point, particularly because the therapist assumes that the patient has understood that he or she is being guided by a scheme, and this is not the case.

We mentioned at the beginning of the chapter how one of the most frequent errors lurks here. The therapist thinks that if the patient has realized the underlying regularities in his or her own functioning as the episodes change, this implies that he or she has realized that he or she is guided by a pattern. Instead, the patient has only recognized her own ideas about herself and others, but she still believes them to be true.

We show in detail how to get over this crossroad and what relational problems may arise. The steps are as follows.

9. Recognize regularities between episodes and describe mental processes according to the schema structure.
10. Assume that such regularities are a sign of the existence of patterns.
11. Make a cognitive inquiry dedicated to finding out whether the patient recognizes the self-image as an idea and not as a fact or as merely a reaction to how the other person treated him or her.

12.   Recognize the transitions between healthy parts and schema-related self-ideas in the stream of consciousness.

13b.   Recognize the link between the emergence of nuclear self-concepts and the activation of behavioral coping strategies or IRT.

Therapy comes to these steps when multiple episodes have emerged, no matter whether from the remote past or collected week after week.

Step 9 is cognitively complex for therapists: they have to figure out what the regularities are among the episodes, then begin to form hypotheses about the structure of the pattern and likewise bring the patient to share in it. We tell therapists, especially the less experienced, that it is not necessary to do this immediately, as soon as the patient has brought sufficient episodes. We can take time, say to the patients we need to think about it and then organize the ideas at home, or ask the supervisor for help. In addition, it is shared work, so it is very helpful for therapists to not only bear in mind with great theoretical clarity the general structure of the scheme but also go through all the steps together with the patient in real elbow-to-elbow, pen and paper or computer work. Here, techniques do not play an important role, and alliance ruptures depend on something else. It happens that while the therapist is working on reconstructing functioning together with the patient, patterns are activated in the latter. She may detach, compete, or deny aspects that were obvious just a few minutes before. As we described in Chapter III, it is simply a matter of noticing this and moving on to work on the relationship rather than insisting that the patient understands the formulation and makes it her own.

Step 10 is accomplished by offering the patient a summary, structured according to the pattern, of what happened in the various episodes, stressing recurring aspects. It sounds like this:

T: "It seems to be important for you to act on your own; we saw this in the recent episode when your wife complained that you had gone to visit the museum in Prague, leaving you and your daughter alone for a few hours. And it seems similar to the episodes in which your mother scolded you when you were playing ball late at night in the middle of the street. In both cases, you are curious, you play, but the other person criticizes you and accuses you of hurting her, at which point you freeze and feel guilty. On the other hand, you sense that your desire to play and explore the world makes sense and then you feel that the criticism and accusations are unfair. This seems to me to be at the root of the outbursts of anger that have worried you and your wife, what do you say?"

The steps we now describe are rigorous and unavoidable; the successful continuation of therapy depends on them. First, the therapist asks the patient whether he sees himself in such a reconstruction and assesses whether the response is accompanied by congruent non-verbal signals. If the patient agrees, the therapist is easily convinced that the former has realized that he is driven by a schema and is ready to work to change.

In many situations, this is not the case! The therapist discovers this when she sees that experiential techniques, for example, guided imagery or role-play, are not working. Or that the patient does not perform homework, either by finding loads of excuses or by simply forgetting it.

What to do to prevent these problems? First, we have to ask patients if they recognize that the regularity is related to their own way of being and not to how others treat them. A good sign in this regard is, for example, when a patient with a mixture of surprise and frustration exclaims, "Oh no, does that mean I'm still dealing with my mother?!"

Decision-making procedures naturally point to this outcome. It often happens, however, that patients recognize regularities and understand that there is a lifelong pattern underlying relationships, but their mind remains focused on the "other does to me" mode. In other words, although they recognize the existence of a tendency toward repetition, their mind is focused on the actions of the other. As a result, they are oriented to hope that they will be able to change how others respond and not their own internal structure, that is, their nuclear self-image.

It is then essential to move on to step 11, which is to make a simple but focused cognitive inquiry about what the patient believes about herself. As in the following example, this involves taking the patient back to one of the episodes and asking her to observe herself from the outside:

Now that you are looking at the 'you' of that moment, what do you think of yourself? Your father looks at you; he is disappointed because the gymnastics test went badly; you feel humiliated, sure. But what do you think about the Renata who failed?

The therapist takes the response as valid only when the patient clearly expresses the cognition, for example, "I think Renata is a mess, a failure."

The crucial step is for patients to move from "I feel bad because I received criticism," a state in which their mind will be focused on preventing the others from criticizing again, to "If my partner criticizes me, I feel bad about it because I partly agree with him."

We repeat that it is about checking that patients no longer think "I suffer because I've been criticized," "the other makes me . . ." But "I suffer because the other criticized me, and it's painful, but the problem is that I think I'm unworthy."

Techniques play an important role at this junction because they make cognitive inquiry embodied and show the patient clearly how the self-concept is internal, accompanied by emotional and somatic correlates.

Attention: now it is crucial to understand our goal; it is not for patients to change their mind! This step is only to make them aware that they have a nuclear self-image they deeply believe in and that it does not depend on what others do but is their own and is stable.

Instead, clinicians often add an element of change, which is a mistake at this time! We should not make the patient realize they have a negative image and correct it, but we should make them say, "Okay, I get it; that's me seeing myself this way."

Having made this clear, let us look again at how to get patients to identify nuclear self-images. The therapist, once she has summarized what looks like a possible pattern, leads the patient to relive in imagery one of the underlying episodes. When the patient gets to the moment when the other responds in a way that causes her pain, the therapist intervenes like this:

> There, now you are faced with your father who has just told you that you are an endless disappointment. Pay attention to what you feel emotionally and bodily – okay, you feel ashamed, you feel an emptiness in your stomach, weak legs. So what are you thinking about yourself at this exact moment?

We enhance cognitive inquiry by working on step 12, that is, by leading patients to oscillate between times when they fully believe the negative self-idea and times when they access positive, benevolent ideas. For example, during the imagery described above, we can ask the patient to first adopt a posture that *accentuates* the negative self-idea, for example, slumped over with hunched shoulders. When the patient feels even more inadequate, sad, or ashamed, we ask her to straighten up, raise her chin, and gaze or widen her shoulders. At that point, we ask how she feels at this moment and what she thinks about herself.

One can also invite the patient to address the other, the father in this case, in a different way, for example, more firmly and assertively. Warning: the goal here is not rescripting! It is always about dynamic assessment. That is, for the patient to realize how the negative cognition about the self – related to what she is now discovering to be a pattern – is just an idea and not reality. She realizes that she has power over her inner world and that, in addition to a negative nuclear idea of herself, she has alternative and positive ones.

Now patients know they are guided by schemas and, therefore, understand that the problem is not how the others treat them, and in a sense, not even how they react, but that they believe that the negative ideas they rely upon are true. Finally, clinicians are allowed to conclude in their inner dialogue, "Well, she has realized that she is being driven by a schema. I can move on to agreeing with her on change operations."

Usually, if we perform these operations correctly, alliance ruptures during the use of the techniques are minimal and no different from those already described. Patients may feel the technique constraining or a source of shame. Instead, it may happen that it is the therapist who initiates a rupture because, if the patient struggles to recognize a negative cognition about himself, the therapist experiences concern, irritation, or frustration and then tries to insist that the patient understands that he is a victim of a pattern. We repeat again: the goal of therapy is to first help patients form a model of their own mind and functioning and only then to use this model as a map for change. If this operation fails immediately, no problem; we will devote as much time as necessary to it and postpone change operations.

If we perform the steps correctly, it is actually likely that the relationship will be strengthened or improved. Patients gain agency over their own mind, understand what therapy is about, which is to change their internal world, and become active in the process. This reinforces cooperation and confidence that the therapy is useful and reduces or zeroes out earlier reactions such as passivity or opposition we described earlier.

In parallel with points 11 (cognitive investigation of the nuclear image) and 12 (oscillating between negative and positive views), it is possible to work to show how coping is activated as a result of the emergence of the nuclear self-image in the face of the other's response: "When the other person criticizes you, you feel ashamed, think you are ridiculous, fear humiliation, and tend to . . ." We point out to patients that perfectionistic control in study and work, emotional dependency, physical overtraining, binge drinking, alcohol use, addiction to internet pornography, or compulsive video gaming, and so on are activated in response to the emergence of the negative self-image, with the painful emotions this entails. For example, a therapist showed a patient how, a moment before accessing a porn site, he had experienced shame as he thought back to the awkward way he had approached a girl. With this knowledge, we have more precise tools to reduce symptoms and improve regulatory skills (Figure 4.1, Box 13b).

Point 13b, then, intertwining with 11 and 12, is an important step in therapy. It is an aspect of MIT we describe for the first time. We describe it through a detailed example whose purpose is to show how the therapist, at various points, helps patients: a) to recognize how coping has been activated as a result of the emergence of the negative self-image; b) to see how they are able to oscillate, guided by the therapist, between negative images and positive alternative images; c) to calm their core pain without resorting to coping; and then d) to discover that the pain depends on the schema rather than on a concrete action of the other.

Rachel is a 38-year-old nurse who suffers from dependent PD and suffered severe physical violence in her family throughout her adolescence. She is returning to dating but is terrified of being humiliated and abandoned, and as a result, she acts impulsively, texting all the time and sometimes checking where the man is at that moment. She has an initial awareness, so she knows that the sense of abandonment depends on family history, but it does not operate in-between sessions. The therapist asks her for an exercise in abstaining from coping for regulatory purposes, starting with the awareness that controlling behavior and rumination depend on the core idea of self-deserving of abandonment.

T: "Next week, it will happen to you that the man with whom you are building a relationship does not respond to messages because he is very busy at work. He has clearly explained this to you. You tend to disbelieve him, suspecting that he is chatting with some girl, and feel humiliated. At that moment, try to pay less attention to what he is doing and instead notice how you are the first to believe you are a woman no one could really be attracted to. Can you try?"

R: "Look, I have it right in my head, I suck! No wonder he's going to look for someone prettier than me."

T: "Good. And that's when the urge to write to him will be at its peak. When you feel it, can you try to resist it? It doesn't matter if you succeed; it is only necessary that you pay attention to what you are thinking and feeling at the moment when you try not to text him. You will tell me in the next session what has happened to you inside. We just want to start to see if you realize that, no matter how much you are convinced you are worthless, you can have some control over actions that then, we know, make you feel even worse."

Rachel fears she will not succeed but agrees. She has realized that out-of-session coping depends on the emergence of an extremely negative self-concept and wants to try to counteract the automatism; she knows that her behaviors are detrimental to relationships.

The next step after the behavioral experiment takes place in session and serves to further enhance regulation and awareness of how certain ways of functioning are schema-dependent.

In the following session, Rachel recounts that she did the exercise, resisted the urge to text but only briefly, and then began writing compulsively. She is also distressed in the session, speaking fast. The therapist is welcoming but firm: "Rachel, I'm here. Don't let the worry get to you; you're ruminating. Shall we work on it together now?" Rachel agrees. The therapist asks her to access a memory of competence, and she quickly retrieves moments of effectiveness while working in the operating room. At that point, he invites her to close her eyes and retrieve the memory of efficacy, feeling it in her body. Rachel feels a sense of strength in her chest. Now she feels worthy; the idea of being doomed to loneliness is gone.

The therapist asks her to recall the moment of distress and tell herself that she is worthless, that her partner will surely betray her for a more attractive girl. Rachel returns to the negative mode but, already, the nuclear idea is less strong; she believes it to be less true. The therapist has her make numerous shifts between the negative and positive images as she repeats in an increasingly loud voice, with her arms spread wide and her chest expanded, phrases such as "I am good, I am capable." By the end of the exercise, she calms down and finds that she did not need to flood her partner with messages. Work will continue to strengthen regulatory capacity and to understand more clearly how her thinking she is worthless is the result of a pattern, an awareness that is only now beginning to emerge.

In Rachel's case, the therapist used a combination of attentional, imaginative, and bodily techniques, and this made it possible to a) achieve the necessary emotional regulation in session to proceed with therapeutic work; b) increase the sense of agency over mental states; and c) move toward an awareness that pain does not arise from what the other person does, but from negative ideas that may not be true, which may leave room for more benevolent images of self and other.

Note that the most advanced steps of the shared case formulation now described already have a core aimed at change. Patients begin to historicize their way of experiencing relationships, access the healthy parts, and begin to work through suffering by deciding to modify their internal world. These are, however, operations that still rest on uncertain ground. Patients quickly return to believing negative ideas about themselves and others to be true. It is necessary to move systematically toward structural change, first making differentiation and the experience of healthy parts stable, and then taking steps to change personality structures.

In other words, we have laid the foundation for moving on to the other section of decision-making procedures, the *promotion of change*. In the next chapter, we will describe them by showing, once again, how patients improve through experiential techniques and relationship work.

Chapter 5

Decision-making and relational procedures

Change promoting

What does promoting change mean in PD? The core of personality psychopathology is the interpersonal schema, which fits with the proposed naming of PDs *interpersonal disorders* (Wright et al., 2022). It is the system of predicting the fate of one's evolutionarily selected core wishes. Because of negative aspects of their own nature, patients predict others will frustrate their wishes. They imagine that "My desire to be liked will meet with harsh criticism because I am of little worth"; "My desire to be cared for will be met by someone who neglects me because I am unlovable"; "My desire to explore and learn will remain unfulfilled because the other does not offer me support and backing, and I am powerless and lacking in resources."

What, then, does the change consist of? First, it allows patients to access alternative core self-images, on which to ground a different system of predictions where wishes have hope of being fulfilled. Consequently, to access ideas such as, "My desire to be liked will be met with a glance of approval, which I deserve because I know I have qualities"; "My desire to be cared for will be met by someone who cares, because I know deep down I am lovable"; "My desire to explore and learn will result in a journey as others will support me and vouch for me, and I can embark on the journey because I am motivated and able to use the resources they offer me."

The focus of change, then, is to help patients realize they are being driven by patterns, begin to read themselves and others in healthier, benevolent, realistic ways, and move through the world differently and more adaptively.

We then show how to act out the various steps of *promoting change* through experiential techniques so that change occurs at the cognitive, procedural, and behavioral levels. We will do this through relentless monitoring of the therapeutic relationship. We illustrate the procedures in Figure 5.1.

PART I

Change promoting: realizing one is driven by patterns and consolidating healthy parts

How to get patients to change their perspective? We saw this in part at the end of the previous chapter, and now we turn to describing it in detail. The cornerstone of

DOI: 10.4324/9781003570967-5

Differentiating
Box 1

Consolidating and empowering
healthy self aspects
Box 2

Treating residual
symptoms,
behavioural
coping and
interpersonal
repetitive
thinking

Discovering how after having accessed the
healthy self, the mind returns to read the
world through the lenses of the schemas
Box 3

Tackling avoided or feared
relational situations
Box 4

Exploring the environment and
pursuing healthy wishes
Box 5

Promoting more
sophisticated and
effective mastery
strategies

Discovering how after behavioral homework the
mind returns to read the world through the lenses
of the schemas
Box 6

Adopting more effective modalities to fulfill own
wishes/Acknowledging own contribution to
interpersonal cycles
Box 7

Forming a mature theory of
mind/Decentering
Box 8

Box 10

Forming an integrated
representation of self with others
Box 9

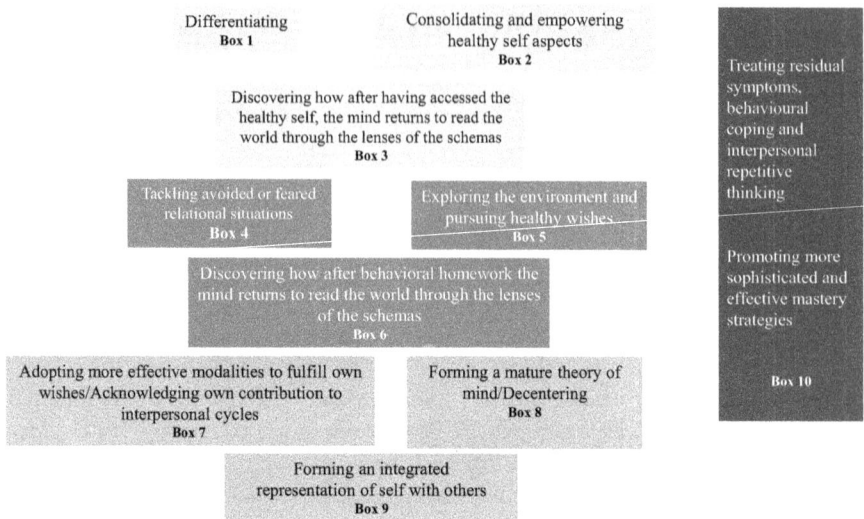

Figure 5.1 Change promoting

overcoming psychopathology and creating the new is the realization that *relational suffering comes from a perspective on the world and not from reality*. That is, it is necessary to bring the patient to state explicitly, fully consciously,

> I realize that when the other person responds to me in a frustrating and painful way, I feel bad about it, and it is a human reaction. But that reaction hurts me so much and stays in my mind and conditions me in my actions because it corresponds to what I think of myself. It criticizes me, and part of me agrees with the negative judgment.

This is both a *cognitive* and *experiential* reading. Patients *know* they are guided by these ideas and *feel* their emotional and somatic correlates: "I know I judge myself negatively, and when it happens to me, my legs tremble and my shoulders hunch."

Likewise, we promote new perspectives on self, others, and the fate of one's wishes at two levels: cognitive and experiential. Patients need, yes, to read interpersonal events in a more flexible, benevolent, hopeful way, but it is important that the change be accompanied by new patterns of feeling and action. Cognitive change alone is useless if it does not travel together with new emotions and, above all, consistent behaviors.

In these passages, we use experiential techniques to their full power for the purpose for which they were designed: to change the reading of events and update the map of the world. That is, to change the interpersonal patterns at the root of PD. Guided imagery, chairwork, and role-play are first choices.

The most typical working procedure begins with the reenactment of a recent or remote narrative episode that the patient feels is emotionally relevant. The therapist first clarifies that working on the episode means changing the internal space and not the responses of real others. When the patient has understood and shared the purpose, he or she has already taken a further step of differentiation: "I am trying to change the way I see myself and others because I have realized that the problem is in my reading and not in the world." The therapist asks the patient to relive the episode as if it were happening now (we will describe how to deliver these exercises in Chapter X). When arousal mounts and emotions are intense enough, it is time to attempt rewriting.

The therapist asks the patient to try to act in the scene in a different way, trying to fulfill the wish and interrupting coping mechanisms such as submission, escape, compulsive caregiving, avoidance, and so on. In doing so, the therapist makes room for the healthy parts and gives them space and power to control the action. When the exercise is completed, the patient has seen that he or she has the power to change perspective and act more freely and creatively.

For example, a patient holds the idea she is *unlovable* and, therefore, deserving of the abandonment she recently experienced. She relives an episode in which she requests presence from her mother, but she is fighting with her father. The therapist asks her to evoke a part of herself that is capable of care. Once she succeeds, the therapist brings that part to interact with the *unlovable* self, to be there for her and to care for her. The focus at this point becomes helping the part of her that sees herself as unlovable to express pain and to discover that the caring part is there! So she can receive care and attention. The patient feels it in her body, experiences relief and warmth, and starts thinking: *I am lovable*: change has begun. She senses that being lovable is true; she has experienced it and felt it in her body. So, she knows that not being lovable is her own idea, one that she has formed but does not necessarily correspond to her nature.

In Chapter 10, we describe in detail the procedures for accomplishing these parallel steps of differentiation and access to healthy parts. Here, we illustrate them through an example. Therapists first complete the shared formulation. Patients begin to discover they are guided by patterns and that they have healthy parts, but they do not yet really differentiate them. The idea of being schema-driven is tenuous, and negative ideas still taste like a bitter truth. Therapists then immediately work to more clearly promote differentiation and access to healthy parts.

Maggie, 32, suffers from generalized anxiety and dependent PD. She enters therapy in despair because the boyfriend with whom she has been cohabiting for three years is showing concrete signs he no longer loves her. In addition to the human pain of loss that seems inevitable, Maggie's anxiety is focused on the idea of not being able to survive emotionally and not knowing how to navigate in the absence of someone who guides her.

In session, the interpersonal pattern is active, although Maggie does not recognize it as such: she sees herself as fragile, does not know her own wishes, and perceives herself as unable to carry on with her life without the partner's support. She worries about the consequences of the separation and ruminates about the mistakes she made and how she could have made things go differently. At times, she calms down, only to plunge back into despair.

At these moments, Maggie associates past episodes; for example, as a child she was always afraid to face new experiences alone, preferring to stay home with her mother. Once, in her primary school years, she decided to practice artistic gymnastics but, as soon as her mother left her at the gym, she felt lonely, fragile, lost, and unable to cope. She pretended to feel sick to get her mother to pick her up. The *lonely and fragile* image won out over the desire to do gymnastics. She only had fun if her mother accompanied her or she was with her best friend, with whom she felt safe. Her mother was, in her words, overprotective and anxious and prevented her from going out to play with friends in their neighborhood because she feared she would get hurt or get her *nice clothes* dirty. The only safe place was home, but there she often felt sad and dull. She was afraid and felt fragile. Nevertheless, she longed to play with other children, but nobody was there to encourage or support her.

From these accounts, Maggie seems aware that her present concerns are the result of a pattern built in the past. But they are not! She does connect the current state of the relationship with her boyfriend to these past episodes, but these associations only feed rumination: "What is my fate? Will I end up again alone and fragile in a dangerous world?"

The therapist then asks her to stop ruminating. He invites her to close her eyes and then asks questions to fill item 11 of the formulation: discovering the negative core self-idea.

T: "Can you describe this Maggie with an adjective?"
M: "Alone and fragile."
T: "How real is this aspect of self? How true do you believe it to be?"
Y: "That's me, that's who I am."
T: "Well then, let me see where in the body this lonely and fragile Maggie is located. Where is the suffering?"

Maggie verbalizes only a sharp pain in her chest. The therapist extends the exploration, and the picture becomes richer: she has shortness of breath, swollen eyes, and a heavy head, a pounding heart, and restless hands and feet.

T: "Would you like to represent this part of yourself using gestures and movements? Try impersonating this Maggie as if you were an actress. Mime her, caricature her. If you want, you can adopt a posture consistent with this feeling."

Maggie is surprised for a moment; then the exercise intrigues her. She stands up and crouches on the carpet in the room, crouching down, and wrapping her arms around her body. Her face expresses fear, with eyes wide and mouth open.

D: "Like Munch's *The Scream*."

Bodily sensations increase in intensity, then they reach a *plateau*. The therapist asks her to regulate her breathing, then to slowly change position and assume a posture and mimicry *opposite to* the previous one. Maggie stands up, straightens her back, opens her arms, and smiles.

T: "Is there a movement that would help you express this new state?"
 [*Maggie hints at a dance step.*]"
T: "How do you feel?"
M: "Mmm . . . it's nice . . . balanced . . . most of all it tastes like freedom [*She appears calmer. Her chest pain is almost gone, hands and feet are still, and heart beats slower*]."
T: "Well, now, how much of the lonely and fragile Maggie lies within you?"
M: ". . . a little. If I think about it, I find it, but . . . no, I feel more solid now."

The therapist asks Maggie to *put on* this part of herself and imagine her acting in the situation she is going through. Maggie sees herself in a scene in which her boyfriend tells her that he has doubts about their relationship and wants to break up.

T: "Try to answer him from this position."
M: "I don't want to break up; it hurts me, but if you want it, okay, amen, I can't help it."

This time, Maggie maintains her connection to her healthy self even at a painful moment. The therapist asks her how true she believes the core idea of being alone, fragile, and unable to cope is. Maggie replies that she is starting to disbelieve it. But she recalls all the times she needed to be supported in exploration and in play, but faced her frightened mother blocking her. At that point, abandoning her desire for exploration in the face of her worried and paralyzing mother, she shut down: she was fragile and could not face the world. As a solution, she adopted avoidance and gave up her desires. Maggie now senses that the past influences her view of herself and others today. She foresees an alternative: contacting desires and following them while feeling solid, balanced, and free, but she finds it difficult.

Work is needed to stabilize differentiation and help her realize that her negative ideas are schema-dependent, and she can make room for the benevolent ideas that have now surfaced. She needs to realize more clearly and stably that the problem is not her boyfriend leaving her and that the solution lies in her hands.

The therapist suggests reliving an episode in guided imagery. She is at a party with her primary school classmates. She plays happily while her mother chats with the other mothers. A little girl accidentally spills a soda on her dress. Maggie is dirty and wet; her mother rushes over and takes her home. In the car, her mother tells her that they would not go to any more parties with *savages* and that she risked getting hurt. Maggie is angry that the party was ruined; it is unfair, but negative images resurface.

M: "It's my fate, I can never have fun; I'm not allowed to doing things like others . . ."

T: "Observe your mother driving, what does she look like?"
M: "She is anxious, lost in . . . dunno what, distant."
T: "How does it feel to see her like this?"
M: ". . . alone."

The therapist begins rescripting to stabilize differentiation. He asks her to open her eyes again and return to the posture they previously staged. Maggie stands up, straightens her back, and opens her arms. She is now in touch with her solid, free self. The therapist asks her to enter the scene, embody this part, and speak to the lonely and fragile Maggie.

M: [*Solid and free*]: "I'm sorry you're sad; you're also right to be angry."
T: "Well, go on."
M: "Do you want to go back to the party? Even with the dirty dress, what do we care – in fact, you know what? We'll get it completely dirty, so we have more fun! [*Smiles. Her need for play and freedom is fulfilled.*]"
T: "How do you feel now?"
M: "I feel happy. I can play, I can mess around, and I'm dirty. Like a normal child, wow!"

Having finished the exercise, Maggie realizes she has rediscovered the part submerged over time by ideas of herself as fragile, dirty, and defective. She understands that her fear of facing the world alone stems not from real dangers but, precisely, from her mother's teachings that the world is harmful. Experiential work has let her feel strong, confident, and vital. She begins to believe these self-aspects to be true and to give them space.

The therapist explores the state of their relationship. Maggie's reaction is unexpected.

M: "At first, it seemed a little strange to me to take those postures; I had some concerns, they seemed difficult."
T: "And how did you perceive my presence?"
M: "At first, when I was getting stuck, that you thought: 'She's not gonna make it!'"
T: "Ah. And then?"
M: "Your voice was calm; I knew you believed in me."
T: "And at that point?"
M: "I realized I could go on . . . I ended up having fun, I was really dancing!"

Maggie reads both the therapist and the exercise through the lens of her schema. However, it is not necessary to intervene since she spontaneously latches onto the non-verbal cues to retrieve a benevolent and encouraging image of the therapist and continue the exercise. We are in the presence, therefore, of pattern 3 of technique-relationship interaction.

It is through asking a question about the relationship during the exercise that the therapist discovers, even more clearly, that Maggie really does differentiate: she briefly reads the therapist in the light of the schema, but she does not believe it and immediately switches to a schema-free perspective.

On this basis, the therapist can confidently proceed to the next steps of change promoting. The task they agree on is that Maggie will try to call to mind the balanced and solid image of herself whenever, in the days ahead, she notices herself getting stuck or ruminating. At that point, she will try to act consistently with her autonomous wishes.

PART II

Discover how, after accessing healthy parts, the mind reverts to reading the world according to the schema to reinforce differentiation and prepare for work on rumination (Figure 5.1, Box 1–3)

After patients have begun to differentiate and recognize how much healthy parts belong to them, it frequently happens that, even during the same session or in the next session, they shift back to schema-driven reasoning. It is as if the previous change never happened. Therapists, as we have noticed during supervision, are often puzzled by this shift, which is why we have added this section to the decision-making procedures. It is a step that requires dedicated attention.

At the end of an imagery exercise, a dramaturgical or body technique, patients notice the benefit, the change in perspective. Everything seems to be going well, but suddenly, rumination begins, and the patient belittles the achievement: "Yes, it's true, here I succeeded, but then in reality . . ."

Immediately, their mood worsens, and the negative self-image – inadequate, unlovable, fragile, powerless, paralyzed, in danger – resurfaces and rings true again. If therapists do not notice the shift, an alliance rupture is just around the corner. For example, therapists may get frustrated and insist on the same technique or add a bodily exercise to return to benevolent, positive feelings.

Sometimes, patients do not voice the rumination but merely show non-verbal signs of returning to the negative state. Therapists do not catch them, try to assign behavioral tasks, and show satisfaction with the change achieved, but patients do not react with the same optimism. Therapists get confused and worried and, metaphorically, press on the accelerator. They insist on experiential work and propose different behavioral tasks. In these cases, proposing the technique generates a rupture, but it is not the technique to blame. The origin of the rupture lies in the error of not noticing that the patient has taken a step back and not acting accordingly.

These shifts, in fact, are the norm, and therapists must perform a simple task: show the patient in real time how he or she has shifted from a healthy way of thinking to the old schema-dependent beliefs and, if so, how he or she has returned to ruminating.

The intervention sounds like this:

> Look how interesting it is! Your mind is very quick to switch from the positive mental state you reached to the usual mode in which you see yourself as incapable (or inept, inferior, endangered, and so on) and the others as critical and dismissive (or threatening, fragile, damaged, and so on), and to agree with it! Do you notice how quick this automatism is?

Or,

> You see, you have just felt secure, active, confident, and now you're back to questioning everything. You fear the consequences of your actions, and you think in terms of "yes . . . but . . .," and this cancels out the positive effects and wears you down.

Only when patients are aware that they have fallen prey again to schema-dependent mechanisms or repetitive thinking can we resume promoting change. At this point, techniques are invaluable (see Chapter 10). We only anticipate that both attentional and somatic techniques allow patients to notice how, by changing body attitude or directing attention voluntarily, they change their mind about themselves and others. For example, the therapist invites a patient to slump down and say negative phrases to himself and then gradually pick himself up and address kinder words of encouragement or appreciation. The patient almost immediately notices a change in mood and regains strength and confidence.

To the same end, we ask patients to retrieve the healthy image evoked in the previous sessions, assume a posture congruent with that image, adjust breathing, and identify the body areas where the healthy parts are located: the feeling of relaxed neck muscles, of calmness and openness in the chest. At this point, we ask them to recall the negative image with all the physical sensations and, after a short time, to return to focus on the body parts where the healthy parts are located.

After a few steps, the patient perceives that the negative image loses power, no longer colonizes his mental landscape, and does not impose itself as true. The patient then experiences the correlates of the negative nuclear image but returns to the idea that it is just an idea, tending to believe it to be true, and that, in fact, another self exists.

In these passages, very often techniques strengthen the therapeutic relationship and increase collaboration with respect to tasks to achieve well-being. This is pattern 4: the technique, already while being carried out, strengthens the relationship because the patient sees the therapist as confident and capable while feeling the benefits of experiential work in real time.

PART III

Dealing with avoided or feared relational situations:
Exploring the environment and pursuing healthy wishes.
Discovering how, after behavioral experiments, the mind
returns to reading the world according to the schema
(Figure 5.1, Boxes 4–6)

The previous step is the turning point of treatment; therapy now aims to change patients' relationships with the outside world. We have led them to realize they are guided by schemas and take on new perspectives. The behavioral experiments so far were aimed at improving metacognition and making patients take action to interrupt automatisms and coping. Patients were able to discover that they were not doomed to perform automatisms branded by their genetics and developmental history and that they have power over behaviors and attitudes.

Now the goal is more ambitious: it is to try to change what the person does and thinks week after week, to put healthy wishes and self-images in the driver's seat and steer toward health, and to give up coping behaviors more and more. In summary, it is the stage at which the patterns underlying PD are rewritten, and patients are brought to think, feel, and act in the world in new ways.

Updating the contract is critical. Therapeutic work now requires increasing levels of activity on the patients' side. Session after session, understanding how the past gave rise to current functioning matters less and less. The real ingredient for change is for patients to intend to act differently in the week following the session.

The greatest difficulties lurk in this step and the next, which is to seek more adaptive behaviors with the knowledge that the old ones were dysfunctional. Following the procedures described here allows them to be addressed with relative ease. In particular, therapists must pay attention to the revision of the contract, especially the tasks necessary to achieve the goals. Revision is also crucial because we are asking patients to act by breaking automatisms, so this is when fears and painful emotions surface. It is essential that patients decide to face them in full awareness.

Sometimes, however, there can be deep disagreement about what it means to continue therapy. It happens when people with intense psychic pain and severe relational dysfunction steadfastly and protractedly refuse to adopt new behaviors that break patterns and promote health. Some do not think they make sense; others remain focused on *the other does to me* and *if only the other* positions, persist in angry or powerless ruminations, or both, and demand that the therapist ally with them.

Others see the path ahead but are paralyzed by the pain they must overcome in walking it: fear of loneliness – "Will I be able to take care of myself?"; fear of criticism or aggression; survivor's guilt – "If I become autonomous, I will abandon my loved ones; they will suffer; I am selfish." These patients know that health is along that path, but they decide not to take that step.

How do therapists act now? They reformulate the contract and assume the position of *leaning forward powerlessness* (Chapter 3). They first clarify, leaving no doubt, that therapy will only generate transient relief in session and refrain from promising symptom and relational change. They gently re-iterate that new actions are required for improvement but that the patient is not obliged to take them. Finally, they make clear their intention to be there, attentive, and available so that their statements do not sound like an ultimatum in any way. Therapists do not promise well-being but remain present.

Let us now return to considering how to proceed when patients agree to engage in therapeutic tasks but problems emerge in the therapeutic relationship. It is common for minor ruptures to occur that require attention. We describe together how to make this step and its potential impact on the relationship:

Agree on a goal consistent with the wish and formulate it in a concrete and actionable way through behavioral experiments

One must focus on what patients would like to accomplish and when they will try. Frequent micro-fractures of the alliance of the *withdrawal* type (Safran & Muran, 2000) occur due to avoidance attempts. Patients accept the task but remain vague about when they will perform it. The therapist does not hesitate: ask the patient when exactly he or she will attempt the task. Jokingly, we often approach the problem this way. Let us imagine that the session took place on a Monday at 4 PM.

PATIENT:	"I might do it in the next few days, then."
T:	"Well, when exactly?"
P:	"I don't know, maybe, let's see, Thursday or Friday?"
T:	"That's fine, but look, our session ends at 4:50 p.m. Can you make it start in about 1 hour and 38 minutes?"
P:	"Whaaat!?"
T:	"Ah, sorry, it's too late. Shall we say in 1 hour and 20 minutes?"

Put more formally, we are talking about situations in which the contract is clear to both, so it is a matter of taking territory away from avoidance and procrastination. The therapist can also voice, again with irony, the underlying anger that the patient will inevitably feel.

T:	"Yes, I know you hate me, you are right. I've realized that I have to give you more. Let's make it 1 hour and 39 minutes, okay?"
P:	"Wow, how nice you are today."
T:	"Very good. I see you agree, and I'm glad."

In other cases, patients may be reluctant to perform the task, and again, the necessary step is to explore the reasons. If reticence persists, we return to the contract. First, we propose tasks that patients evaluate as easier. If they refuse these as well, it is necessary again to adopt *leaning forward powerlessness*: "I understand that you don't feel like going away, leaving your suffering mother at home . . ."; "I realize that going out with your friends, even though your husband criticizes you and holds a grudge, and you fear abandonment, is challenging . . ."; "I know that resisting sending the message to your ex comes at a cost . . ."; "I realize that introducing a food that you have always avoided so far is difficult."

All these sentences are completed with, "But if you decide not to do it, how can I help you? What therapeutic tools do I have?"

If patients agree to reformulate the contract, it is easy for the therapeutic relationship, after this withdrawal rupture (Safran & Muran, 2000), to improve due to the beneficial effects of the exercise, related to pattern 5 of technique-relationship interaction.

Review in-session behavioral experiments

The next session includes a reflection on the outcome of the exposure. Did the patient try to pursue the healthy wish or refrain from coping? Did she succeed? Experiments at this stage continually generate narrative episodes in which, again, to explore thoughts, emotions, and somatic sensations. Typically, a set of healthy aspects surfaces, and a return to the pattern occurs. With this information, therapist and patient update the shared formulation, that is, the map that guides treatment. Indeed, the therapist points out to the patient how her mind goes from moments of good functioning to moments when the schema still exerts its power. However, he shows her how, at various times in the new episodes, the patient has had agency over her mental functioning and can continue to exercise it.

Using experiential techniques in session to enhance behavioral experiments

We need to support patients in such important and, at the same time, delicate transitions, where well-being surfaces but suffering is reactivated. Experiential techniques in session are invaluable in consolidating the results of behavioral experiments or in overcoming the problem that prevented them from working. It may be that the patient has agreed to an experiment, but it has generated a micro-fracture related to pattern 2 of technique-relationship interaction. At other times, the patient has not performed the task and, in the next session, is dejected, closed, and afraid of disappointing the therapist; at still other times, he becomes irritated because he thinks that the therapist has proposed the task superficially, neglecting his pain or objective difficulties.

The therapist first works on the relational breakdown. If it is a closure rupture, the goal is to make sure that the patient is confident that the therapist will not be disappointed or judge him for not doing the task. In the case of a hostile rupture, the therapist must bring the patient to realize that he proposed the task for good reasons, knowing that it would be a difficult and painful exercise.

At this point, therapists are likely to discover that the healthy parts of a patient are not solid enough to deal with exposure in real life. It may, therefore, be helpful both for the progress of therapy and to reconsolidate the relationship, as well as to have an imaginative exercise focused on anticipating the behavioral exposure and mentally simulating it. Therapists thus have a way of bringing up negative ideas and emotions such as, "I am not capable, and the other person criticizes me"; "If I do this, the other will suffer, and I feel harmful and bad." Then, the therapist goes back to evoking the healthy parts until the patient can act consistently with that wish. The therapist brings attention to the somatic aspects of the healthy parts and the core idea of self that emerges when the patient relives it and experiences it in the body.

For example, we say, "Now you feel curious and feel like telling your partner that playing in the band with your friends is important to you. Where do you feel the sensation?" The patient may notice his fingers moving in anticipation of playing a song on the guitar or feeling active. The therapist then asks him to keep these sensations in mind, savor them, and say what he thinks of himself at that moment. If he answers something that sounds like "motivated, happy," the therapist asks him to dwell on these feelings for a moment longer and simulate in his mind the moment when he will tell his wife that he cares about playing in the group. The therapist anticipates that he will be seized with feelings of guilt for harm done or fear of being criticized and abandoned. In this way, the patient already knows that during guided imagery the pattern will resurface. At this point, the therapist invites him enact the new behavior several times in his imagination until the vital part of himself prevails and is no longer overwhelmed by the core idea of guilt, harm, and abandonment.

It is easy at this stage for the use of techniques after experiments to consolidate the alliance, in accordance with the type 4 pattern, whereby the patient perceives the therapist to be solid, supportive, and trusting.

Sometimes, however, even a few moments later, the pattern is reactivated, and suddenly, the patient is back to perceiving the therapist in a schema-dependent way. This is pattern 2 of technique-relationship interaction, in which the proposed exercise or its execution causes a micro-fracture that demands attention. Patients may perceive themselves to be disappointing and imagine the therapist to be critical, bored, and eager to break off the relationship.

In addition to the possibility of micro-alliance ruptures, it also happens at this stage that, after experiencing positive moments consistent with wishes and after interrupting behavioral copings that were hitherto almost incoercible, patients return the following week to schema-dependent functioning (Figure 5.1, Box 6). Therapists should be aware that these transient relapses are completely normal and predictable and should therefore not be frightened or worried, ignore them, or pressure the patient to continue functioning well. Any of these reactions would initiate a relational breakdown, and the cause would be schemas related to fear of failure, guilt for harm done, fear of peer judgment, or compulsive caretaking. These tendencies need to be recognized, regulated, and curbed, as described in Chapter 3.

At this point, the therapist points out the relapse to the patient, normalizes it, and moves on again to redefine goals and tasks. She shows with even greater clarity that the path to health is made up of moments when the old schema-dependent modes regain control, often under the influence of events that occurred during the week. And there is no reason to worry, remembering that therapy from this point on is no longer focused on understanding already known mechanisms but on empowering the new and healthy that is surfacing.

Psychological health is the goal of a journey of knowledge, but, more importantly, it is about training and new learning: clinicians must be aware of this and remind the patient frequently.

When the above steps are successful, patients have come to the following realizations: (a) that they are being driven by schemas of which they know the triggers; (b) that they react to schema-related pain with maladaptive coping that they begin to see as unhelpful and harmful; (c) that they have many healthy self-aspects that are intact but still labile; (d) that, precisely because of this, they need to be trained and consolidated; (e) that they have agency over both their mental states and their behaviors; and (f) that patterns can regain control and transiently take on the flavor of reality again, but they know from the experience of previous months of therapy that these are transient fluctuations and they just have to actively counteract them.

At this point, patients are ready for the next steps: improving adaptation to social relationships, understanding others more richly and articulately, and minimizing behavioral coping and repetitive thinking. Relational breakdowns are also possible here.

PART IV

Adopt more effective ways to realize wishes and recognize one's contribution to interpersonal cycles: Improve theory of mind, decentering, and integration (Figure 5.1, Box 7–9)

Reality is not always our friend. Therapists must know that change in real relationships is not an accurate measure of therapeutic progress. Reasoning in these terms is a mistake because it leads us to measure our results on the plane of reality, which obscures the structural change already taking place. A very reliable indicator is when patients face the same negative reactions as the real other but realize that these do not depend on their own faults and shortcomings but on how others reason; thus, they suffer transiently, but patterns are not reactivated.

For example, patients looking for work improve because they started looking for it and not because they find it. Patients who dream of fulfilling romantic relationships improve because they try to get dates or choose people different from the past or, at least, if they choose partners who seem carbon copies of previous, dysfunctional ones, they break away from them sooner or with less pain. If they live in a painful relationship, as children, partners, or colleagues, and decide to maintain it, they suffer less in the face of others' gestures and attitudes.

This means that the psychic structure has changed, and reality can still hurt, but it is a burn that lasts only the time needed to cool it with ice and medicate it. There then remains some pain in the background and no more.

However, we all have the right to seek a full life, one with meaning, and for us to achieve it, reality matters. At this point in treatment, therefore, it is correct and necessary to agree with patients that to achieve goals on the reality plane, they must follow different paths. It is essential that they realize that they are adopting relational modes that do not work and often alienate others. Based on this awareness, they try to act differently. It is therefore a matter of patients using more sophisticated interpersonal skills based on a richer understanding of others and realizing their own contribution to dysfunctional interpersonal cycles.

The time is ripe for agreeing with patients that their future is even more in their own hands. Realizing important goals and getting rid of symptoms or drastically reducing them depends on their actions. The contract must be reformulated again, because patients are going to take more responsibility for therapeutic progress. Therapists now heavily involve them in experiential work, both in session and especially outside, and this time, the measuring tool is also reality. Patients then use their now well-developed metacognitive knowledge about themselves and others to deal with complex relational situations, satisfy desires, and solve problems and conflicts. It is, therefore, a matter of promoting advanced forms of metacognitive mastery in the relational domain (Carcione et al., 2011). Continuous reality monitoring is required, and it is possible that, despite the effort, results may be disappointing, so that it is easy for patients to perceive the therapist as distant, critical, disappointed, or resigned. It goes without saying that the risk of relational ruptures is high.

The tools to be adopted are the same as in the previous section; only the goals change. Until now, we have aimed to take power away from negative schemas and make room for healthy parts. Now, it is about affecting reality and interpersonal relationships. We bring patients both to recognize how their own communication patterns can negatively affect others and to adopt different, new behaviors tailored to the context. They will make attempts and reason with the therapist whether these are more effective or make them feel better.

A typical case is emotional dependence. We ask patients to adopt less surrendering and submissive and more autonomous and assertive attitudes. And then ask themselves,

Once I act differently, does what I fear really happen? Does the other criticize me, abandon me or suffer? Or am I better off, and is the impact on the other person different from what I thought? Or am I better off anyway, and, even if the other reacts more or less as I expected, is the effect on me different, bearable?

In this case, chairwork is very useful. The patient, moving from one chair to another, plays herself and the other and observes how she feels and thinks in the two positions. The game continues until she contacts her desire in a sufficiently stable way and experiments with expressing herself clearly and firmly. Here, it is permissible and necessary for therapists to explicitly support tendencies toward greater interpersonal effectiveness, albeit keeping in mind that their judgment is partly subjective.

Equally useful is role-playing; here the therapist offers feedback on the newly adopted communication modes that seem functional and will, hopefully, be so in reality. The therapist, while performing the role-play, repeatedly asks the patient for feedback on how he or she feels at various stages: Does personal efficacy increase? What are the bodily sensations? Do thoughts change according to the sentences the patient says and how she says them? We will describe these in detail in chapter 12.

What impact do these exercises have on the therapeutic relationship? It is possible that the proposal generates fractures because patients feel pressured both to act and to evoke painful moments. They may feel criticized and blamed because they fear failing. Strategies for dealing with alliance ruptures are similar to those in the previous section. We add here that it is easy for active work to strengthen the alliance at this stage because patients perceive the therapist as even more supportive of their goals, and, when behavioral experiments are successful, the sense of shared joy, like a goal scored in a team sport, is vivid. This is pattern 5 of technique-relationship interaction: improvement in relational life strengthens the therapeutic relationship.

Once again, remember that the success of behavioral exercises is almost always transient. The therapist should not be surprised if, in the sessions that follow, patients relapse. Work on PD requires training and repetition: moments when patients act healthily and understand others more maturely are followed by moments when they function as at the beginning of therapy. Theory of mind becomes limited again, and patients do not decenter and again end up attributing schema-dependent ideas to others. The therapist must see these relapses coming and return to work from the point of decision-making procedures at which patients are at this very moment. Therapy is a kind of Goose Game, and if patients are late in treatment and tell us that they have gotten worse and are in pain, the therapist starts again from the question from which it all stems, "Can you give me an example?"

The therapeutic contract is fundamental at this stage. It is a time when therapists can cause relational ruptures because they are driven by the impulse to make patients' lives more like their own idea of what a healthy life should be. What do we mean? Sometimes, patients are satisfied with forms of adaptation that we consider problematic. They persist in relationships with partners they have described to us as frustrating, flat, cold, judgmental, cynical, and unfaithful. They stay in their jobs not because they love them but because they do not want to risk going down new paths. They continue to act out submission, renunciation, and perfectionism coping despite knowing how unhappy it makes them. Yet their lives seem acceptable to them, and if they still involve suffering and sacrifice, they have nevertheless chosen them. As one patient, a sports shop owner who lived with a woman who physically assaulted him on a few occasions, told us, "Despite her being a whirlwind, with all her destructive rage, she is better than the frost I was raised in."

We consider it mandatory that therapists do what patients now ask from therapy. If they choose to discontinue it in full awareness of their own patterns and the consequences of not pushing themselves further, it is not a dropout. It is merely the result of a conscious decision to live in what they consider the best ecological niche possible.

The most advanced operation from the metacognitive point of view is to integrate self-parts. Here, patients are aware of the schema-dependent aspects of self, but these have now become nothing more than non-pathological personality traits and styles. They are aware they have vulnerabilities, the *unfinished business* (Greenberg, 2002), and know they can resurface. At the same time, they are aware of their healthy aspects and put them into practice. They realize how, depending on circumstances and possible stressors, old functioning can emerge for a while, but it comes with less suffering and leaves room for mental states of well-being and the ability to regulate pain. It is, therefore, a matter of accepting one's own self-multiplicity. Joint reformulations, including in the form of drawings or diagrams, are useful for this purpose. We ask patients to write a letter (Ryle & Kerr, 2002) describing how they saw themselves at the beginning of therapy and how they portray themselves now, pointing out progress, any remaining areas of work, and, indeed, the *unfinished business*, the life issues they know they will have to work through from time to time.

Therapists act as a vicarious memory: when negative moments resurface, they remind patients that they are normal and how they have repeatedly gone through them and overcome them. Although this part (Figure 5.1, Box 9) is basically treatment termination, we actually perform it several times at various levels of complexity during therapy. So we ask patients with some regularity, say every one or two months, to take stock of how they were before, how they see themselves now, and how they think the therapeutic work has helped them; to keep in mind both what is still not working today and what is working.

Experiential techniques can play a role. A role-play or guided imagery, for example, helps the patient recognize the oscillation between one aspect of the self and the other. In these steps, ruptures in the relationship are rare or minor. It is necessary for therapists to be accurate in formulating functioning in its entirety and to have a validating attitude. They must show understanding and acceptance for the once problematic areas that still occur, even if in a less harmful way. Finally, they must point out what good has emerged and the active role patients have played in building their own well-being.

PART V

Promote effective and articulate mastery strategies: Treat residual symptoms. Interrupt dysfunctional behavioral coping and repetitive thinking (Figure 5.1, Box 10)

Patients have come a long way: they have improved access to internal states, understood the meaning structures that cause them pain, and realized that pain persists because of an internal cause. They have succeeded, at the same time, in accessing the healthy parts and discovered they can be guided by them toward meeting relational or autonomy wishes. They have learned to recognize their own contribution in generating and maintaining interpersonal cycles and to make richer, more articulate, and realistic assumptions about what goes on in the minds of others outside of their schema-driven readings. In short, they know in which direction well-being is and they move along that path.

They have understood the origins of symptoms and found that, no matter how pervasive and persistent they were, they have the power to control, reduce, or get rid of them. They know that symptoms are underpinned by purposes, beliefs, and components that are automatically activated and die hard. They have already changed their minds about many things: they do not give truth value to negative ideas about themselves, and, regarding repetitive thinking, they no longer believe that, to solve problems, they must ruminate.

What is missing? We need to bring patients to learn to modulate their subjective suffering in different ways and to face social problems through increasingly complex mastery strategies. Patients with PD often resort to dysfunctional strategies – for example, self-harm and substance abuse – to regulate emotions. In social relationships, they lack the tools to act effectively and adaptively, such as negotiating their goals with others, flexibly modifying their goals as the relational context changes, or complying with rules and norms. This is something that has already begun in part with the procedures described in Boxes 7–9 in Figure 5.1, when we help patients break dysfunctional cycles and use a richer, more mature theory of mind.

It is now a matter, as a final step, of building problem-solving strategies based on a more articulated awareness of one's own internal states and those of others: "What do I do if my partner leaves me? How do I handle the pain of a loss or a problem at work that risks igniting serious conflicts and diplomatic incidents that would backfire on me?" The therapist helps the patient construct a varied and flexible set of mentalistic strategies through a combination of anticipatory imagery, role-play, and behavioral experiments.

Moreover, at this stage, some symptoms still persist, perhaps reduced in frequency or intensity, or reappear because of relational triggers. Well, it is time to work continuously to reduce dysfunctional coping and symptoms as much as possible. Some automatisms are written in body and mind, sustaining habits that are hard to make disappear. In the final stages of therapy, work is aimed at counteracting, reducing, and, when possible, eliminating them. It is necessary, however, that patients agree with this plan and are willing to undertake the necessary work. Change comes at a cost: they have to recognize their tendency to ruminate and decide to stop and nip, if possible, repetitive thinking in the bud, knowing that this will result in a transient increase in negative feelings. They have to address contexts that still generate social anxiety, discontinue behaviors such as perfectionism and procrastination, and consequently accept exposure to anxiety, guilt, shame, or fear. For example, a patient has to refrain from compulsive caregiving, knowing that this will make her feel guilty and consider herself 'mean'.

It always starts with reformulating the contract. Lynette, 25, suffers from dependent PD, which has been at the root of severe emotional dependence and OCD since she was 13 years old. Lynette spent a lot of time in the past trying to neutralize intrusive thoughts and images in which her sister or other loved ones died violently. Dozens of times a day she would see the picture of her sister burning, ending up crushed in the furniture of the house or skewered on the spikes of the gate. She would respond to these obsessions by retracing her steps, looking at the object that had stimulated the picture (stove, cabinet, or gate), and striving to retrieve a picture of her sister alive and smiling. At this point, she could go on with her day, but in the meantime, she had lost time and felt exhausted.

At the end of therapy, dependent PD and emotional dependence are overcome, but OCD still recurs. The therapist intervenes in this way.

T: "Lynette, I would like to propose something to you. Tell me what you think. You have made incredible progress; you have practically overcome your historical, emotional dependence, you have distanced yourself from the woman whom you let enslave you. You are autonomous, you travel, you have changed job and are freely considering if this one suits you. However, when the symptom comes back, you almost treat it by glossing over it, 'I just had some obsessions, no big deal.' The point is that when you say that, then within a few days the obsessions take over, and you are sick. We have already seen you have power over the anxiety that pictures of your sister dying in excruciating torment generate in you. We know you are able to stop the obsessions with the tools you have learnt. When you interrupt rituals to assure yourself you are not the cause of your sister's death, you feel guilty for a moment, but within seconds, guilt disappears. In short, you are very capable of counteracting OCD; we have seen this many times. Now, we know that every time you experience a tense situation, the intrusive images come up again, and that is normal. It's just that you still adopt obsessive behaviors, and you do it in a self-indulgent way as if it's something not so harmful, right? But we know it's certainly harmful! Can we agree that, in the final part of therapy, you will be vigilant about obsessive behaviors and try to resist the temptation to enact them? It will not be easy, but it is important to know that you need to be alert to such behaviors at all times, you cannot indulge in them. Yes, of course, there will be a price to pay: you will transiently feel a little more anxious and guilty. But then you will feel better, much better. What do you think? Do you want to do it? Of course, you can fail, you will sometimes enact rituals to make sure your sister is alive and well, especially when you are under stress. But what matters is that you notice them and immediately say to yourself: I will try and counteract them! Do you agree?"

Similar interventions apply to patients who show residual signs of subjugation, self-harm, and aggression, or who indulge in behaviors that may rekindle alcohol and substance abuse or compulsive video gaming. These patients may return to seemingly healthy eating behaviors but hide a relapse of the eating disorder, or return to overwork driven by perfectionism. In all these cases, therapists reformulate the contract and agree with the patient that they have to commit themselves to recognizing these tendencies as problematic and counteracting them (Chapter 13).

Problems in the therapeutic relationship can be reactivated. A possible rupture in the working alliance is just around the corner. Patients sometimes do not agree with the steps needed to get rid of residual pain or do not want to deal with the pain the exposures generate. It is also possible that they read the firmness with which therapists show the means/ends relationship between active work and suffering reduction in light of a dominance/submission pattern. None of these is a good reason to desist from explaining to patients that if they want to get rid of as much residual suffering as possible, active work is essential.

If patients do not agree or simply do not want to pay the price, therapists will have to anchor themselves in the position of *leaning forward powerlessness*, which here takes a well-defined form: accepting that the treatment ends with the patient being satisfied with the results while they still see problems. If the end of therapy is not yet in sight and patients bring back the re-emergence of suffering to the session, therapists must, every time, really *every time*, ask, "I see that you are suffering. But we said you don't want to work on it, right? What can we do then?"

Above all, however, in these closing moments of therapy, patients are grateful to therapists for their determination to work actively. Yes, inwardly, they may protest, as one does with a coach who forces us to train despite fatigue and sore muscles. But they know that insistence is for good and, above all, that theirs is a relationship between equals: it is the patient who has asked the therapist to adopt the position at the same time of *caregiver* and *coach*. The therapist is a spur: a reminder that health, like any human activity, requires effort, repetition, and commitment. The goal is healing, a new way of living one's life.

Chapter 6

Narrative episodes, early access to healthy parts, and dynamic assessment

Awareness of internal states and cognitive-affective-somatic processes

One of the first steps for the shared formulation of functioning is to collect auto-biographical memories (Figure 6.1, Box 1). It is one of the bases for knowing a patient's subjective experience (Figure 6.1, Box 2) and immediately afterwards reconstructing the causal links between events, thoughts, emotions, somatic states, and behaviors (Figure 6.1, Box 4).

Episodes should involve relationships in which someone is present interacting with the patient and predominantly frustrating his wish. These are scenes in which a patient relates, for example, that she felt lonely when her husband did not take care of her in a time of need, or when another patient showed a project to the boss and received dismissive criticism instead of the praise hoped for, and so on. Therapists need to dig deep into an episode to allow the patient to begin to find out how she feels and thinks in certain situations; so they ask questions aimed at exploring cognitions and emotions in the various passages of the story.

In this way, one obtains material about the internal world closer to raw experience. Patients' initial description passes from something like: "When I was with friends, I was tense and left" to

> As my friend said he had doubts about my proposal for the vacation, I got anxious. I imagined that he would think I didn't get anything right as usual, and I felt ashamed. I let it go because I was afraid he would blackball me.

Before recounting an episode, the patient may say, "When I come home and see my son talking back to me, I can't stand it; I swear, I regret giving birth to him." After describing the episode in detail, thanks to targeted questions, his story sounds like this:

> The other day, I came home, and my son was on the couch; I greeted him, but he talked back to me. This made me feel sad because I wanted to be greeted with affection. I'm afraid he doesn't consider me a good father, but then I think I am, and I get angry at how he behaves.

DOI: 10.4324/9781003570967-6

| Collecting specific autobiographical memories
Box 1 | Identifying the elements of subjective experience
Box 2 | Early access to healthy self aspects
Box 3 |
| Reconstructing psychological cause-effect links
Box 4 | | Dynamic assessment: Behavioral homework and experiential techinques to improve monitoring
Box 5 |

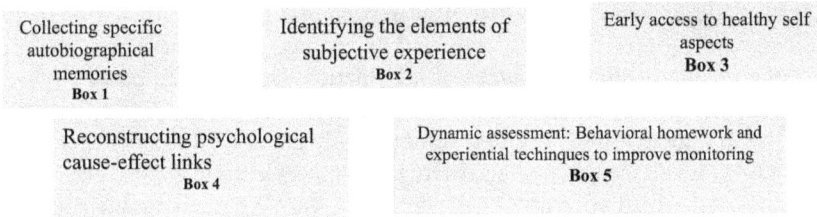

Figure 6.1 Reading the internal world

Moving from generalizations to episodes is important for improving metacognitive monitoring, often lacking in PD. In addition to fostering greater awareness of the internal world, detailed analysis of episodes promotes the recovery of agency over mental states. Patients often describe their own mental state as a necessary and inevitable reflex to the actions of others, "the other does to me" mode: "I'm angry with my boss because he didn't allow me a vacation; he mistreated me, he didn't listen to me." They do not realize the importance of their interpretation of the event and what cognitions led them to react. What did a patient think of herself at that time?

Helping a patient understand what thoughts her aggressive and careless boss activates in her is difficult but essential. We aim for descriptions such as, "I see myself as inept, someone who can be put in the background, vis-à-vis him, whom I see as overbearing and disinterested. He is unfair, but eventually it is I who see myself that way." We aim at giving patients knowledge and power over their internal states, "I see myself this way. However, I could try to see myself differently."

Collecting narrative episodes is essential for overcoming tendencies to intellectualize and theorize about oneself and the world. These are modalities that lead patients to express themselves in terms of value judgments and thus offer no room for intervention: "The idea of going to class at the university makes me sick, the Italian university system makes me sick, and the world equally so, and I am unfit for this world."

In the abstract, intellectualized mode, patients hardly describe their emotions: "I feel tired of this relationship; when we are together, time does not pass. Yesterday, I was wondering if, as a couple, we have a future, and I didn't know what to answer." In many circumstances, patients fail to move from generalized narratives such as, "My father treats me badly; I always get angry with him when I come home," to identifying a specific episode defined in time and space.

What role do experiential techniques play in facilitating the exploration of episodes and the shift from abstractions, intellectualizations, or repetitive thinking to autobiographical narratives? How do they facilitate access to the cognitions and emotions underlying suffering and dysfunctional behaviors? We first show how we intervene when the style is intellectualizing and then when patients begin the session in the grip of repetitive thoughts about relationships.

It is useful to focus on the body (the *second lake*). In the absence of specific autobiographical memories, the body and its actions, posture, and prosody in the flow of speech are valuable sources of information. Gestures and posture indicate emotions and moods that we mark and explore. For example, we ask a patient speaking in a generalized way to dwell on bodily states and observe them mindfully: "As you told me that having sisters and brothers is useless, you lowered your head and intertwined your hands. What do you feel? What emotion accompanies these gestures?" By inviting patients to focus on posture and movements as they speak, we help them discover emotions and related cognitions. Once identified, we move on to ask them about the autobiographical memories in which they experienced them. The path, then, starts from the non-verbal, reaches out to emotions and cognitions, and heads on to narrative episodes.

Another way to improve access to the inner world is the use of role-play, enactments, or structured or unstructured guided imagery. Starting with an episode, we create in-session conditions that activate arousal as the patient relives a relational experience.

Sometimes, where the episode is missing, the therapist creates it on the basis of somatic emotions and sensations and what little cognition has emerged: one patient recounts that *for as long as she can remember,* her mother would show herself to be hurt and disappointed whenever she was autonomous, but she cannot recall specific episodes or identify emotions beyond anger: "It's always like that, I would ask her if I could go out with friends, and she would make faces at me. I would get pissed off but still stay home." The therapist has several technical possibilities: she can ask the patient to "sit" the mother in an empty chair and ask her to interact with her. Or he can arrange an enactment in which he himself plays the mother "making faces" while the patient says she wants to leave. The patient's arousal grows; she sees her mother in front of her, and the possibilities for the inner landscape to be enriched increase. It opens the way to understanding that, for example, she wants to feel free and, in the face of her suffering and critical mother, perceives herself as guilty and powerless. The therapist can also ask her to visualize her mother in her imagination, describing her face, tone of voice, clothing, or posture, and then ask, "What do you think and feel now that your mother . . .?"

From the outset, decision-making procedures require a therapist to foster in the patient an awareness that he or she has healthy, functioning, vital self-parts (Figure 6.1, Box 3), that is, characters in his or her internal theatre (Hermans & Dimaggio, 2004) who think of themselves as lovable, valid, free, effective, included in the group, and so on. Techniques are powerful here. We try to help the patient recall experiences and states of the self that, although present in his inner world, nevertheless remain in the background compared to the negative self-images that occupy much of his inner landscape. After the patient has recalled a scene in which the protagonist is a healthy character from his internal theatre, we use bodily, dramaturgical, or imagery interventions so that he re-experiences it on a somatic level, as well as telling ideas and emotions. If a patient re-experiences an episode in guided imagery, we intervene as follows:

> You went along with you desire to go out with your friend, although your husband disagreed. Let's try to feel in the body how you feel as you go out; what emotions and thoughts is it colored with? Let's try to fix better in our mind what happens when you act in accordance with what you like? Shall we term this part of you in some way, to evoke it in the future?

Sometimes, patients with PD have difficulties recalling moments or relational situations in which they experienced themselves as strong, capable, or lovable. In such cases, we can "build" the healthy self in session with the help of experiential techniques: for example, by moving from a curved and atonic posture to an upright and strong one, a patient may discover herself stronger and more capable of responding to criticism. With calming breathing, through centering or grounding exercises, we evoke states of well-being and security in which it is easier to access self-states such as "safe," "free," and so on. In short, we promote the experience of the healthy self from the body and, from that state, consistently evoke positive cognitions and emotions.

Dynamic assessment (Figure 6.1, Box 5 and Chapter IV) is the fourth lake in which to explore cognitive-affective-somatic processes through experiential work. It helps in describing internal states, circumventing the frequent tendencies to ruminate, intellectualize, or generalize.

One of the reasons patients fail to report episodes and speak abstractly or fail to identify emotions and cognitions in an episode is the massive reliance on coping, which shields them from suffering.

The therapist, once these few readable cognitive-affective contents are emphasized, reactivates some scenes, real or created as needed, with the techniques. The purpose is to increase arousal and find a gateway to the inner world. For example, Lucy, a 50-year-old woman with obsessive-compulsive PD and generalized anxiety, complains of fatigue, depression, and anxiety. She feels overwhelmed by family and work tasks she takes on her shoulders: she has sacrificial tendencies, and the fatigue is reality-based. Sacrificial tendencies are a typical coping mechanism, but the therapist does not understand what Lucy is protecting herself from. She says only that it is natural for her to go along with others' demands. For the purpose of the dynamic assessment, the therapist proposes a role-play:

> Would you like it if I try to ask you for a favor, asking you, for example, to get those books from the top of my bookshelf because I need them? Of course, you don't really have to do it. You can stop for *a moment before* acting when you feel the urge. I am interested in understanding what moves you, what thoughts, what emotions. How you see me when making this request and how you see yourself.

Lucy agrees. The therapist asks her to get the books, and Lucy tightens her lips, "If I don't do this, I get anxious . . . you need . . . I see myself as a bad person if I say no . . ." New material has now emerged for us to explore. We specify that as we implement practices such as this, we carefully monitor the relationship, as we will see later.

In other cases, we offer patients homework assignments with attempted coping abstention: "What happens inside you if you stop for *a moment before you* pick up your cell phone and call your partner to tell him you are angry because he has neglected you?"; "You try to turn down an invitation to have a coffee from a man with whom you are flirting, but you know you are not really interested. What happened to you at that moment?";

> You're at dinner with your friends, had a pizza, and now you're tempted to binge. You can try not to; I know it's hard, but it's okay even if you just try for a moment. Then tell me what happens to you
>
> Fioravanti et al. (2023)

The goal is not behavioral change, which would be premature, but to increase arousal and note emerging cognitions and emotions.

The interweaving of experiential techniques and therapeutic relationships during the first steps of the procedures

Techniques play a key role in the steps described. We ask a patient for active involvement, often from the very first therapy sessions. What can happen to the therapeutic relationship at these moments? Suggesting that the patient talk to an empty chair in which he "sees" his father, stand up for a grounding exercise from which to contact the healthy self, or talk with the therapist playing the role of the critical leader are operations that can generate stress. Patients may feel ashamed at the idea of being ridiculed and obligated by the therapist, who appears overbearing to them, and may feel the exercise is useless since no one, therapist included, can help them.

Scanning a scene with guided imagery or asking patients to try and refrain from coping during the week can have an impact on the therapeutic relationship. During the exercise, or already at the mere idea of performing it, patients easily experience negative emotions. Moreover, at this stage, they cannot abstain except with great effort and only sometimes. They may experience it as a failure, fearing being criticized by the therapist or disappointing her. In contrast, finding relief from anxiety through a grounding exercise or discovering more about themselves through imaginative exploration of their inner world generates feelings of hope and trust in the therapy and the therapist, strengthening the alliance.

The therapeutic relationship may thus experience friction or even difficult impasses that require metacommunication and repair work, as we shall see in the next sections. In other cases, the same practices strengthen the alliance.

Collecting autobiographical memories: enactment to activate subjective experience and enhance awareness of mental states

We now describe how techniques and the relationship are intertwined when the therapist attempts to bring a patient with an intellectualizing style or repetitive thinking to retrieve specific episodes and accurately describe what she is thinking and feeling.

In the following example, the therapist uses the enactment technique, which generates both an impact on the therapeutic relationship and schema-related transient reactions fostering metacognitive monitoring.

Sibyl, a 28-year-old student, suffers from avoidant PD. She seeks help for anxiety that prevents her from showing up for exams. She tells of always feeling tense in front of others and avoiding contact, fearing ridicule. She cannot define her internal state better than "tense" and "fear of ridicule." When asked to recall any incident in which someone ridiculed her, Sibyl cannot answer, "I don't remember, I always had this feeling and this fear. Sometimes it happened, at school, they made fun of me because of the way I dressed and my glasses, but I can't say more than that." In addition, Sibyl is distant; her face shows no emotion and her voice is flat.

The therapist explains to Sybyl that she will use an enactment to activate her emotions and to understand clearly what she thinks and feels if someone ridicules her. She will tell her something slightly critical about her glasses and asks her to pay attention to what she thinks and feels in her body when the therapist criticizes her. Sibyl replies that the experiment is fine, nods but barely conceals her embarrassment. The technique-relationship interaction pattern 2 is now active: the beginning of the technique has generated negative emotions and thoughts that need to be explored and a rupture that needs repairing. Sibyl probably constructs the therapist as critical or dominant. How does one act under these circumstances? The therapist notices the non-verbal signals and asks her what is going on. Sibyl, blushing, says she is afraid of making a bad impression and is ashamed to be seen as ridiculous: "I don't like being criticized." The therapist replies that it is precisely this feeling that she wants to deal with and would like to soothe. Sibyl notes the therapist's calm and benevolent tone, breaks out of the pattern, regulates her embarrassment, and agrees to begin the experiential practice.

T: "Sibyl, I don't like your glasses; they look old-fashioned. [*After a few seconds*] How do you feel now?"

S: [*Blushes, stuttering*]: "I feel just like I felt then, ashamed; I know you were pretending when you told me this. However, the first thing I thought was, "You, too, like the others." I'm feeling a little ashamed."

The therapist continues exploring internal states. Sibyl is now able to say that she would like people to like her, but there always seems to be something wrong with her, and consequently, she protects herself by avoiding them.

S: "I understand how strong the shame is. So strong that I can't do anything, I want to run away."

T: "Sibyl, you really got so active! The fact that I told you it was fake, what does that make you think? By the way, your glasses are cute!"

S: "I realize by now that I have a wound that bleeds even when no one is there to mistreat me."

Thanks to this passage, later in the session, Sibyl understands she hopes others will like her but remains convinced that it will not happen. She understands she sees herself as awkward and ridiculous every time she meets someone and now knows clearly that "tense" means shame and anxiety at the prospect of experiencing it. We notice that Sibyl has transiently reached a higher metacognitive level, begins to differentiate, and realizes she is the one who has the tendency to fear judgment even when others do not express it. Thanks to the technique, a healthy representation of relationships, at least of the therapeutic relationship, has emerged: now Sibyl does not see the therapist as critical but as solid, supportive, benevolent, and even capable of helping her to experience emotions that she always avoided. Let us summarize: in this sequence, the proposal of the technique caused a micro-rupture that required stopping until it was repaired, which was done easily. It is, therefore, interaction pattern 2 (Chapters 1 and 4). Then, during execution, she changed her mind about the therapist and the relationship was consolidated, thus moving to pattern 3.

When patients start the session with repetitive thinking

Some patients begin therapy or sessions using IRT. They brood, for example, about how an exam or job presentation might go, predict negative outcomes, and experience anxiety or sadness. The clinician immediately shows patients that the repetitive mode is a mechanism that offers no solutions and accentuates pain. The clinician proposes that they engage in certain operations designed to reduce repetitive thinking itself (see chapter 8). IRT, however, prevents therapists from accessing the contents of experience in the flow of relationships, and therefore, in addition to interrupting it, they have to invite patients to recount episodes.

Improving access to the experiences within episodes

(Figure 6.1, Box 2)

Narrative episodes do not guarantee that the internal experience is readable. Even in recounting interactions well located in space and time, access to thoughts and emotions can be difficult. Therapeutic operations are needed to improve metacognitive monitoring (Figure 6.1, Box 2). MIT requires intervening to develop this capacity in several ways (Dimaggio et al., 2015, 2020), including experiential techniques. Among non-experiential interventions, therapists recall targeted questions, psychoeducational interventions on emotions, and the use of illustrative videos depicting similar situations for the purpose of activating the patient's mirroring and accessing probably inhibited painful emotions. A therapist can, in addition, increase monitoring by revealing certain aspects of the patient's self, both in terms of moods and by sharing personal episodes, so as to function as a model that leads the patient to open up.

Remember that self-disclosure, to be effective, must be specific, limited to showing the painful component of the therapist's experience, and not include references to how the therapist solved the problem. The purpose is not to suggest solutions but to open an avenue of access to internal states through mirroring, devoid of the idea that suffering means being fragile, wrong, or inferior. It is necessary for a therapist to monitor the impact of the disclosure on the relationship: how did the patient experience this opening? Usually, the reaction is beneficial, and the relationship is strengthened. A patient easily thinks: "I feel understood; it has happened to the therapist, too." Monitoring the impact of disclosure is crucial since the patient may also react negatively: "There, she has the same problems. What if she is fragile and unable to support me?" Therapists ask for feedback so that if residual relational problems emerge, they can work to repair them (Safran & Muran, 2000).

Early access to healthy parts (Figure 6.1, Box 3)

We encourage access to healthy parts from the very beginning, an operation that begins to give patients confidence and hope and awareness that they have vital and creative internal aspects. We attempt to bring out benevolent self-representations in which patients accept themselves, consider themselves valid, competent, and lovable, or see their own limitations without too much severity. These self-concepts are obscured by schemas, which lead them instead to notice mostly negative elements. Perseverative thought processes then colonize the mind, with the sole effect of reinforcing negative emotions and taking away space from the healthy parts. In addition, behavioral coping, such as avoidance or aggressive protest, and the way patients contribute to interpersonal cycles prevent them from entering positive states, which consequently remain nourishment-free.

Working to bring out the healthy parts right away aims to identify positive elements that we will include in the structured summary of the episode first and in the formulation of the schema later, as we will see in the next chapter. We want to help the patient see that when a wish is turned on for, for example, care, a positive image exists within them, such as, for example, "I am lovable." But quickly, in their mind, a negative content image imposes itself that obscures the previous one, such as, for example, "I am alone, and no one will take care of me."

How do we help patients notice the healthy self-aspects? What happens to the relationship as the therapist tries to evoke them? It is common that as the therapist invites a patient to notice positive self-aspects, negative representations of self with the other immediately surface. If the therapist offers them an experiential exercise, the patient may read themselves and the therapist through the lens of the schema: "I feel ridiculous," "I won't be able to do the exercise," "He expects too much from me," "He is asking me for something absurd" and so on. The therapist may be read as distant, cold, overbearing, disinterested, and so on. In other, more frequent, cases, the patient accesses a healthy core, which results in an improved relationship: "Therapy gives me confidence, makes me feel better."

Let's look at an example in which the use of techniques promotes early access to the healthy self and has a positive impact on the therapeutic relationship from the beginning. This is pattern 4: the technique immediately generates relief, and the relationship improves.

Isabella, a 50-year-old elementary school teacher, is married to an engineer with whom she has always had an adversarial relationship. They have three adult children. She presents traits of dependent and avoidant PD. She appears kind but dull. She sought help because of a month-long major depressive episode. She is on leave from work, feels lacking in energy and motivation, spends her days at home doing nothing, and constantly ruminates about the futility of her life and how lonely, bored, and inept she is. Isabella, convinced that she cannot stop ruminating, fears that she will go mad. She is no stranger to depressive states. When they happen, she oscillates between sadness and despair at feeling neglected. This triggers conflicts with her husband, who, too busy with work and hobbies, ignores her. Going back to historical memories, Isabella reconstructs that her desires for exploration and play were frequently frustrated by her parents, who were caught up in other things. Boredom, shutdown, and sadness were hers even in childhood.

She describes herself as shy and lonely, has few friends, and prefers to stay at home. She has no hobbies, and when she is not working, she throws herself on the couch and broods: there are many things she would like to do, but she feels that everything is useless.

However, during one of the first sessions, she spontaneously recounts that she went for a walk in the countryside to pick blackberries. The therapist, with the aim of identifying positive elements early on that she can include in the formulation, encourages her to dwell on positive feelings and cognitions. As she describes them, Isabella relaxes and gets revitalized. The therapist asks her if this is a new experience or if she has similar memories. She recounts that, as a teenager, she walked for hours in the countryside and felt good. In recalling memories, she seems even more relaxed, and the therapist points this out to her. A distant memory surfaces spontaneously: Isabella is eight years old, and she is in the garden alone, as she often was. It starts to rain; she fears she'll have to go inside, but doesn't feel like it. She runs to the garage, grabs some galoshes and a raincoat, and goes back to play in the rain. She is amused; she even likes doing it on the sly. The therapist smiles with relish and proposes that Isabella see this memory in guided imagery to help her better feel the vital, playful part of herself and know more about it. The imaginative technique, in this case, helps reinforce aspects that have already emerged in the conversation.

Isabella is in the garden, playing alone. It starts raining; she regrets having to go back inside. The idea comes to stay there and cover up: "I like the rain!" The therapist nods, amused, so Isabella dresses appropriately with galoshes and a waterproof jacket and goes back to the garden, feels the rain, and is happy and full of energy.

She remembers making up a song and singing it. She also remembers jumping in puddles, amused that it was a forbidden thing back then. We anticipate that in imagination one should not allow room for associations. Otherwise, the patient turns away from experiencing the scene as if it were happening here and now. The therapist, therefore, invites Isabella to sing and imagine jumping. Initially skeptical and somewhat embarrassed, Isabella does so. The therapist invites her to stop and describe what she felt in her body at that moment when she was there singing in the puddle. Isabella describes a sense of lightness; her breathing is calm. She feels the smells, the noises, and the coolness of the air, the rain on her face.

T: "How do you feel now?"
I: "A kind of joy, a strange thing."
T: "And what do you think of this child feeling joy and jumping and singing?"
I: "She is lively, I like her."
T: "Does she seem like a dull, lonely child?"
I: "No, she is a child who can do it."
T: "Now go back to the initial moment. It's about to rain. She knows she has to go back into the house and return to being bored alone in her room. Can you do that?"
I: "Yes."
T: "How are you? What signals does the body give? What is it thinking? Does it feel anything?"
I: "Everything heavy . . . the legs, the head, the energy is gone, my goodness how flabby."
T: "Okay, great. So now go back to the time when you were singing and jumping through puddles. How are you doing?"
I: "Happy again, it's nice; I feel like I can hear the rain now."

What was the purpose of this operation? The therapist now has healthy parts that she can include in the structured summary of the episode and later in the shared formulation of functioning. Let us see what the structured summary of events sounds like, although it is an operation that we will describe in chapter 7.

T: "Isabella had a desire to explore and play, which she felt was hers, beautiful, vital, like singing in the rain. But it was short-lived for her; she was immediately caught up in the idea of being alone, with no one to keep her company, and at that point she shut down."

As we have said before, the use of techniques requires constant monitoring of the relationship, even in these cases where the effect is clearly positive. The therapist asks Isabella what she noticed about the exercise and how she felt its presence.

I: "I had forgotten what joy is . . . I feel alive; this exercise is amazing. The transition from one to the other then really amazed me; with imagination, I changed my mood. It made me do something lovely."

At the beginning of the exercise, Isabella already had trust in the therapist, which enabled her to accept the imaginative exercise. In the end, she finds that, thanks to the technique, she is better off: the effectiveness of the therapeutic intervention improves the alliance, and it helps her to discover that the therapy works and consolidates the bond; it is a technique-relationship interaction pattern 4. Experiencing the therapist as supportive came as a surprise to her and served as a corrective emotional experience. Isabella used to suffer because, when she had a desire to explore and play, she could not find anyone to play with her. Now, she begins to discover that it is possible to play under a benevolent gaze. Through this gaze, she discovers that there is a vitality within her that she has forgotten. These will be the elements on which the behavioral reactivation that will help her overcome depression will be based.

Reconstruction of causal links (Figure 6.1, Box 4)

Through exploration of narrative episodes (first lake), material gathered by observing non-verbal behavior (second lake), reflection on the relationship (third lake), and dynamic assessment (fourth lake), the patient's internal world has become more readable. It is now necessary to know the logical processes and mutual cause-and-effect links between thoughts, emotions, somatic reactions, and behaviors. What thought triggered an emotion and behavior? How did an emotion, for example, anger, settle in the mind, foment angry thoughts, and trigger rumination on wrongs suffered? How does a relational antecedent lead to dysfunctional behavior that generates a relational difficulty that is followed by a symptom? Very often, patients with PD and post-traumatic disorders struggle to reconstruct psychological cause-and-effect processes. Experiential techniques make a valuable, sometimes decisive, contribution in revealing them.

Laura is 40 years old and suffers from covert narcissistic PD and complicated grief. She lost her partner to illness two years earlier, presents with generalized anxiety and depression, and has sudden outbursts of anger. She asks for help to reduce symptoms that she traces back to the grief of loss.

During one of the first sessions, she recounts a recent painful episode. Laura went through her partner's treatment with the help of a couple of friends. Her parents live outside Rome and told her they could not come and help her. The day after her partner's surgery, Laura was driven home by a friend. Her mother called her. At the end of the brief phone call, Laura punched the window of her friend's car. To the therapist, Laura could only say, "I'm pissed off at life."

To the therapist's questions, she responds by saying that she was angry about her partner's condition and nothing more. But how did the phone call trigger such anger that it led her to hit the window of a car that was not even hers? What was the trigger? What was the cognition? Did she feel other emotions before the anger? How did she feel after the punch?

The therapist proposes guided imagination for her to discover her cognitive-affective processes, but Laura refuses. Her face shows a mixture of anger and contempt.

L: "Doctor. What is there to understand? My life is over; it's a fact. What is the point of talking about it? Can you help me change it? Of course not! I live very well as it is, without anyone, since my trust in mankind is low. Wisely. I don't think you can do anything else."

Laura's face is red with anger. The therapist feels useless and powerless; the experiential technique may have generated a rupture in the alliance but more probably brought to light a preexisting one. However, the therapist does not succumb to her own reactions, does not let criticism stop her, and invites Laura to explore the rupture.

T: "Laura, okay, don't worry, we don't have to do anything. But what's going on? I'm very interested in what you're feeling. What did my suggestion to do the exercise provoke in you? How did you feel at that instant?"
L: "I'm angry. I feel that you are a kind and caring person, but what can you do to solve my situation? Can we change the world? Can we bring my partner back to life? The only one who cared for me? Yes, I am angry with you, I am alone, it is a fact, end of story. Can she do something about it? Can anyone do anything about it? No. Then why delve into it? Just to make me feel worse?"
T: "I understand better now. No one can help you, including me. In fact, if we approach the pain, it makes it even worse. This feeling must be unpleasant and frustrating, right?"
L: "Well, your tools are useless. You can't do anything for me, this is is how I feel and this is how I will stay. It makes me very angry, so let's change the subject; otherwise, I feel bad."

Laura has described her internal world better, and some cause-and-effect connections have appeared, related to the therapeutic relationship. But she remains frozen in her anger toward the therapist and in turning away from her. The therapist returns to feeling useless and cornered.

T: "Laura, I would like to help you, but I don't know how. I can't get close to you; in fact, you want to keep me at a distance."

The therapist says this with a smile, trying to convey calm and hope. Laura pauses for a long time and looks into her eyes. A long period of metacommunication begins, and eventually, they repair the break; Laura is connected again.

L: "Doctor, what should I do about this feeling of loneliness?"
T: "That's a good question. What if it becomes our goal? I mean, exploring if there is something we can do when we feel lonely and in need of help. It might be difficult, I know, but are we willing to try?"

Laura nods. The therapist proposes again that she review the episode in guided imagery. Laura agrees and, during the experience, realizes that the punch was the consequence of disappointment in her mother. In the phone call, she seemed distant and disinterested; Laura felt lonely, sad, and worried that she would not be able to take care of herself in the future. At this point, she thought that her mother was unfair and that she should have acted like a mother and not a stranger. So she threw her fist at the window. The therapist points out to her how much clearer her inner world is now and also how the anger in which she lingers obscures her ability to read herself and communicate how she is to others, and how anger triggers repetitive thinking that only makes things worse.

Summing up: the therapist proposed using guided imagination. Laura read the proposal in light of the pattern: "I need care, a part of me deserves to receive it, but the other does not help me because he is incapable and selfish." This leads her to contact the negative image of a lonely and unlovable self that makes her feel sad and worried. At the same time, the other appears unjust, and this generates anger, which in turn generates aggressive behavior and the tendency to push others away. Now Laura is aware of the steps she made; the cause-and-effect links are clearer to her.

As regards the technique-relationship interaction, pattern 1 has been carried out: the technique generates a rupture that requires interrupting the experiential work and repairing the rupture. Although feeling attacked, useless, and powerless, the therapist did not react on this basis. She quickly realized that she was about to fall prey to her own patterns; she had recently talked about this in supervision. She then adjusted in real time and thus did not activate an interpersonal cycle. She would have done so if she had insisted on the technique. Instead, she metacommunicated, repaired the rupture, and then regained agreement on goals (soothing the pain) and tasks (using guided imagination to better understand the internal world).

Improve understanding of the internal world through dynamic assessment (Figure 6.1, Box 5)

Dynamic assessment (Figure 6.1, Box 5) is a process and set of technical operations that aim to understand the patient's inner world through active, experiential interventions. It includes in-session techniques, such as guided imagination, even without rewriting, as well as dramaturgical and bodily exercises. It is also most useful to suggest behavioral experiments in which we ask patients to refrain from coping. The purpose during dynamic assessment is not to reduce symptomatic or dysfunctional behavior but to curb protective automatisms, for example, avoidance, complacency, perfectionism, aggression, dysfunctional eating behaviors, and so on. Remember that copings have, predominantly, the function of reducing negative arousal: when a patient adopts them, emotional experience drops in intensity, and reading the internal world becomes difficult or impossible. The therapist asks the patient to try to stop before acting out the coping and notice what happens in his stream of consciousness. We clearly explain to a patient that it is not important for him to be able to refrain from coping; it is enough for him to try and observe himself just enough to learn more about his inner world at such moments.

Let us see, with an example, a dynamic assessment that begins with a body exercise and continues with the proposal of a behavioral experiment. A relational breakdown emerges, and we show how the therapist deals with it.

David, 30, suffers from avoidant PD. He works in a pharmaceutical company and lives alone. He is depressed, has no social contacts, and stays at home most of the time. He asks for help both to overcome his depression and to have a richer and more satisfying social life. He has some acquaintances, mostly related to his big hobby, cycling, but with rare exceptions, he avoids participating in group outings. He has only occasional sexual relationships and never establishes an intimate and lasting romantic relationship. Avoidance coping is so pervasive that David does not know how he feels or understands what he fears. The avoidance is now structural and embodied; the therapist recognizes it in prosody, voice, and posture: he speaks in a low voice, his head is bowed, and his shoulders are hunched forward as if hiding. The therapist points out these bodily aspects to him and asks if he adopts certain postures for a specific reason. David replies that he is more comfortable this way; he feels safer. The therapist has access to one more cognitive element. However, she is missing a lot of information: what is David protecting himself from? What negative emotions and thoughts has he learned to avoid by adopting a posture that makes him safer? It is coping, yes, but to protect himself from what . . .? To find out, the therapist begins the dynamic assessment and asks David to change his posture: "Lift your head up, open your shoulders, try to speak in a fuller voice." Then, she explores the stream of consciousness connected with the idea of no longer being hidden. As soon as David tries to move, he blushes with shame and says he feels uncovered, exposed. Access to the inner world begins to be possible. David understands that his hunched posture protects him from unpleasant emotions that he still struggles to name; however, he speaks of discomfort, of a tension that is activated in the presence of anyone, even the therapist.

Much information is still missing: how do you see yourself, and what do you feel in these circumstances? What is the negative self-image? What desire does he feel is frustrated by others' responses? What does he fear will happen? To fill these metacognitive gaps, it is necessary to continue the dynamic assessment, and behavioral exercises with attempted abstention coping are perhaps the most powerful tool. In fact, when the patient tries not to use a pain-protective mechanism, almost automatically arousal rises, and consequently, cognitions and emotions emerge and become more readable. Precisely because of the expositional nature of behavioral exercises, it is possible for them to cause relational ruptures, partly because we are usually at the beginning of treatment and the therapeutic relationship is not yet solid.

The therapist proposes that David accept an invitation to lunch from colleagues. She explains to him that the purpose of the exercise is just to give himself a chance to accept, and even if he refuses, the exercise will have achieved its purpose: to read his inner world. David should, in this case, just dwell on the moment before he says no to his colleagues, understand the reasons and emotions of the moment, and report them in the next session. David agrees but arrives late for the next session.

He sits down, pale, his face tense. He feels dazed and speaks with difficulty. The therapist asks him what he is thinking and feeling. David, after long turns of phrase, says he did not want to come because he did not accept the invitation.

D: "I feel like when you go to school and you haven't done your homework . . . I even thought about quitting therapy . . . it's too much work for me. Except I didn't understand the point of the exercise [*a hint of protest anger emerges here*]. I mean, I have difficulty being with others, and you propose I be with others. I mean, but if I'm not able, how am I supposed to succeed? Maybe I need one of those things, right, when people lay on the couch and talk? Maybe that way I would understand things I didn't know."

Anger is more evident; a confrontation rupture is taking place (Safran & Muran, 2000). The therapist reminds him that the exercise also foresees rejection of the invitation; it was only important that he rejected it, not automatically but by observing what happened, precisely, a moment before avoidance. She adds that she is intrigued by his reaction, "It seems to me as if you expect a reprimand or punishment at the slightest opportunity." The therapist is calm, validating, not helping to activate interpersonal cycles, and David relaxes. He says that he actually overreacted in seeing her so critically, and that he always has so much anxiety when he has to meet others, including the therapist. He always has the idea that he will be misjudged. He recalls other details about the carrying out of the homework.

D: [*Lowering his eyes*]: "I was very eager to accept, there was also a colleague I like. However, I got scared that I didn't know what to say . . . In the end I stand there, I don't speak, they look at me, I shut up like an idiot and these people think: 'What did he come for . . .?' It was stronger than me, I said I had a commitment and so goodbye! In short, a disaster."
T: "What are you feeling as you tell me this? You have also lowered your gaze"
D: ". . . Shame . . . you will be disappointed in me. I mean, you gave me the homework, and I didn't do it."
T: [*Smiling*]: "But sorry . . . then you did the assignment right! That was what the exercise was for. To try it, to fail quietly, but to see what excitement came out in you, and for crying out loud, you're damn right it came out! And to realize what you were thinking. I mean, you did it beautifully."
D: [*Relaxing, he hints at a smile*]: "Ah. So I wasn't wrong?"
T: "No way, you were great. That's what we wanted!"
Now that he sees her curious and attentive, rather than critical, David is open to listening to the therapist's rereading, a beginning of the structured summary of events, a step we will show in the next chapter.
T: "What happened with the homework also happened with me. You want to meet other people but you believe that you are clueless and that others will think you are a klutz, to be generous. And so that is why you avoid it, to

protect yourself from shame. Anxiety at the idea of making a bad impression drives you."

D: [*Nodding*]: "It makes me sad on the one hand, but I'm relieved. I'm understanding better what's happening to me."

The homework then generated a rupture that the therapist intercepted and repaired. Shame at being inept and fear of reproach led David to think about quitting therapy. David understands that the task elicited transient negative emotions and thoughts related to the idea of being the one who always makes mistakes, and so he constructed the therapist as critical, disappointed, and, simultaneously, useless. Although he did not show it, in the background David had a positive representation of the relationship with the therapist, and this allowed him to return to talking about his intentions. Meanwhile, his perception of the therapist, now seen as solid, supportive, validating, and able to be there for him even during an emotionally intense transition, has changed. Overall, then, we see a sequence in which a breakdown in the relationship that creates problems in task performance is followed by its repair: this is pattern 2 of technique-relationship interaction. After the repair, David discovers the beneficial effects of behavioral exposure, and this increases his confidence in therapy: this is pattern 5.

When, with the operations described here, we gather information about the inner world of patients, we move to formulate the schemas jointly. It is a job composed of several steps that we will describe in the next chapter.

Chapter 7

Identify the narrative structures underlying the episodes

We have shown how to bring out information about patients' inner worlds: what they think and feel and what drives them to act. Here, we work to organize, again in a shared way, the psychological material according to the structure of the maladaptive interpersonal schema. We do not talk about patterns yet because the observations are based on one or a few episodes and on the analysis of non-verbal markers. However, this information should already be summarized according to the underlying rationale: people suffer by fearing that due to their structural problem, that is, their negative self-image, their wishes will remain unfulfilled because others will frustrate them.

If patients get used to reading their experience in terms of "Psychotherapy guides me toward the expression of a healthy and vital desire; I'm not just here to dismantle my pathology," they face the process with more hope and become proactive: "If I act in new ways, I can change, at least a little, my future."

What structure do we use to help patients understand their own experience in an organized way? We have been inspired by the Core Conflictual Relational Theme method (CCRT; Luborsky & Crits-Christoph, 1990) but reworked in a specific way (Dimaggio et al., 2015, 2020).

The structured summary of events

We use material that emerged from the narrative episodes, the non-verbal channel, and from the *4 lakes* in general (see Chapter 4), and we summarize it to include the nuclear wish, the other's responses, particularly the dominant negative one, and the self's response to the other's response. The latter element includes information that will help us understand what the core self-images are, particularly the dominant negative one, and let the patients realize how they obscure the positive ones.

The clinicians' purpose is to give voice to what patients begin to understand. They lay it out to the patients and check to see if they can read things the same way so that there is a shared knowledge base on which to design the next steps. Therapists then lay out the structured summary of the episode. They anchor themselves to reality data and begin to highlight the psychological and mentalistic aspects

DOI: 10.4324/9781003570967-7

Structured summary of the episode
Box 6

| Evoking associated autobiographical memories, past or collected in the weeks after the session
Box 7 | Further exploration of inner states into associated episodes through experiential techniques
Box 8 |

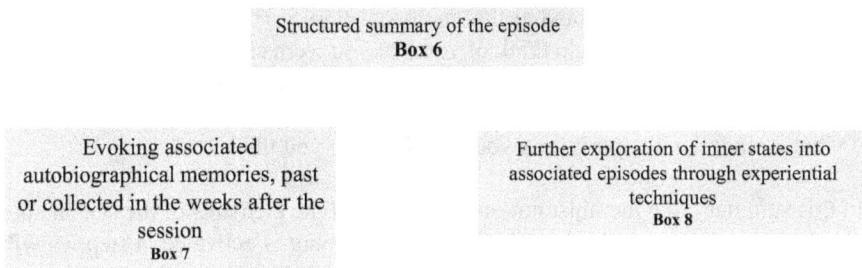

Figure 7.1 Recognizing underlying regularities in relational functioning

of the incident: "It seems that the desire to . . . moved you"; "So, when the other reacted like that, you thought X and felt Y" (Figure 7.1, Box 6).

When they talk about others, patients often describe their behaviors and mental states, but we still don't understand how they represent them: "He neglected me, he got angry." Instead, we need to ask how they read the other: "So would you describe him as . . . disinterested? Tyrannical? Cold?"

In this way, we begin talking not so much about the concrete others but in terms of the role the patient attributes to them in the drama unfolding in their own internal theater. That is, how they construct the others in a schema-dependent way.

Once the summary is formulated, the therapist asks for feedback with simple questions, such as, "Does this all add up to you?" and "Do you feel that I summarized well what happened and what you experienced?"

We recommend doing this step jointly with patients, using pen and paper or on the computer. Therapists outline the general structure of the pattern, for example, drawing blank boxes on the paper: "This is the desire that moves you. Here is, as you see, others, and here is how you react when . . ." Then they recall the passages of the episode and invite patients to fill the boxes jointly: "Here we try to understand what moved you. When you turned to your friend, were you driven by the desire to . . .?"

Thanks to the structured summary, an initial transformation takes place. A patient described the episode like this: "I was at a party, and I was feeling bad, agitated. Then I drank and sat in a corner, and after a while, I left without saying goodbye to anyone; I felt lousy."

After elaborating on the internal states (Chapter 6), the therapist summarizes the episode according to a psychologically meaningful sequence that sounds like this:

Yesterday you were at a party, you hoped to be welcomed and included in the group, you even felt able at first, but you saw the others as different, you saw them as comfortable, and you started to feel like a fish out of water. At that point, you felt ashamed, different. It was no longer important to be part of the group but to feel appreciated, and at that moment, there was no hope; you were was convinced that they would think of you that you were clumsy. The idea of being so was real and unbearable, and so, to calm down shame you drank. But you still felt sick, laden with shame and guided by the conviction that you would never feel included in the party, and you left. What do you think?

In this summary, the therapist not only highlighted the elements of the schema but also began to illustrate the processes by which coping is activated, a step we will describe in the next chapter. In this passage, therapy is about starting from stories which patients do not recognize the plot of and turning them into a narrative with a clear, organized, and easily recognizable structure. Now we look at a movie in which the main character's motives are obvious and his or her actions understandable in light of what he or she thinks. Summarizing the narrative correctly and sharing it is crucial because it prepares patients to evoke the associated memories in a way that we hope enables them to retrieve episodes more easily.

The search for recurrences: evoking associated memories in the past or in episodes in the following weeks

Once patients find themselves in the episode summary, therapists look for other memories to explore jointly (Figure 7.1, Box 7). They are guided by the narrative architecture of the interpersonal schema described in Chapter 2. This is a delicate step that requires precision because it will most likely take therapists quickly to the heart of the problem in a way that will make shared formulation and treatment planning easy.

We proceed with attention. Therapists repeat the structured summary in its entirety and then ask patients to evoke episodes that they feel are similar. Patients may be free to associate memories from any element: the wish, the other's response, the self's response. Our way of asking for associations is distinct from techniques such as *affect bridge* (Rafaeli et al., 2014) or *floatback* (Browning, 1999). In these cases, therapists ask only to recall memories in which patients have *felt* that way. However, it is a type of request that is likely to evoke memories unrelated to the nuclear schema. Emotions, in fact, are not specific to one motivational system: sadness can be caused by loss, defeat, constriction, or duress, just as anger can stem from abandonment, rank, sexual disappointment, and restriction of freedom. Moreover, clinicians cannot be sure if they are asking for *affect bridges* starting from primary emotions, such as sadness and shame, or reactive emotions, such as some forms of anger that arise to protect against emotional pain (Greenberg, 2002). Clinicians cannot easily decide which emotion is nuclear. Moreover, asking only about the emotion does not train patients' minds to think about their own unfulfilled wishes. It is one thing to ask "Do you remember an episode in which you were sad?" and another to ask "Do you remember an episode in which you wished that . . . but the other instead . . . and at that point you felt sad?"

So, we elicit associated episodes like this:

Can you think of other scenes in which you needed to be cared for and valued, and the person from whom you expected protection failed to do so and left you alone? A situation at the end of which you were sad, or angry, or both?

Alternatively, clinicians may ask,

Where did you learn that your need, your desire, is doomed to being neglected? Where do you get this heightened sensitivity to signals of criticism, so much so that they are so easily activated with such emotional intensity? Is it possible that it is something you know well, that you experienced in relationships that were very important to you, perhaps while growing up?

In the face of these questions, very often, patients recall memories, making schema reconstruction possible. Ideally, these should be developmental memories, but this is not essential. MIT does not rely on systematic reconstruction of patients' life histories, nor is it interested in the etiology of the disorder, which often remains unknown. What is needed is for patients to come to understand that the way they think, feel, and act is due to schemas with which they read relationships and which do not necessarily correspond to reality.

Recall that memories are not as important as memories, but as windows into the structure of internal functioning. Memory is a predictive tool: it serves not to tell us who we have been but who we will be tomorrow, how we should behave, and what we expect (Solms, 2021). They are maps of the world that need to be continually updated. Personality psychopathology, in some respects, consists of a defect in updating maps. Consequently, to formulate the schemas we do not necessarily need core episodes that occurred in childhood. We need emotionally charged narrative episodes that occur at any time.

Guided by this concept, clinicians, instead of becoming depressed, know what to look for when patients do not remember the past. They precisely summarize the elements of the episodes already collected and invite patients to pay attention to moments in the following week when something will happen that includes more or less the same elements. So, new episodes will emerge that patients will recount in the following session.

Or, phrase the question more openly: "Do you notice if something emotionally significant happens to you." With this question, both associations and new problem areas may emerge that will then need to be reexamined in detail. Indeed, it is possible, even likely, that patients suffer from numerous maladaptive schemas. Thus, the various dysfunctional areas gradually emerge, sometimes even more severe or important than those from which therapy had started. In each case, the therapist looks for memories in the future, week after week.

Recall the reason for this step: to obtain episodes that patients feel are associated with the starting one to arrive at a shared understanding of regularities. What characteristics must the episode now surfacing have? It goes without saying that we imagine it has broadly the same structure. Other elements probably emerge, such as new responses of the other and new responses of the self, but they are grafted onto a plot that we have already recognized in the original episode.

But does the evoked episode have to have exactly the same structure as our summary? No, and often the memory that emerges is different, not only in the plot but also in the starting wish. It is, therefore, underlain by a different core self-image. How then do therapists behave? Do they remain dissatisfied and insist until they get an episode photocopy? No, absolutely not. As much as we have presented to the patient's memory and associative functions a precise, affectively charged plot, we cannot predict what will emerge.

It is crucial that patients *feel* the association as emotionally relevant. The therapists' task is to understand what the connection is between the present episode and the associated memory.

Often, the past episode is the one in which the core schema really lurks. The recent episode, we are going to find out, unfolded from a secondary wish activated for the sake of maladaptive coping. What does that mean? We explain with the most classic example: the recent episode is articulated around social rank. The therapist summarizes it, asks for an associated memory, and the patient, saying "I have no idea why, but this scene comes to mind," recounts an episode in which the core wish is attachment; she needs care but describes the other as suffering or distant.

What is the connection between the two episodes? Reasoning together, the therapist and patient discover that she now suffers in the present because the other criticizes her, and the frustrated wish is social rank. But at the structural level, satisfaction in rank had become important because showing brilliance in school was the only way to get her mother's attention and see her eyes shine, moving her from disinterest or suffering. However, the pain of being unappreciated is important because it represents the failure of coping, the purpose of which was to maintain the proximity of the other. The patient's nuclear problem is that when she needs care – it is the domain of attachment – the other (her mother) is absent, and as a result, the patient sees herself alone. Of course, we come to this kind of understanding not in the confines of our own minds but by reflecting on the episodes together with the patient.

Therapists begin by noting, "It's a strong episode emotionally . . ." then summarize the storyline again according to the schema structure, and then continue, "How does what you just told me seem related to the episode we were starting from?" At that point, it is the patient, with our metacognitive scaffolding, who tells us what the psychological connection is.

Whether we have obtained an episode similar to the original one or one with a different storyline, which requires the connection work just described, the request for associated memories does not end with evoking the past memory. To complete the sequence, we need to ask "Now that we have reconstructed the episode that happened at that time, can you help me better understand how this knowledge is helpful to us in understanding what makes you feel bad today?"

MIT therapists are never interested in knowledge for its own sake! We always want patients to know that the process of understanding is for a purpose: addressing a problem, healing a scar, fulfilling a wish. We must be especially vigilant because the seduction of understanding the present in light of the past is powerful. We seem to have discovered the keys to suffering, to have been good archaeologists, to have unlocked ancient mysteries. That may be true, but if we do not connect this knowledge to purposes to be achieved in the future, it remains useless.

Relational ruptures may emerge in these passages but are unrelated to the use of techniques. Patients may refuse to explore the past because it seems useless to them, a mere intellectual exercise. In that case, therapists acknowledge the rupture and work to repair it (Chapter 3). Sometimes, on the other hand, the surfaced memories are traumatic or simply very painful: patients try to remember but become blocked and emotionally detached. Here again, it is necessary to explore the state of mind in the moment, ask patients how they perceive the therapist, and work to both regulate emotions and repair the rupture. Only then will it be possible to return to explore the associated memories.

When we ask people to pay attention to the following week's episodes and try to refrain from coping, there is room for some alliance breaches.

Christine, 32, an office worker, suffers from dependent PD and bulimia nervosa. She seeks help to cope with the depression that has gripped her for several months. She feels sad and dejected because she sees herself as physically unattractive and fat, and soothes this suffering through binge eating. Binges, in turn, make her feel sadder and think she is a failure. She ruminates about her incapacity and then obsesses about how to lose weight, often resorting to self-induced vomiting or fasting, which often culminates in further bingeing. At that point, she feels like a wreck, ashamed, and so locks herself in. Depression mounts.

In one of the first sessions, while reviewing the food diary to track the mental state prior to a binge, Christine tells the therapist about coming home sad and opening the fridge: "to console myself." The antecedent of sadness is in an afternoon of shopping with her mother. She was trying on a dress, and her mother commented, "Nice skirt, too bad about your big thighs, or it would look suits you well." Christine became angry, but upon investigating the details of the incident, it emerges that the moment her mother criticized her, she felt ashamed and thought she was clumsy. Anger was the secondary coping emotion triggered by the thought. "It's unfair for my mother to treat me like this; she should appreciate and encourage me." Christine thus seems to access internal states easily, and the storyline is consistent. The therapist summarizes the episode.

T: "So, you would try on a dress you liked and hope your mother would tell that you looked good. Instead, she was dismissive. You then saw yourself as awkward and ridiculous, first ashamed and a moment later angry at the unfair humiliation. At home, you thought back to the episode, and at that moment, a sense of abasement prevailed, a mixture of shame and sadness. At that point, you went to look for something in the cupboard to console yourself. Right?"

Christine agrees, and the therapist asks her if she can think of any episodes like the one just summarized. Christine acknowledges that she often feels this way, but other episodes do not come to mind. When associated memories do not surface, we resort to *dynamic assessment*: therapists propose a coping abstention task, in this case, from binge eating. The goal is to better investigate the relational and psychological antecedents of the binges week by week so as to trace any regularities.

During the next session, Christine shows irritation when the therapist asks her how the attempt went, but shortly afterward, she blushes and lowers her head. She then attempts to change the subject. The signs of a relational rupture are macroscopic, so the therapist places the rupture at the center of the dialogue.

T: "What happens now? I feel like my question gave you I don't know . . . irritation . . . . Anyway, it didn't please you. Would you like to tell me about it?"

C: "I don't feel so much like talking about homework. Is it really necessary?"

T: "Sure, if you want . . . but I need to understand what's going on with you now . . . you know, we told each other that what's going on between us is important. What has been bothering you?"

C: [*After some hesitation*]: "It's no good – I feel lousy even in front of you, I mean, I went on a colossal binge."

T: "Does that make you feel . . .?"

C: "Ashamed."

T: "Of course, if you think I'm judging you, it's natural to be ashamed. Listen, have you noticed anything in my behavior? Is there any sign that I might criticize you? Even now, how do I seem to you?"

C: "Well, not really, though . . . you're thin . . . but . . . no. I'm the one who feels that way about anyone."

Now it emerges how there was a relational rupture preexisting dynamic assessment, which has now become more pronounced. Christine, in noting that the therapist is thin, reads it in the light of the social rank motivation: she sees herself as inferior in front of a woman who, for her, represents the ideal model she believes is unattainable. From this point of view, dynamic assessment was diagnostic: it made it possible to identify a problem in the therapeutic relationship that would have damaged the treatment if it had gone unnoticed.

However, this is a type 2 technique-relationship interaction: during the execution, the patient constructs the therapist in a negative way and then interrupts the task. The therapist works to overcome the break, and when the patient is free from social rank, she proposes a new coping abstention exercise, which this time Christine accepts with curiosity. In the next session, she recounts trying to resist another binge but failing. This time, however, she lingered on the internal state a moment before opening the cupboard and noticed that she was down in the dumps.

Exploring the causes, it turned out that she had gone to the doctor because of episodes of tachycardia, and he had prescribed an electrocardiogram. Christine was worried and hoped to be comforted by her mother. Instead, the latter had only told her harshly that it was all due to being overweight and that she should diet. It emerges, then, how underlying rank was a frustration of attachment.

We cannot speak of a schema: Christine is unaware that these episodes unveil a psychic structure, but the common plot of the episodes is evident. She needs care and hopes to receive it, as is normal. Her mother, on the one hand, ignores them and, on the other, considers her vulnerability a sign of ill will and therefore criticizes her. This leads Christine to see herself as inferior, and she at least seeks appreciation as coping once she has given up being cared for.

Shed light on internal states in associated episodes through techniques

Once new episodes are collected, we are likely to be accessing potentially rich areas of psychological information relevant to case formulation. They are like a mine to which access must be found because metacognitive monitoring is often lacking in PD and patients with post-traumatic symptoms. It is likely that the episodes that surfaced show only limited aspects of the internal experience at first telling. It is also possible that we have understood what patients thought and felt in the source episode but failed to do so in the associated one, either because it is a remote one or because coping processes emerge at its surfacing, ones which we are unaware of.

Moreover, even if monitoring is good, therapists may spot holes in the storyline and ask themselves: "What thought generated that reaction? In the recent episode, the patient didn't react like that. There's something new, but I can't understand what." At that point, they become curious, and to fill in the gaps, they may resort to techniques (Figure 7.1, Box 8), again for the purpose of dynamic assessment, just as they did for the initial episodes (Chapters 4 and 6).

So far in the decision-making procedure, we have guided patients to elicit narrative episodes whose psychological content we explored. We then collected associated memories and analyzed similarities with the first episodes.

The next step brings us closer to the cornerstone of treatment: bringing patients to recognize that regularities in episodes are not the result of chance or the malevolent, stinging influence of the outside world. Instead, they are signs of stable and crystallized ways of making sense of relationships. In short, regularities are due to the presence of maladaptive interpersonal schemas, and we want patients to understand this. We will see in Chapter 9 how to proceed.

Therapy, however, in these passages or in general in its initial moments, is not just about gathering the material that will allow the discovery that suffering and relational problems depend on schemas. Patients enter therapy laden with symptoms and enacting a multitude of dysfunctional coping. Think of Christine's eating disorder symptoms, Mariella's complacency, or many others that are often the reason for seeking treatment: self-harm, gambling, aggression, substance use, and so on.

Therapists do not wait to understand the existence of schemas to act on symptoms and coping, partly because that is what patients are asking for and need: to reduce suffering or counteract harmful, sometimes dangerous behaviors. This is something we dedicate ourselves to from the beginning. We are aware of a difficulty, though: metacognition is poor. We attempt to be helpful, but we rely on limited psychological information. In the next chapter, we will see how to act.

Chapter 8

Reconstruction of coping and beginning work on symptoms when metacognition is poor

Symptoms and dysfunctional behaviors comorbid with PD must receive clinical attention from the beginning of treatment. The therapist, from the outset, works to understand symptoms in light of the various steps of the shared formulation of functioning. We show how to deal with such symptoms and problems, which are the result of the systematic application of dysfunctional coping strategies – either behavioral or repetitive thinking (Figure 8.1, Box 13a) – when patients' metacognition is impaired. Some symptoms and coping mechanisms also occur as a response to the activation of schemas, and in Chapter 9, we explain how to deal with the portion of suffering that is a direct expression of the self's response to the other's response.

Coping and symptoms

Symptoms and dysfunctional behaviors are the reason why almost all patients seek help, and they have to be addressed from the start of therapy for several reasons: a) it is what the patient is asking us to do; b) reducing pain, even to a minimal degree, is crucial; c) symptom reduction reinforces the alliance and trust in the therapy (Westen et al., 2004). Moreover, as patients begin to take action to reduce symptoms, they gain agency over their mental states and, at the same time, veer toward cooperation: "Therapy also works because of my contribution." But how to deal with symptoms when patients do not have good metacognition and do not know that they are guided by interpersonal schemas, and when the case formulation is still incomplete and not yet agreed?

First, the therapist should expect only a partial response because patients: a) do not yet have sufficient metacognitive monitoring; b) lack awareness that suffering comes primarily from an internal source, that is, from their own maladaptive interpersonal schemas, and that they are thus still in a state in which they believe that the pain they experience is caused by others, and not by their own way of reading events and by their underlying negative self-image; c) have little agency over their own mental states and are thus either in the "I have no power and the other makes me . . ." position or in the passive "if only the other would . . ." position; d) lack

DOI: 10.4324/9781003570967-8

Identifying behavioral coping and repetitive
thinking

Promoting low metacognition stragegiesto deal
with symptoms and problematic behaviors
Box 13 a

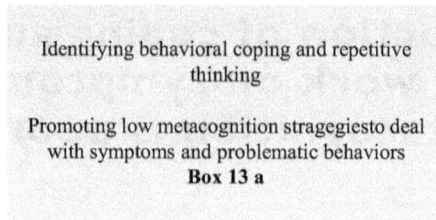

Figure 8.1 Treating coping and repetitive thinking when metacognition is limited

awareness of healthy self-aspects that could guide them toward more functional reactions and behaviors.

Early work on symptoms and maladaptive behaviors has three transdiagnostic targets: 1) behavioral coping, 2) emotional dysregulation, and 3) IRT. Regarding IRT, we describe a detailed intervention procedure and show how it often triggers behavioral coping. Dismantling the former will thus reduce the latter.

Early work on dysfunctional behavioral coping

When patients have little ability to describe their internal world, behavioral interventions are very helpful. Empirical support for them is extensive. Think of exposure tasks in anxiety disorders or exposure with response prevention in obsessive-compulsive disorder. For the sake of space, we only focus on two behavioral interventions in the context of MIT procedures.

The first is used in eating disorders (ED), very often comorbid with PD (Dufresne et al., 2020; Martinussen et al., 2017). Some behavioral interventions are crucial at the onset of ED treatment, for example, self-monitoring of weight (Kelly-Weeder et al., 2018; Waller & Mountford, 2015), food diary (Fairburn et al., 2003) and nutritional counseling (Ozier et al., 2011). All these interventions are part of MIT as applied to ED (MIT-ED; Fioravanti et al., 2023). These are, we repeat, interventions suitable for patients who struggle to describe their emotions and have no awareness of the role of interpersonal schemas in both eating symptoms and relationship problems.

The second is behavioral activation, a key, empirically supported intervention to treat depression (Lewinsohn, 1974; Martell et al., 2022) and of great importance as a transdiagnostic treatment element (Dimaggio & Shahar, 2017). It includes psychoeducation, self-monitoring of daily activities, goal and value setting, scheduling of daily activities (for example, going out for regular walks), and, finally, subjective evaluation of activities performed in terms of engagement and enjoyment. In MIT, we use it both to address depressive aspects and to enhance the sense of agency, which is frequently impaired in PD (American Psychiatric Association, 2022).

We present an example in which the associated symptom was an ED. It is evident how symptom work was immediately intertwined with problems in the therapy relationship.

Silvia, 34, employed, suffers from avoidant and schizoid PD and binge eating disorder and is treated with MIT-ED (Fioravanti et al., 2023). The therapist explains to her the reasons for filling out the food diary. It helps to understand whether the reported binges are physiological, therefore due to excessive restriction, or emotional. The emotional ones are a form of coping triggered by the activation of schema-dependent core ideas probably surfacing because of some relational event. The diary, therefore, allows exploration of the cognitive-affective antecedents of binges, especially if metacognitive monitoring is severely lacking. The diary also helps to identify which foods patients avoid, so as to plan dietary normalization.

However, Silvia does not fill it out, reports eating behaviors vaguely, and shifts the focus to problems in her relationship with her mother, which she believes is the main cause of her pain. During one early session, she reports having the "worst" binges ever, so the therapist asks her to explore the food diary to understand its cognitive-affective antecedents. Silvia stiffens: "I didn't have time . . . I had a big fight with my mother. I would like to talk about that."

The therapist realizes that she is in the midst of a relational rupture. It is pattern 2: the execution of the technique causes a rupture that requires repairing. The therapist first validates Silvia's stance: if she wants to prioritize the fights with her mother, it means that her mind is focused on painful emotions emerging from that interaction. However, she suggests considering that the arguments are a trigger for her binges. Silvia relaxes, changing her attitude. The therapist explores how Silvia felt when she told her that filling out the diary was an essential part of therapy. Silvia now acknowledges that she is ashamed of how she approaches food, and that is why she did not fill out the diary. She was afraid that the therapist would judge her for her inability to control binge eating and scold her "for not doing her homework."

Nonadherence to the task is, therefore, not dependent on prioritizing arguments with the mother but on avoidance. The therapist has probably just passed a relational test (Gazzillo et al., 2022; Weiss, 1993). In not filling out the diary, Silvia has unknowingly tested the beliefs: "If she finds out what I did, she will judge me badly" and "If I don't behave, she will scold me." The therapist, on the other hand, does not scold her and is, in fact, open about talking about the relational problem as a priority. When they then broach the topic of binge eating, the therapist is curious, and Silvia realizes she lacks judgment. At the end of the session, after the test is passed and the rupture repaired, the therapist asks Silvia if she agrees with jotting down, during the week that follows, whether she notices that binges are in any way connected to the fights with her mother.

This time, Silvia fills out the diary, and they find that two out of three binges are triggered by arguments with her mother. In subsequent sessions, Silvia has almost always filled out the diary, and when she has not, she accepts discussing the reasons in session. In parallel, she accepts the other behavioral aspects of therapy for ED; for example, she contacts a dietician to plan a more correct diet (for a detailed description of this case, see Fioravanti et al., 2024).

Beyond the former example, clinicians can tailor interventions to the symptom: they can use, for example, graded exposure in case of anxiety disorders, exposure with response prevention in obsessive-compulsive disorder, behavioral activation for depression, self-regulation strategies for self-harm, and so on.

Early in-session work on emotion regulation

Many patients, still lacking good metacognition and with sketchy case formulation, enter sessions dysregulated or lose control while talking about painful episodes. The therapist listens to them and validates them but intervenes as soon as possible with techniques to calm them down. If patients do not regain control over emotions, the session is useless.

The approach we take is based on three aspects: 1) agreeing with patients that the dysregulation needs to be addressed and developing a plan to reduce it; 2) acting at a bodily level with regulatory goals; and 3) monitoring the therapeutic relationship. Of course, mindfulness and attention regulation strategies also have a regulatory impact, but we will describe them in the next section.

Sharing the action plan

When suffering is intense, the therapist listens and allows patients space to express its contents. Then, the first technically oriented step is to call their attention and ask them if they want to be helped to calm down. This usually requires a lot of presence and firmness because patients continue to talk with the idea that pain cannot be soothed. When therapists have captured patients' attention, they invite them to think about how to calm down.

In Jade's case, the therapist tries to build a working alliance from the beginning. He is not directive but instead invites Jade to decide whether she prefers to be just listened to or to work actively. In this way, agreement on the techniques to be used is easier, and most relational breakdowns are prevented. This way, Jade can regain agency over her pain and begin to realize that she has an active role in therapy. On the other hand, the therapist frees himself from the difficult position of having total responsibility for treatment. Now, Jade and the therapist share a plan, an initial contract: to experiment together with the aim of reducing her illness. Now that she has an emotion-regulation capacity, Jade begins to calm down.

Acting on the body

Now, there are the conditions for technical action. The therapist does not have the information to trace Jade's suffering back to schemas they have reconstructed together previously; metacognitive monitoring is poor. He does, however, hold a contract: when Jade loses control and her arousal is too high, she has agreed to do something. Under these conditions, we teach patients some exercises to calm themselves down, such as regulating breathing rhythm, relaxing contracted voluntary muscles, and modulating posture.

One of the causes of dysregulation is the lack of even the simplest levels of integration between mental states (Carcione et al., 2021). This is a frequent phenomenon in borderline PD and complex PTSD. Patients move from one mental state to another, and each time, they completely identify with what they are thinking and feeling at the moment, forgetting that just before, they had a different perspective. They are often surprised by the abrupt transitions between different states of mind (Horowitz, 1979), do not understand the reasons, and become disoriented or frightened. They go from transient states of calm to others where they are suddenly anxious or nervous without awareness of the reason.

Ilaria suffers from borderline PD and speaks of her partner with a mixture of anger, anxiety, and despair, her eyes veiled with tears.

I: "You have no idea the bad things he's been doing to me at work . . . I want to leave him. I can't stand him anymore; I even told him so."

T: "The episodes are unpleasant, but until last session you told me you loved him very much."

I: "It made me fucking mad! I'm not okay at all with it; we're sleeping one on one side of the bed and one on the other side . . . I don't understand any of it."

The mix of despair, anger, and confusion is noticeable. Moving on, Ilaria recounts events in a haphazard way; the therapist cannot grasp what she wants to communicate. This is another sign of difficulty in integrating mental states. Meanwhile, Ilaria's suffering becomes tumultuous.

Promoting an initial awareness that mental states are all part of the self is necessary to foster emotion regulation. We help patients move from perceiving transitions between states as sudden, unmotivated, and senseless to something that is part of the stream of consciousness and will simply have to be understood together. Ilaria's therapist intervenes with this goal in mind.

T: "Ilaria, stop for a moment, listen to me. We know that all of a sudden, you pass from a state of relaxation and well-being to feeling prey to the fear of getting sick or being abandoned or betrayed. At that point, you are sick because of the thoughts you have, but you also think you're crazy; your head isn't working. We now instead begin to realize that these are all aspects of your experience that belong to you, and we need to understand how they are connected. We will do this together. Now, however, it is necessary for us to re-establish some calm; otherwise, we will not be able to think properly. Would you like to?"

Ilaria agrees, and they start working on somatic regulation. When she is calmer, the therapist asks her to recall two or three memories of herself with her partner, of different, almost mutually opposing, affective tones between them. Ilaria recalls one at work, when her partner was being combative and treated her disrespectfully, almost contemptuously; then another in which they were in sync and joking; and finally, a third in which he cared for her.

The purpose is not to help her understand whether it is good to leave her partner or not; that would be a gross mistake. We work at a much more basic level: to make her experience how different memories elicit profoundly different, sometimes opposite, mental states and to enable her to hold them together simultaneously in consciousness.

The therapist then shows her how she experiences a transition between states and that in each, she has contrasting thoughts and feelings about her partner. Nevertheless, they are the same couple. In this way, Ilaria discovers how, in a relationship, it is possible to move between even very different ideas of the self and of the other. She also realizes how each state is consistent with the context: when her partner disrespects her, she is angry; when they joke, she is cheerful; if he cares for her, she feels protected. Awareness of how these transitions are physiological helps her calm down.

While regulating Ilaria's mental state, the therapist, therefore, promotes basic levels of integration, even in the early stages of therapy, when complex metacognitive operations, such as understanding patterns and differentiation, are still far away.

Working on interpersonal repetitive thinking: an eight-step procedure

We now show how to curb IRT use and mitigate symptoms when metacognition is low by following an eight-step procedure. The order in which the later steps are described is flexible.

1. Assessment of coping strategies

During the reconstruction of the first narrative episodes, therapists try to identify the elements in interpersonal patterns. In addition, they reconstruct the coping strategies patients enact and what triggers them. These are often a response to a relational exchange; for example, a patient reacting aggressively to abandonment. At other times, coping precedes the other's response: for example, a patient anticipates criticism and avoids the situation in which it would occur, does not show up for an exam, or does not give a "like" on Instagram to a girl he fancies.

2. Determine the temporal sequence between immediate and late cognitive-affective reactions and between primary and secondary coping

A relational event generates immediate schema-dependent pain: "He neglected me, I think he doesn't love me, I feel sad"; "She criticized me, I don't deserve it, I get angry." This is followed by immediate coping: "If he doesn't love me, it's useless for me to seek him out, I shut down"; "I can't accept unfair criticism, I retort angrily."

Then, there are the delayed reactions used intentionally and goal-driven. For example, "She criticized me unfairly, she wanted to humiliate me. I don't answer her right away, I wait for her to speak and, as soon as I can, I answer her sarcastically so she learns."

Typical examples of delayed, goal-mediated responses are those of Mary, a woman with paranoid PD, who spent time suspecting, ruminating, and, even days after the activating episode, protesting or filing complaints against neighbors she was convinced made noise to disturb her.

So, a good reconstruction of the narrative episode must, in the self's responses to the other's response, include both *immediate* and *late* cognitive-affective coping. This assessment makes it possible to recognize which dysfunctional coping is primary. Sometimes, these are behavioral copings, often acted out impulsively, automatically, and without any reflexive effort. At other times, they are repetitive thoughts that begin immediately after the event, as in the case of Angie, a 28-year-old woman with covert narcissism: "Why did he treat me like that? Why didn't he respond to the message? What is he doing? Is he chatting with another girl?"

Another coping, however, is a result of IRT: Angie's boyfriend does not respond to a message, and she first broods; then, when a mixture of jealousy and abandonment, her anxiety becomes unbearable. She starts with a cascade of phone calls and text messages, and when the boyfriend responds, covers him with protests and insults.

It is important to understand the architecture of coping because it underlies much suffering and relational dysfunction. For example, part of patients' depression is schema-related, stemming, for example, from anxiety and shame at being humiliated and seeing themselves as unworthy; another part, however, is the outcome of monitoring others to check whether they are critical, of worry about impending criticism. Sadness and shame are the core emotions, generated directly by maladaptive structures, while depression is the final outcome of the combination of primary negative feelings and the effects of continuous attention to potential criticism and worry about being humiliated.

3. Identify the purposes of IRT

Once patients have understood the link between IRT, dysfunctional behavior, and suffering, we need to identify why they used it. This step is similar to procedures for eliciting so-called *positive metacognitions* (Wells, 2008). These are rigid, dysfunctional beliefs about the idea that repetitive thinking is helpful: "I can only get better if I fully understand why my boyfriend broke up with me"; "I have to predict what might happen, what they might do to me, and how it will allow me to avoid getting ripped off"; "Ruminating allows me not to repeat the same mistakes and hurt others," and so on.

Clinicians must also be aware that IRT has a short-term purpose that the patient is unaware of. It is a protective automatism to prevent emotional pain. Indeed, when patients try to stop ruminating or monitoring threats, negative emotions immediately increase. For example, if a patient ruminates to reassure himself with respect to something that makes him feel in danger, not doing so will cause him to temporarily feel even more vulnerable. The therapist, therefore, has to explain that he ruminates not only to prevent future harm but also to avoid experiencing anxiety and feeling vulnerable.

How to elicit the goals that support IRT in patients with lower metacognitive functioning? One recommended avenue is experiential, for example, with imagery or chairwork.

With imagery, we proceed as follows.

a) We ask patients to identify an episode, as recent as possible, in which they ruminated (or worried or monitored threats, etc.);
b) We guide patients to focus on the moment in the episode when they felt the need to allocate attention to a certain topic. In many cases, this brings attention to unpleasant scenarios: events that have happened or their life condition (*rumination*), possible relational dangers (*worrying*), or looking for possible dangers in the environment (*threat monitoring*). In other cases, they focus on pleasant scenarios, hoping to achieve a desired scenario: "If he only were with me in Bruges" (*desire thinking*).
c) We wait for the emotions to be activated and for patients to recognize them. Once they emerge, we ask them to dwell on that specific scene in the story that unfolds in their imagery.
d) We explore the scene: "What is the active desire right now? What would your mind like to achieve?" These are examples of valid responses: "I want to understand why things went the way they did so I won't repeat the mistake"; "I want to get revenge for an offence or get an apology"; "I want to reassure myself that I won't take any risks in the future"; "I'm trying to absolve myself of a fault"; "I want to feel energized so as to ward off a sense of emptiness."

Incomplete answers are like "It's like I'm trying to figure out if I did the wrong or right thing," or "I want to understand why my boyfriend broke up with me." Why are they not good answers? Because they do not include the end or the purpose precisely.

Once she understood why her boyfriend left her, what would the patient get? Therapists want an answer to this question. So they can ask "Okay, and do you want to understand it in order to . . .?" possibly cooperating in seeking the answer. For example, the incomplete answers above need content such as "In order not to feel guilty," "So as not to think I'm dumb," and "In order to reassure myself that I won't be alone in the future."

Alternatively, therapists can use chairwork. These are the steps we suggest following:

a) We ask the patient to place on a chair the part of himself that implements an IRT. For example, he can identify the part that ruminates self-critically, or the part that worries, or the part that wishes, and so on.

b) We have the patient sit in the chair where the part of himself engaged in IRT is and ask him to imagine and embody its perspective, motivational setup, posture, facial expression, and tone of voice. For example, Steve, an avoidant young adult with social anxiety, impersonated the worrying part, taking on the movements and prosody of the character *Fear* from the cartoon *Inside Out*.

c) We interview the patient, empathizing with the part engaged in repetitive thinking. In the interview, it is important that we reconstruct the historical development of that part, with questions to it such as "How long have you been cohabiting with Steve?"; "What episodes in Steve's life have invited you to come on the scene?"; explicate the problem detected from the IRT's point of view: "What is wrong with Steve?"; "What would you change?"; "Are there other things about Steve that you don't like?"; understand what the patient feels by embodying the IRT: "How do you feel about seeing Steve like this?"; "What worries you most?"; and finally, understand the function of the IRT: "What was its purpose when it became part of Steve's life?"; "What is it now?" The answer to this last question is what we were looking for to identify the *purposes* of IRT.

Usually, chairwork continues, and patients move to the chair where they play the part that "undergoes" the IRT. This is preparation for the next step.

4. Examine the immediate and mid-term consequences of IRT

First, a recent narrative episode in which the patient used an IRT is evoked, and an attempt is made to understand what the effects were. Patients thus come to discover that IRT worsens mood, increases emotions such as anxiety, shame, guilt, and anger, reinforces a negative self-image, and lowers self-esteem. In this way, they become aware that because of their repetitive thinking, they end up adopting behavioral coping: perfectionism, workaholism, avoidance, aggression, submissiveness, emotional dependence, and so on. They also understand that, as a result of IRT, they adopt symptomatic behaviors: alcohol and drug use, binges, self-harm, and so on.

We can look with patients for the consequences of repetitive thinking during chairwork, completing the procedure begun in Step 3, where we invited patients to position themselves in the chair in which they embody the part of the self that is the *victim* of IRT, for example, of self-critical rumination, anxious worries, or desire thinking.

At this point, the therapist summarizes what he has understood about the IRT:

We have seen that the self part that criticizes you, even if it makes you feel bad, has understandable motives: from your point of view, it acts for good: it would like to make you more successful or prevent you from making a bad impression and being excluded. However, this part is also contemptuous of you; it considers you clumsy and defective. How do you want to answer it? Address it directly.

At this point, the patient may realize that the intention with which he adopted IRT to, for example, protect himself from looking bad, has the paradoxical effect of making him feel inferior and ridiculous in his own eyes. He also discovers that he has a chance to counteract this thought process, which he now sees as a maladaptive part of himself sitting in the chair, an internalized other to whom he can retort.

5. Strengthen agency over one's mind and weaken negative metacognitions

Changing one's mental functioning requires *feeling* that it is possible and *believing* that it is possible. Feeling it is possible is about agency over mental states. The sense of poor agency is an embodied, preverbal helplessness (Dimaggio et al., 2009): not being able to obey one's own mind without knowing why. Then there are negative metacognitions, the idea of not being able to influence the course of one's thoughts, for example, to stop a rumination (Wells, 2008). Negative metacognitions contribute to patients' resistance to counteracting IRT.

Getting patients to understand that they ruminate not because they cannot direct their thinking but because they are guided by specific goals, and are driven by metacognitions. Trying to make patients aware of their diminished sense of agency over their mental states is an important moment in therapy. To break down negative metacognitions about IRT's uncontrollability and to develop a sense of agency, we use experiential techniques, which we illustrate with examples.

6. Promptly identify and stop IRT when it occurs in session

It often happens that patients spend the session time ruminating aloud, often starting immediately. One way to stop rumination is to ask for a narrative episode instead of keeping on talking generically. This is the first step in the procedures: moving from abstract semantic language, typical of repetitive thinking, to autobiographical memories (see Figure 4.1). It is one of the reasons why the basic MIT question is "Can you give me an example?" Insisting on episodes already counteracts IRT. But it is also essential to get patients to recognize *the form* of their thinking, their thought processes, for example, ruminating or worrying. Without this awareness, they will not be able to engage in the deliberate and intentional work of counteracting it.

After the first few sessions, when therapists have collected episodes and begun to understand the structures of the interpersonal schemas, it is therefore crucial to promptly place the *thought process* at the center of clinical attention, label it as dysfunctional, and block it. When therapists first embark on this path, they begin with careful metacommunications and then jointly explore ongoing repetitive thinking.

Rita, 39 years old, dependent PD, tends to interpersonal rumination and worry. Here's how the therapist intervenes.

T: "I see you in a lot of pain, and I am sorry for you. You can communicate your pain to me, and that's good; you make me feel it. I was noticing one thing, though: the situation you are talking about certainly hurts you, but the way you talk about it seems to make you suffer even more. If you think about it, you kind of recount the facts, kind of start to reason about it, to figure out whether what you did was right or wrong, whether what the other person did was her fault or you were the one who behaved badly. Then you go back and tell a piece of the story and try to figure out what is going to happen to you. You usually see bad things coming. The effect is that anxiety increases; you almost despair. On the other hand, when I succeed in anchoring you to telling me about just one specific incident, pain is there, of course! But I feel like pain is more tolerable. You're aching, but I don't see that despair in your face; you don't twitch your lips with tension. Is this something you notice as well? More importantly, does your mind work this way at home as well?"

R: "But doctor, I do this 24/7. Only when I work do I have some peace."

This shared awareness makes it possible to update the contract and give priority to the attempt to stop worrying in session.

T: "Since this way of thinking about yourself feeds the pain and confuses you, is it okay if I interrupt you every time you start to reason like this?"

R: "Look, I give you carte blanche. In fact, you have to interrupt me! Because when my head starts, I don't know how to stop it."

We adopted this style the first few times we showed patients how they tended to worry in session. The phenomenon recurs naturally, and we gradually intervene more and more immediately and decisively. A few sessions later, Rita resumes alternating narrative episodes and IRT. The therapist is brusquer this time.

T: "Excuse me, Rita, I understand your distress, but right now, you are again activating that way of thinking that we noticed in recent sessions. If you now give way to rumination, you will be worse off than when you came in. We saw that, and the session will be useless. Do you remember what we said to each other last time? Do you authorize me to interrupt you?"

In subsequent sessions, therapists step in earlier, even seconds after rumination begins, applying energy, presence, frankness, and a good dose of irony.

T: "Rita, you are ruminating again!"

R: "I know, but it's just that he acted like that, and I would like to understand . . ."

T: "Oops, you're ruminating further. If you want, I'll let you do it for the next 4873 hours; no problem. At the very least I'll go home, cook a plate of pasta and come back, because you're staying here anyway, right?"

Usually, patients notice their own tendency and realize that talking this way makes things worse. As a result, they try to interrupt themselves, not least because they realize that their therapist will not listen to them forever!

7.   Evoke in the patients a part capable of resisting and controlling repetitive thinking

This part will attempt to deal functionally with times when the mind is caught up in painful memories and worries, pursues out-of-reach or unhealthy desires without reflection, or is lost in daydreaming. Like any work on healthy parts, we use experiential work extensively. The first choice tool is imagery; alternatively, we use chairwork.

In imagery, starting with the reenactment of a real situation, a moment when IRT was triggered in response to some painful interaction, therapists invite patients to evoke a self-image capable of coping with suffering without ruminating. This is precisely a matter of imagining a self that, in the presence of negative emotions, "resists" and does not give in to the intention to think and rethink. It restrains itself from determining its own worth based on the judgment of others, from reviewing its life to find evidence of personal worth and yet finding evidence to the contrary, from trying to predict worst-case scenarios to figure out, in vain, how to be 100% safe, and so on.

Therapists are not satisfied if patients generically figure out what behaviors to enact instead of worrying, such as calling a friend, thinking about something else, or doing something interesting. They want patients to imagine how to regulate their internal state in a precise situation: What could they actually say to themselves? Where could they allocate their attention instead of ruminating? What posture would help them? It is important that patients evoke in session a self-image that is attractive, agentic, strong, and capable of acting in unpleasant circumstances.

If we use chairwork, we proceed as follows: we have the patient sit in a third chair, placed in front of those chairs where the part of the self that adopts IRT and the part that undergoes it are located. In this third chair, the patient tries to impersonate the healthy self. We give him the time he needs to stabilize the healthy part, help him retrieve it from memory, and invite him to "wear it," taking on its posture, expression, and gestures.

Once the patient feels the sensory pattern of the healthy self in his body – for example, straight back and strong legs – the therapist invites him to talk to the parts he imagines in the other chairs. The therapist urges him to encourage and offer support to the part that suffers and to set limits on and contain the part that ruminates, worries, or is caught up in desire thinking.

The most delicate moment is this: the therapist supports the healthy part, encourages it, and spurs it to intervene energetically towards the parts placed in the other chairs. The risk is that patients, in the guise of the healthy part, interact with the other parts like psychologists or schoolteachers, giving common-sense advice but without really participating and, in the end, without believing the things they say.

Therapists need to stimulate the active participation of the healthy part by asking it, for example, how it would talk if there were two loved ones in front of it, two friends, for example, one frightened or humiliated and crushed, and the other critical or hyperprudent or vindictive. The aim is for patients, after chairwork is completed, to clearly perceive that there is a part of themselves capable of dealing with problematic emotions, even intense ones, with presence, firmness, and flexibility. Once they have trained these parts in session, they can use them when they find themselves engaged in repetitive thinking.

8. Propose homework to pinpoint the moment when they start ruminating or worrying

Repetitive thinking usually flows unconsciously: patients do not notice they are absorbed in a dysfunctional scenario. When metacognition is low, they do not realize that they are focusing their attention on an unsolvable problem, on a desire that they will never fulfill, on a catastrophe, and so on. They do not even realize the reason triggering the chains of thoughts, and, most importantly, that after a while, they are more sick and the problem has not been solved anyway. For this reason, the first homework is aimed at making patients aware of when they start ruminating. When they succeed, we also ask them to try to understand what triggered IRT and how long they use it for.

This is crucial: if patients do not notice when they start thinking repetitively, they cannot stop! Clinicians must be clear that even when patients recognize in session that they are using a certain IRT, it is by no means certain that they will notice it during the week. And so they will have to train themselves to catch it in the bud: during the week, self-observation tasks are indispensable.

Subsequent homework related to how to dismantle IRT in daily life takes place mainly in the change promotion phase when metacognition has improved, and we will see it in chapter 13.

Problems in the therapeutic alliance during the initial treatment of symptoms and coping

We work to reduce both symptoms and coping, both behavioral and cognitive-attentive, while carefully monitoring the therapeutic relationship, especially when patients have limited metacognitive abilities. Therapists find themselves in a bottleneck. On the one hand, they feel the pressure of symptoms, dysfunctional behaviors, and repetitive thinking, all of which require fixing, as they generate suffering and relational problems. In some cases, patients' behaviors are dangerous to them and their close ones: restrictive anorexia damages body and metabolism, overtraining increases risks of injury, and extreme sports used as coping for feelings of emptiness or inferiority put life and physical integrity at risk. Substance use, alcohol, and domestic violence are harmful.

On the other hand, however, therapists do not yet know the psychological cause-and-effect processes leading to the problem behavior, much less the interpersonal patterns that are at the root of it. Typically, the therapeutic relationship is unstable, still undermined by schemas that are easily activated. Therapists need to find a balance between being effective and being aware of the limitations of their interventions.

Difficulties often arise early in the formulation of the therapeutic contract. Consider patients with restrictive anorexia who often disagree with the goal of regularizing food intake and regaining weight (Fairburn et al., 2003). The same is true for some who use substances (Miller & Rollnick, 2012). In both cases, dysfunctional behaviors are not just coping but have become egosyntonic.

Daniel, 36, suffers from covert narcissism and borderline PD and has asked for help in regaining control over alcohol and substances, which have led him to risky behaviors and caused him trouble concentrating on work on days when his consumption is highest. In the second session, the therapist tries to figure out what reasons there could be for him to reduce his alcohol and substance use so that the necessary tasks can be agreed upon. Daniel compiles a list of very good reasons to keep drinking! The therapist is wrong-footed but quickly realizes that there is no point in insisting that he cut down. He immediately moves on to redefining the contract from a position of what we term leaning forward powerlessness. Therapists here clarify that without a contract they are not able to help patients (powerlessness), but while doing so, they display clear verbal and non-verbal signs that they are motivated to help, if only patients offer them some leverage (*reaching the other*).

T: "Daniel, I don't see reasons for you wanting to quit or cut down. I have not heard a single one. On the other hand, I must say that you are convincing me to use substances! [He *smiles along with the patient.*]"

D: "I know doctor! But I like drinking – with friends if the restaurant is good. While everyone is drinking crazy red wine, should I say 'No thanks, just water?'"

T: "No for heavens' sake! [*Ironic*] Listen, I really need to avoid becoming the one who prescribes the right thing for you to do, or else we just need a couple of sessions and, wisely, you'll feel bugged and send me to hell. I just need to understand: you contacted me about reducing alcohol use, but now you are not asking me it anymore. Can we talk about this again next week and, in the meantime, focus on a treatment goal you consider reasonable?"

This way, the therapist avoided alliance ruptures both in the bond and working components. Daniel came out of the session pensive and doubtful, but the relationship was good. The therapist probably passed a test: the patient was moved by the exploratory system and feared that the therapist would adopt a coercive or worried position, both aspects of the others connected to his family history, as becomes clear after a few sessions. The therapist did not embody the role of setting limits and judging, so it is likely that he allowed the patient to feel respected in his desire to explore. In the next session, Daniel slumped in the chair:

D: "Doctor, you have to help me. I got high and things ran out of control! I can't take it anymore!"

The intertwining of the therapeutic relationship and early behavioral tasks

When we assign behavioral tasks, relationship breakdowns lurk even more since behavioral coping either protects against painful states or is egosyntonically pursued as pleasurable or rewarding.

In the case of eating disorders, particularly anorexia, negotiating with the patient to change an attitude about weight requires a series of steps (Fioravanti et al., 2024). The premise is that there must be a therapeutic contract about the use of the tools, both in daily life and in session: filling in the food diary during the week and reviewing it together with the therapist; tracking weight in an agreed way; using a weight chart and monitoring the disorder maintenance mechanisms, such as excessive and compulsive exercise, binge eating and vomiting, use of laxatives and diuretics, or other body check mechanisms.

Normally, patients want to work on ED but are afraid of regaining weight. If they are unwilling to regain weight, it is necessary to agree that they will not lose weight and, in the meantime, work on the ED maintenance mechanisms. We emphasize that psychotherapy with ED can begin only if patients agree to some of these goals at an early stage. If the BMI is less than 15 or eating behavior is so dysfunctional as to prevent effective outpatient therapy, it is necessary to refer patients to inpatient admission.

If patients agree with these preliminary goals, it is possible to attempt the first behavioral exercises, which are strongly exposure-based. Relational breakdowns are, despite contractual agreements, lurking. How do we prevent or minimize them? It is essential that therapists: a) identify the disorder maintenance mechanisms that produce the most discomfort for the patient: for example, she is exhausted by her own tendency to run every day to stay underweight. This is a behavior that is beginning to be egodystonic. At this point, it is more effective to agree on a task of abstaining from this coping than to ask her to assume more calories; b) read the food diary with the patient and identify at what times she has not used one of the usual maintenance mechanisms or has voluntarily enacted a healthy behavior, for example, she has eaten less restrictively or added an avoided food.

This is a core intervention from the MIT procedures described in Chapters 4 and 6: early access to healthy parts. In the case of ED, it is easier to find them in areas unrelated to eating. For example, a patient is asked to identify moments of lightness, leisure, involvement in hobbies or social activities, and contact that state of mind. She now tries to anchor herself in that healthy part and see if she can adopt a less restrictive eating behavior from that perspective. In some cases, healthy parts concerning the relationship with food emerge, and the therapist immediately notices them, validates them, and explores them: "What did you think and feel that, at that moment, allowed you to eat something extra or to enjoy a food with pleasure?" She then explores its relational antecedents: in fact, something positive often happened in relationships, a sign of a breach in the patterns.

Anna, 18, suffers from restrictive anorexia nervosa (BMI: 17.5) and avoidant PD. She soon makes it clear she has no intention of regaining weight; she was pushed to enter therapy by her concerned parents. The therapist proposes behavioral work for her with two elements: committing not to lose further weight; 2) filling out a food diary as a dynamic assessment, that is, understanding why she considers restricting necessary and how it affects her relationship with food day by day. Anna agrees on both tasks.

Thanks to the diary, it emerges that controlling weight and body shape supports the social rank motive: at such moments, Anna feels strong and valid, and this is the only area where she has this self-image. In general, when faced with the need for appreciation, she only faces her mother's devaluing and hypercritical response or her father's absence, and both confirm that she is unimportant. For her mother, thinness is a quality, something her daughter can brag about in front of her classmates. Her eating behavior is thus aimed at counteracting the core idea of herself as inept and insignificant. She implements this very rigidly, both in controlling her calorie intake and through exercise. What Anna has completely lost is the sensory pleasure of food.

Realizing that the request to increase caloric intake would only lead to a breakdown, and since her BMI does not signal an impending health risk, the therapist looks for moments when eating has kept its pleasurable aspects, untethered from the rank system. Anna fills out her diary regularly, and an episode emerges: she is at the home of her loving and caring paternal grandmother. Anna tastes a teaspoon of meat sauce while the pot is on the stove; when she talks about it in the session, her gaze softens. The therapist catches the expression, points it out to her, and asks her what it depends on.

A: "My grandmother loves me."

The therapist now understands that attachment is also frustrated, but at least her grandmother cares for her. She finds that when Anna's attachment need is met, she sees herself as lovable and cared for and stops caring about rank. This allows her to pay less attention to food rules and connect to a pleasurable sensory dimension. Because of this awareness, it is possible to plan a behavioral experiment with a new purpose: to suspend control over food, not to regain weight but to expand contact with healthy experiences related to sensory recovery. The sense of amiability is the state of mind that will allow this new path to be traveled.

A similar difficulty can be found with domestic violence perpetrators suffering from PD. In this case, the intention not to act violently is a MIT precondition (Misso et al., 2022; Pasetto et al., 2021). Under the pressure of dysfunctional relationships, maintaining this intention can be difficult, and when therapists insist on the centrality of attempting to abstain from coping, there can be relational ruptures.

A pattern 1 interaction is common: the therapist asks to refrain from verbal aggression or controlling behaviors, and the patient immediately objects, does not see the point, finds it unfair, and gets angry with the therapist.

Lino, 55, is separating from his partner, and one of the reasons is his verbal and sometimes physical aggression. Now, however, he faces a problem: his ex-wife has custody of their 11-year-old daughter but engages in behaviors that put the latter at risk. Upon careful assessment, Lino's concern appears well-founded. When his wife engages in further behaviors that are risky for his daughter, Lino is seized with intense anger, driving him to insult and threaten his wife. The therapist validates him and tells him he understands the instinct to protect his daughter; for a father, it is normal, and it is a sign of love. But at the same time, he reminds him that these behaviors are harmful for him first and foremost because they could jeopardize the possibility of seeing the little girl regularly. Lino gets angry.

L: "And what should I do? Should I leave my daughter in the hands of that bitch who doesn't give a shit? Do you think I should stay home and do fuck all while my daughter is in danger of someone taking advantage of her?"

T: "I know, wait a minute. Of course you are worried and angry, even angry at me, I understand that. It's just that if you're convinced that it's helpful to yell, threaten your wife, and meet her in person when she's with your daughter, then I'm worried. Do you think that would solve the problem? Isn't there a risk that it would lead to a, perhaps dangerous, escalation?"

The therapist validates the anger arising from Lino's concerns about his daughter's well-being and simply notes the risks associated with persisting in aggressive behavior, in a calm, nonjudgmental manner. Lino changes his attitude.

L: "No, it would be a mess. She is crazy, and doesn't give a damn about her daughter. And remember, if she has a chance to hurt me, she takes it."

T: "So, we know it would be useless and maybe harmful, right?"

L: "I don't know what else to do."

Lino does not consider aggression as reasonable anymore and begins to realize that it is just a sign of a desperate need to protect his daughter in the absence of better alternatives. The therapist, at this point, proposes to him a two-step task. The first is to attempt abstention from aggressive behavior solely on the basis of the need to prevent the inevitable harmful consequences. The second is in-session regulatory work. Only if Lino succeeds in calming himself can they think about the reasons underlying his aggression in a more metacognitively complex way. Now Lino agrees to curb aggressive behavior. In the next section, we describe the regulatory strategies the therapist uses in session (Pasetto et al., 2024).

The interweaving of the therapeutic relationship and early work aimed at emotional regulation in session

The use of regulatory strategies must also come through attention to the relationship. We illustrate how the therapist proposes strategies for Lino to calm down and the impact this has on the relationship. Despite being unaware of the role of schemas in activating his reactions, Lino decides to restrain himself out of awareness of the negative consequences. The therapist tells him again that he understands how difficult it is to resist the impulse to act and suggests that he use some exercises to calm himself down.

T: "So, we have seen that it is difficult to resist the impulse to attack and insult your wife when you imagine your daughter alone at home and in potential danger. But we also know that following the impulse would be futile and harmful. Do you agree?"

L: "Yes."

T: "Perfect. Let's recap: our job is to help you calm down when you feel that urge. To accomplish it, I would say the first thing is to train you in session to use some tools to calm yourself, what do you say?

L: "Okay!"

T: "First, we have to do something unpleasant. Basically we first have to piss you off. Because if we calm you when you are already calm . . . it's pointless, you see?"

L: "Yes, I got it."

T: "Of course, if your anger increases too much, tell me anytime. If I can, I'll help you carry out the exercise; if not, we'll stop, and it's no problem [*Lino nods*]. Can we go back to a moment when you imagined your daughter in danger? A moment in which you just pictured that something bad might happen to her?"

L: "I'm already nervous, holy shit."

T: "All right! So you'd get the urge to grab the phone, call your ex-wife, insult her, threaten to go and take your daughter away from her by force – correct? What do you feel? What do you think now?"

L: "That I would yell to her face until she asks for forgiveness!"

T: "This is it, I would say. Close your eyes, try to go back to that moment and tell me when you visualize it. Try to not just remember; imagine it's happening now."

L: "I'm there, I'm on the couch in my house . . . My daughter is alone at home, left on her own. Her mother is out getting drunk; anything could happen to my daughter . . ."

T: "Do you see a particular picture? A specific danger?"

L: [*Thinks about it, wrinkling his forehead, narrowing his eyes*]: "Nothing specific, but she's getting hurt. That bitch is going to be drinking and being a slut."

T: "What would you like to do now? Call her, cover her with insults . . ."

L: "Go fucking home, be with your daughter. If not, you'll fucking regret it!"

T: "Here's the anger! But you can't go, though; you can't insult her. How do you feel?"

L: "Shitty, like a dog on a leash."

T: "Very clear. Now, the hardest part. Try to say where in the body you feel the anger, and the sensation of being a dog on a leash!"

L: [*Takes a while, looking inside*]: "In the chest . . . here [*points*]."

T: "What kind of sensation?"

L: "Pressure . . . and in the head. Wait, even the stomach, like gastritis, burning . . . My heart is beating. Holy shit, I'm so nervous!"

T: "Great! Don't react, Lino, breathe regularly noting the pressure in your chest, in your head, the burning, but don't stop breathing regularly, inhale, hold, exhale, can you? Breathe in . . . good . . ."

L: "It's tough."

T: "In what way? What do you feel in the body?"

L: "Always agitated. Less pressure on the chest, less throbbing . . . the stomach keeps on burning . . . breathing better."

T: "Good, keep breathing deeply. Now put your feet firmly on the floor, press them down, and pay attention to the contact with the floor. How do you feel?"

L: "My breathing is more regular, less agitated, better."

T: "Is the impulse to insult your wife, to threaten her, still present?"

L: "Hm . . . it's rising again . . ."

T: "Normal. Breathe regularly, inhale deeply, send out the air . . . your feet are in contact with the floor, how's the urge?"

L: "Now it's less."

The exercise continues. The therapist asks Lino to think back to his lonely, endangered daughter. Lino's negative emotions mount again, and the therapist asks him to repeat the regulation exercise. This time, he calms down more quickly; by the end of the exercise, he is well regulated.

The therapist asks him if the next time he knows his wife is leaving his daughter alone or otherwise in a risky situation, he thinks he can use this exercise. Lino believes he will be able to, and so in fact he will. In fact, the work is successful, and already after a few sessions, Lino has stopped aggressive acts, which do not recur either during treatment or at a 3-month follow-up (Pasetto et al., 2024).

But what impact did the experiential work have on the therapeutic relationship? It seems that everything takes place in a good alliance atmosphere, which was the case for the most part. But at the end of the exercise, the therapist asks Lino how he felt about his presence.

L: "At first I was going to tell you to go to hell! You want me to stop protecting my daughter?! What?! Then I realized that you just wanted to help me."

In the subsequent sessions, Lino is happy with his new regulatory skills and trusts the therapist. Pattern 3, therefore, occurred first: a micro-fracture happened during the exercise but did not prevent it from being carried on successfully. Then, pattern 5: the success of the experiential practices consolidated the relationship.

The intertwining of the therapeutic relationship and work aimed at disrupting IRT

Experiential work on repetitive thinking at the beginning of therapy can have an impact on the relationship for the two reasons stated: IRT arises from a protective intention, for example, worrying to prevent danger. Stopping it generates pain that patients try to avoid. Experiential techniques, on the other hand, start by focusing on scenes laden with negative emotions, and this can generate suffering that, in turn, can trigger alliance strains. Patients may open their eyes, interrupt a task, or question it: "What's the point? How can going back to those memories make me feel better? Does it change my life?"

Sometimes, a rupture occurs regarding treatment goals, as in the case of Linda, who suffers from avoidant PD and covert narcissism.

L: "Yes, what we do is very interesting, even useful . . . In fact, I am even better when I do the things we do here. But I want to go deeper, into the symbolic, dream dimension . . . I want to sink into my suffering and find the meaning of life there."

Obviously, this was an elegant and intellectualized attempt to involve the therapist in ruminating with her so as not to deal with her serious relational issues. The therapist did not accept Linda's proposal and had to move to renegotiating the contract, with success after some further struggles!

A crucial element in dealing with IRT is to recognize its occurrence in session and interrupt it (step 6 of the procedures described earlier). What can happen when the therapist interrupts patients' ruminations and asks "Can you give me an example?"

Henry, 34, suffering from narcissistic PD, is a philosophy assistant lecturer and has asked for help because of depression and writer's block: he cannot complete an article he has been working on for six years. His narrative style is imbued with intellectualization and rumination: as he speaks, he looks up as if to intercept hovering thoughts. The result is that the therapist becomes confused, not understanding what to work on. Henry has suffered emotional rejection; the therapist intuits that that may have been the proximal trigger of his malaise. But understanding how the rejection really led to the malaise is impossible. The therapist then asks him to recount a specific episode related to his relationship with the girl.

Henry, however, is not convinced that a simple "factual episode" will explain why he suffers. The therapist clarifies the rationale for why the episode can help him precisely to better understand his inner world (Chapter 4). Henry seems to agree and recounts an episode. The therapist attempts to move to the next step: exploring its psychological content. Henry responds by returning to intellectualizing and ruminating.

H: "You ask what I felt when Lisa rejected me . . . Well, look, if you mean in terms of *stimmung*, I would say that there my relationship with otherness became radicalized. It is as if there is a self that lives in the *praesentatio* [*he uses Latin words*] and, at the same time, a self that diffuses, perhaps eclipses, in the *retensio of* a past that basically no longer belongs to me."

T: "Henry, I swear, I don't follow you. I mean, I don't understand almost anything of what you felt, what emotions you experienced. What is it that prevents you from telling me things more clearly? In your opinion, is the problem me not understanding your language when instead I should understand it? Or is there something that makes it difficult for you to communicate more simply what you thought and felt when Lisa rejected you?"

H: "It's confusing to me, but I realize that . . . Yes, this is an important point . . . At work, I am precise . . . very . . . but when I am with others . . ."

T: "What's going on?"

H: "That it's bad. I realize that I should live in the present, but what is there in the present that is worth being present for? Every moment presentifies the utter meaninglessness of being there. What am I doing here? Why am I compelled to be here? Not here by you, I mean . . . But perhaps yes, even here by you. The hollowness of things is everywhere, and so ins this consulting room too. I should commit myself to writing the article, but even that – what's the point? And then I wonder . . ."

T: [*Interrupting him*]: "Wait, Henry, do you realize that, right now, your way of reasoning is taking you back and taking us back to the same stalemate you've been in for years? You're talking abstractly again, but more importantly, this is rumination! Do you recognize it? If this method had been effective, you would have resolved your block a long time ago. I would like to look for a different way of dealing with problems, but you seem to want to keep ruminating! In fact, this way does not involve me in therapeutic work. Could it be that there is something you don't like in my method of exploring life episodes?"

The therapist's intervention reveals that there was no agreement on tasks!

H: "I will be frank, yes! Don't take it personally, but the method you follow is inherently authoritarian."

T: "I appreciate your frankness. With the same frankness, tell me: did it bother you that I interrupted you just now?"

H: "I have to say yes! You do not allow the expression of articulate and complex thought."

T: "I can't blame you. In fact, I've been trying to force you to talk in a way that doesn't belong to you. I'm sorry if it upsets you. But the problem is that I only know this way of working. Of course, I could go along with you, follow your reasoning. I would be interested, your language and arguments make me curious. We could reason together about the existential dimensions of being in the world. But I assure you, your problem will not change one iota, pretty sure of that. You feel bad, you will feel bad. Actually it's your call, how do we want to proceed?"

When asked by the therapist to move from intellectualization/rumination to telling narrative episodes, Henry sees this as tyrannical. Now that the pattern has emerged, the therapist explains that the reason is not to dominate Henry, but to be clear about his own inability to be useful under certain conditions. The intervention resolves the rupture; Henry agrees both to philosophize less and to narrate episodes.

In summary, patients often ruminate or worry out loud in session. They need to be stopped! Will relational ruptures emerge? Probably yes, but this is no reason not to stop them. If an intervention is essential, and this one is, relational ruptures should not be prevented but repaired when they surface.

Many dysfunctional symptoms and behaviors and many personality disorders

The work we have described covers only a very small part of what happens when, at the beginning of therapy, patients with any PD and limited metacognitive abilities have symptoms and enact maladaptive behaviors. Clinicians are faced with the task of taking action to reduce both, but can neither rely on sufficiently developed metacognition, which would allow the use of flexible mastery strategies adapted to various life contexts, nor rest on a rock-solid therapeutic relationship.

The intertwining of symptoms, behavioral problems, and PD takes various forms, many of which require symptom-specific interventions. Sometimes, the target is behavior, for example, graded exposure for agoraphobia, exposure and response prevention for OCD, management of self-harm, and so on. Sometimes, the target is emotion regulation. At other times, the target is repetitive thinking.

Dealing with all the forms of interaction between symptoms and PD, and all the ways in which experiential techniques can trigger ruptures in the relationship, would require a volume of its own. We hope, with the procedures and examples illustrated, to have provided clinicians with the rationale for intervening in this interweaving that is often, at the beginning of therapy, difficult to manage. In Chapter 13, we will return to work on the interactions between symptoms, dysfunctional behaviors, and schemas but with greater levels of metacognition. There, the relational ruptures will loom less, and the range of strategies available to the therapist will be broader.

Chapter 9

Reconstruct functioning and recognize the Interpersonal pattern as such

The completion of the shared formulation

PART I

Patients have drawn a detailed map of their internal world. They recognize cognitions and emotions within interpersonal episodes. They know, for example, they have been driven by a desire for exploration or the quest for status and have faced figures who hinder or criticize them. They are able to recognize that in the face of the other's response, they have negative thoughts – "He humiliated me, neglected me, deceived me" – and that these have generated emotions such as sadness, shame, anger, guilt, or jealousy. They can describe how the other's reaction triggers cognitive-affective chains that, in turn, trigger repetitive thinking and dysfunctional behaviors.

Patients have associated narrative episodes with the early ones they told. Some have evoked past memories, while others have had difficulty retrieving historical episodes, and their therapists have invited them to pay attention, week after week, to events that seemed consistent with the problematic episodes recounted during early sessions. In each case, therapists and patients have a collection of relational scenes and have to discover the underlying plot. How to act at this point?

Reconstruct regularities according to the interpersonal schema structure

Techniques play a less important role in this step. Ruptures sometimes occur with therapists reasoning out loud to reconstruct functioning, while patients withdraw, criticize, and deny aspects that were obvious just minutes before. Schemas are at work in the therapy relationship.

At other times, therapists get the reconstruction wrong, and patients do not see themselves in it. Therapists have to understand whether an alliance rupture is unfolding or if they just made a mistake. In the first case, they have to attend to the therapy relationship; in the second, they have to correct the formulation.

That said, reconstructing regularities between episodes (Figure 9.1, Box 9) is cognitively challenging for therapists, who try to place the elements of the various episodes collected so far into the boxes of the diagram, which are still empty:

DOI: 10.4324/9781003570967-9

Reconstructing regularities among episodes **Box 9**	Hypothesize that regularities correspond to underlying interpersonal schemas **Box 10**	Identifying which coping strategies are triggrered by the response of the self to the others
Explicitly identify the core self-image and make sure patients consider it an idea and not a fact **Box 11**	Recognizing the shifts between healthy and maladaptive ideas about self and others **Box 12**	Strategies to tackle coping and maladaptive behaviors when metacognition is low to medium **Box 13 b**

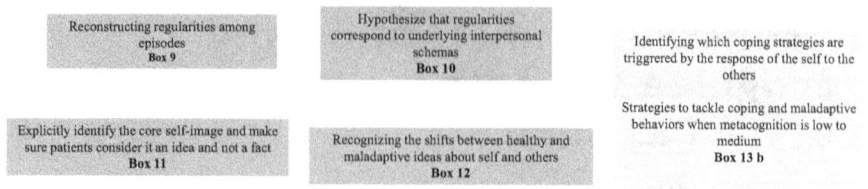

Figure 9.1 Formulation of maladaptive interpersonal schemas.

"What is the primary wish? Is there another wish with a coping function? What is the negative core image? Did I notice a positive image even though it surfaced only at certain times?"

Therapists must know MIT schema structure perfectly. But there is no need to ask too much of their cognitive skills! Therapists, especially the less experienced ones, with the schema structure in mind (Chapter 2), can use pen and paper or the computer to fill in the boxes of the schema together with the patient. It is a totally joint task, and therapists correct their assumptions through patients' observations.

We identify the dominant images of self and other, and name them together with patients using a vocabulary they feel is their own so that they can recall them easily. For example, the therapist and patient may agree that when a critical character emerges, it will be the *Professor*. One patient tends to enter states of low value that then activate dependent behaviors; in her words, "Whatever, doctor, every once in a while the *simp* appears." A patient with avoidant PD talks about the *loser* self, and when the healthy part emerges, he calls it the *Jedi Knight*.

The time is ripe for identifying the regularities in the plots of narrative episodes (Figure 9.1, Box 10). In this step, however, therapists, with great frequency, make a mistake that complicates or jeopardizes therapy. If patients acknowledge that such regularities exist, it does not mean that they have realized they are guided by schemas. Therapists confuse the two operations and find themselves trying to change a patient who still does not differentiate. We now show how to share the underlying structure of the stories so that patients understand that they are visualizing internal functioning, not describing a bitter, hostile reality. In the first example, our colleague makes a mistake: she moves in, convinced that the patient has realized that he is being guided by schemas, and he is not. In the second, we will show the correct procedure.

The first example comes from our colleague's therapy with Andrew, a 34-year-old engineer with covert narcissism and avoidant PD. In the third session, Andrew tells an episode consistent with previous ones.

A: "The head of the committee said my project doesn't convince him. And if he doesn't give the OK, it will never pass. I got angry, it's unfair, he has absurd standards, but basically he doesn't understand anything . . . I wanted to convince him, but it's impossible, he's not one to change his mind . . . I was about to go and rub it in his face: you're wrong! Then I reconsidered, ok, I say my bit, and then what? I have just made myself an enemy of the boss and of half the committee who are frustrated placemen who are dying to break someone's legs." I got disheartened and gave up.

T: "At that point, what did you do?"
A: "I called myself a jerk. I should have seen the objections and the problems coming, and reason more . . . as a politician . . . predicting the next moves . . . I told my girlfriend I didn't feel like doing anything and started videogaming. Five hours. And I didn't even notice that time passed! I felt out of touch, a perfect jackass. At work, a disaster. My girlfriend sooner or later won't stand me anymore. I messed it up."

At this point, the therapist summarizes the story in a way that is similar to the others from the first sessions.

T: "Look, Andrew, there seems to be a recurring plot in your stories; shall I try to summarize it and reason about it? So, you are driven by a desire to do a creative project, you like it, and you even get passionate about it. But then someone, out of incompetence, envy or selfishness, gets in your way. At that point, partly, you have a very healthy proud reaction; you feel unfairly blocked; things are wrong to your eyes. This makes you angry; you would like to fight back. However, you immediately switch to feeling helpless: 'I can't do anything about it.' Then you reconsider, ruminate on it, and try to figure out where you could have acted differently, but in the end, you blame yourself and find no solution. Then, exhausted, you isolate yourself and just want to turn off your brain, and that's what videogames are for. It also works, you relax, but it is a kind of seal on the sense of helplessness. What do you think about that? It sounds very similar to the episodes you told me about your family, doesn't it? Your mother always distrusted you, and you were always worried while your father was tearing everything you did into pieces, and you felt he was doing it out of provocation and defiance. As if he couldn't stand that you had accomplished more in life than he had. Does the similarity come back to you, and does this plot seem to characterize the stories that give you pain?"

Andrew recognizes himself in this description. What happens at this point? Frequently, therapists confuse patients' ability to recognize themselves in the shared reconstruction of regularities with the understanding that they are guided by a schema. This is almost never the case! We see this in the following passage. The therapist is convinced that Andrew now knows that he is guided by a schema and moves accordingly. Wrong.

The therapist tries to engage him in guided imagery: in the scene, his mother forbids him to leave the house to play football with friends. The goal is to help him overcome a sense of passivity by anchoring himself in the creative aspects of his work. The therapist first leads him to recall moments when he feels vital and motivated, and Andrew succeeds. During imagery, she invites him to anchor himself in this part to tell his mother that he cares deeply about playing football and is not as fragile as she thinks. Andrew tries to say this, but his voice immediately becomes tinged with anger. He expresses it to his mother, who is offended. Andrew gets even more angry: "She's always like this, trying to make me feel bad, and she even succeeds."

The therapist asks him to locate guilt in the body.

A: "It's like an iron ball in the chest."
T: "Try grabbing it with your hands, pulling it out, and pulling it away by extending your arms."
A: [*The contracted face*]: "It's heavy – too much – I can't [*shakes head, opens eyes, interrupts imagery*]."

What happens? The therapist assumes Andrew understands he is schema-driven. But for him to be guilty of making the other suffer when he asserts his autonomy is a fact! Andrew cannot accept thinking of himself as bad and prefers to give up his own desires. Likewise, he believes he is unable to overcome criticism and skepticism. He therefore remains stuck in anger: "Only if you stop suffering and if you decide to give me permission will I be free."

Andrew becomes depressed, shuts down, and complains that therapy is pointless: we are in a relational rupture. Was it caused by imagery? Very likely no. The reason is the error in the formulation! The therapist started imagery without Andrew knowing that the purpose was to rewrite a schema. He thought the problem depended on others and was implicitly convinced that the purpose of imagery was to help him change the reactions of real others. But he thought that was impossible: his mother would never change. For him, his mother is not yet a critical, suffering character in his inner theatre. She is a real, stubborn, immobile mother.

Only supervision helps the therapist understand that it is first necessary to get Andrew to think: "My idea that, if I am autonomous, Mom will suffer and eventually leave me alone is simply an idea." At that point, change operations begin.

Many therapists find themselves in identical dead ends, with a technical error leading them there. In metacognitive terms, they mistake a fairly good level of integration for differentiation. Patients articulate their cognitive-affective processes within a series of relational episodes, perhaps occurring at different times in life and with different people.

Therapists take it for granted that recognizing, even in an agreed-upon way, the existence of regularities in episodes indicates that patients have realized that they are schema-driven. They infer that patients have understood that the problem lies not in reality but, precisely, in their own subjective way of considering interpersonal relationships. That they can say *my loser part* and *the stern, uncontentious character*, knowing these are just actors in their inner theater. Therapists thus begin to come up with behavioral experiments and experiential techniques to encourage plot change, resulting in systematic, protracted, and frustrating failure! The techniques are not the cause of the relational breakdown. The problem is the error in the formulation.

Confusing the understanding of one's own mental processes described in the narratives with the awareness of being guided by a schema is, we repeat, one of the most frequent mistakes. For this reason, we added these steps to the decision-making procedures: *Explicitly identify core cognition about the self and check whether it is an idea or a fact* and *Recognize shifts between healthy parts and negative representations* (Figure 9.1, Boxes 11, 12).

In this way, the next step, the real therapy turning point, can be accomplished, which is to bring the patient to say "Gee, reality hurts, sure. But the reason I'm suffering so much and my life is stuck, unsatisfying, unhappy is that I am the first to view myself and others negatively, take it for true and act accordingly."

Recognize that schemas are internal structures and not descriptions of reality: Identifying the nuclear self-image through cognitive inquiry

Once we have reconstructed the underlying regularities of episodes, we really move on to the shared formulation. We now get patients to understand "Okay, this is the way I read events, and it is my way, not simply a description of how relationships go." We lead patients to a form of pre-differentiation, which is by nature unstable and evanescent. It is, however, the point on which to anchor subsequent change-promoting operations.

The crucial action that will bring patients to understand they are guided by schemas is cognitive in nature. It involves explicitly exploring whether it is clear that they are describing their inner world and not reality. We use simple, clear, and straightforward questions.

We have described what passes through your mind in many situations. Can you see that it is the way you predict how things will go and interpret events? I mean, I know that you felt hurt by your father's criticism, and now whenever your boss, a friend, or boyfriend criticizes you, you suffer a lot. On the one hand, you feel lousy again, but on the other, you sometimes get angry, which, in a way, is good because you don't agree with them; you think criticism is unfair. What I would like to understand is whether we are clear that our work is not focused on bringing others to change their attitude but to help you believe their criticism doesn't mean you are wrong or flawed. To anchor yourself in a more positive idea of yourself, which we have seen you have. It's about, in short, understanding that we don't want to work on how others treat you, at least not now. For goodness' sake, it's obvious that we want you to have a life as good as possible, and we will certainly work on that later. The point is to help you see yourself differently and to give less weight to others' negative reactions. To spend less time scanning the environment to see if criticism is coming. What do you think? Do you agree to turn treatment in this direction?

The most important element in this passage, the keystone of MIT, is to bring patients to observe themselves in a scene. We get there through cognitive inquiry, asking direct questions. We reflect on the narrative episode, or we bring patients to review the episode in imagery, role-play, or chairwork, and we ask, "What do you think about that self that you have in front of you now?" We aim for patients to move beyond thinking: "The other person makes me . . . considers me . . ." and instead say out loud "I think of myself that I . . ."

Laura, 23, is a humanities student and suffers from obsessive-compulsive PD with traits of covert narcissism, and obsessive symptoms related to fantasies about hurting her parents. During the first sessions, the therapist reasons about episodes related to her conflictual relationship with her mother. Laura is angry because she feels judged and would like support and encouragement instead. She is hanging out with friends that her mother does not approve of. The plot of her stories revolves around her desires for autonomy and social rank. When Laura is guided by her own initiatives, such as hanging out with some friends or choosing a university, her mother responds with blame and moral contempt: "Ah, you're hang out with that person? Can't you see the family is talked about in the village" or with pain and guilt "If you are seen with that person you'll bring shame on us, your father and I will be hurt, but then again what do you care?"

Laura protests, trying in vain to change her mother's mind. She is focused on her mother's attitude:

She makes me feel like crap, unworthy, dirty, a runaway. Apparently, I'm a disgrace to the family. I mean, geez, I just want to live my life, why can't she and her freaking middle-class Southern values understand that!

Anger indicates that a part of Laura believes her own autonomous goals are valid and worthy, and her mother is unjust. The result, however, is that she is stuck in the position of a victim who deserves approval and support from a judge who, instead, is unfair and self-righteous. Focused as she is on her mother's reactions, she remains paralyzed. Exploring the episodes, it becomes clear how part of the block is the image of the suffering other that makes her feel guilty and harmful and activates her compulsive caregiving. This is a pathological form of inverted attachment: caring for the caregiver for the sole purpose of maintaining relational closeness.

The therapist notes that Laura does not have internal change as her goal. She just believes that her mother should treat her differently and that that is the only way to get better. The therapist asks her whether the idea of harming the other and the paralysis only affects the relationship with her mother or happens in other situations as well. Laura acknowledges that they happen often. Shortly before therapy began, she started dating a boy who, after finishing cookery school, started working in a res-taurant. She flirts and is witty, jokes with the boy by WhatsApp text, and teases him about being assigned menial tasks: "Gordon Ramsay will pat you on the back for how well you slice onions!" The boy responds resentfully. Laura jokes again, and he takes offense. He lectures her about how he "works his butt off," calls her spoiled, and stops responding. Laura does everything she can to make amends, but he offers no leeway; they no longer see each other. She does not grieve the loss. But then, in the days that follow, she agonizes over having hurt him, ruminates over her own *mistake*, and accuses herself of being stupid, disrespectful, and insensitive. For days, she has been sad, refuses invitations from friends, and skips class. She realizes that this was one of the moments when she realized she needed psychotherapy.

The therapist now has associated memories. Evoking associated memories does not mean looking for past memories connected to proximal ones (Chapter 7). It is about evoking memories that patients feel resonate with the summary of the narrated early ones. In this case, Laura started from historical memories and, by association, retrieved a recent episode.

The therapist has the material to take the next step: understanding with the patient that regularities depend on a schema (Figure 9.1, Box 11). He summarizes the regularities the two episodes share.

T: "There seems to be a recurring pattern in your stories. You often act spontane-ously and autonomously. You have a desire to explore the world by going to study what you want in a city you love. You want to make connections with kindred spirits. You have a cheerful sense of humor and use it when you flirt. Do you find yourself in my words so far?"

L: "Yes, however, then things don't go well."

T: "Wait a minute! Don't mind now about the consequences, let's do it later. Have we so far described anything about Laura?"

L: "Sure!"

T: "Good. So, you hope to encounter support. Or encouragement? Which of these aspects resonates most with you, that is, what do you hope the other person will do?"

After a brief negotiation over terms, Laura concludes that she is looking for someone who makes her feel free to be the way she feels.

T: "Okay. The point is that the other person doesn't only leave you free! The others make you suffer or feel ashamed, as in the case of your mother and the aspiring chef, right?"

L: "Eeexactly! Are you telling me that I express myself badly, that I'm tactless?"

Laura here is still focused on how others describe her and therefore imagines that the therapist is also criticizing her. After solving the problem in their relationship, the therapist moves on to the most important question in MIT: *explore core cognitions about the self.*

T: "Laura, now imagine yourself facing your boyfriend telling you that you have offended him. And so you are bad. I ask you if that is what you think of yourself."
L: "My mother and aunt always tell me that."
T: "Their opinion. What is yours? Do you believe it?"
L: "Doctor, at this point, yes. What a pain in the ass, though!"

Laura now swings between positive and negative core beliefs, but her focus is still on the other's reactions. Her hope is that her mother, aunt, and boyfriend will react differently and support her instead of "making me feel like a bitch." She is still not differentiating.

T: "Right. So, on the one hand, you search for support and, said from another perspective, you would like them to stop making you feel like crap, to stop telling you that you should stop doing as you want. You would like them to stop telling you not to hurt others, right?"
L: "Yes, my goodness, and what am I doing wrong?"

Although Laura has a good metacognitive awareness of her own functioning in relationships, her mind remains in the "the other does to me" and "if only the other" modes. She imagines that only when they stop painting her that way can she get better and follow her own autonomous, spontaneous drives. Further inquiry is necessary to bring out her core self-beliefs, and imagery is a very suitable tool. The therapist will first bring up the arousal related to a scene where they criticize her and then ask her what she thinks about herself at that moment.

They agree to reenact the message exchange with *the aspiring chef,* as they ironically call him. She closes her eyes and relives the scene. The therapist makes her dwell on the beginning of the episode so that she notices the positive moments and savors them: the attraction, the excitement, and the flirting atmosphere. To help her get in touch with these aspects, the therapist echoes Laura's voice: "I'm having fun, this guy interests me. Would you like to repeat these words?" Laura repeats them and clearly appears vital and pleased.

The scene unfolds; Laura writes witty messages and is amused, wanting to get into the game of mutual poking and prodding that so often characterizes flirting. The therapist asks her to pay attention to the moment when the *chef* becomes resentful. Laura is surprised: "What did I do wrong?" At this moment, the positive image begins to falter; her face is gloomy.

T: "What's going on?"

L: "I guess I fucked up. I should have been more careful; after all, I don't even know him. I got too familiar, my mother always tells me so."

T: "Hold on, hold on, Laura! Never mind what your mother thinks. Refocus on the scene and reread the chef's resentful messages aloud. How do they affect you?"

L: "That I am a bitch."

The therapist marks Laura's negative ideas about herself in a harsh tone of voice, almost as if he really means it:

T: "I'm a bitch. I'm insensitive, I hurt people."

It is a technique we frequently use to transiently raise arousal and make patients fully aware of the emotional distress associated with certain ideas about themselves. It is effective; Laura lowers her gaze. The therapist immediately returns to himself.

T: "What do you think of yourself right now?"

L: "What's wrong with me? I am really so insensitive."

T: "How much do you believe it? Try looking at yourself from outside the scene: what do you think of this Laura who wrote messages that made the other suffer?"

L: "She's a real bitch."

T: "Perfect. I ask you again: how true is that for you right now?"

L: "Quite a lot."

The therapist stops the imagery. First, he explores the state of the therapeutic relationship.

T: "How did you perceive me during the experiment?"

L: "Good."

T: "Can you tell me more?"

L: "That you were trying to . . . to give me a better understanding of how I function."

T: "I'm glad. Look, at one point, I said bad things about you, almost as if I really meant them. How did that affect you?"

L: "For a moment, I was getting pissed off!"

T: [*smiles*]: "Because you rightly thought I was a bastard and was cheaply insulting you."

L: [*Laughs*]: "That's right. I got the point right away, though. No, no, well, it helped me, I realized how much I believe in some bad things. I mean, yes, doctor, I know you don't really mean them."

Through this inquiry, the therapist finds that the technique interacts with the relationship according to pattern 4: reinforcing it. There is a brief moment, actively sought by the therapist, of pattern 3: the technique generates a brief rupture with the patient experiencing negative ideas and emotions for a moment. The rupture, however, gets solved spontaneously, and work continues productively. At this point, the therapist completes the cognitive inquiry aimed at exploring the core self-idea.

T: "This all sounds interesting to me. I think we are discovering something. Beyond what others – your aunt, aspiring chefs – think, you are the one who has this negative idea of yourself. When others judge you, you are sometimes down on yourself and sometimes rebel. But in the end, the point is that you are the first to consider yourself insensitive. Right? What would you call this Laura?"

L: "Insensitive!"

Here Laura now really knows that she has a negative core schema of herself and has moved from the "the other makes me" setup to "I have an idea of myself as insensitive that I tend to believe to be true." The *Insensitive One* will become the name they use to describe this character in her inner theater.

Making this idea less true and making room for alternative self-images become the therapeutic goal. Laura now knows that the goal of therapy is not to convince the world to support her autonomy but to consider the idea that she is insensitive less true and realize that it is no more than a character in her imaginal world.

We reinforce and stabilize this step by interweaving it with the next one, namely, noting the swings between positive and negative images. Before describing the next step, however, let us look at an example in which the cognitive inquiry aimed at identifying the core self-image leads to a major relationship rupture. Reformulation of the contract will be necessary.

Marianne is 38 years old and suffers from paranoid PD, along with an eating disorder in which she alternates between restrictive anorexia and bulimia nervosa. She also presents with social anxiety, and when she reveals to her therapist that she uses alcohol and benzodiazepines to soothe it, she is adamant that she has no intention of giving up these regulatory modalities or of refraining from using psychotropic drugs without psychiatric counseling.

She owns a big clothing store. She has been in therapy with a colleague from northern Italy for two years to overcome the grief of losing her father, followed by her separation from her husband. She asked for separation because her husband was passive and switched off and did not desire her sexually, but she still sees it as a failure. Thanks to therapy, she has worked through her grief, but she does not allow herself to enter a new relationship. She thinks paranoically that men will exploit her, interested only in her wealth, so she avoids them. All this is reinforced by the idea that she is fat. She alternates, as we mentioned, restrictions with binges followed by excessive physical exercise. The therapist asks her to regularize her eating behaviors, but Marianne categorically refuses. Beliefs about food and body shape have a family basis; her mother suffers from anorexia, her brother from bigorexia, and her father himself had orthorexia and was obsessed with thinness. Despite justifying her obsession with healthy choices, she speaks of her own body and those of others with visible disdain. She dresses oversize, does not expose herself, avoids showering at the gym, and rejects suitors, driven by the belief: "I'm fat, they cannot like me. If they're after me, it's all about money."

A few months pass. Marianne feels lonely and would like a romantic relationship, but giving herself a chance is too risky. She and the therapist come to recognize that the problem is precisely the *ugly and fat* core self-image facing *contemptuous* others. To the therapist's surprise, Marianne believes it to be completely true: physical appearance is the yardstick of all society. The therapist discloses that she has had similar fears and suffered from them, but this does not make Marianne more malleable: "If you change your mind, you are deluding yourself." The therapist explains that it is not important to change her mind; she just wants to show Marianne that she understands her perspective. Marianne remains rock-hard: "The world only thinks about how thin or fat you are and judges you by that."

Over the course of several sessions, the therapist shows Marianne how this depends on the dismissive behavior of both her parents and her brother and that she now fully adopts their views.

M: "It's true, I see myself as they taught me to."
T: "Yes, very good, Marianne. And how do you feel about that?"
M: "That they are right."

Associated memories also therefore fail to lead her to question her core self-image. After a few more months of therapy, she acquires a modicum of critical distance and accedes for a few moments to a more benevolent self-idea; she knows that she is able to guess what clothes will go in that season and that she is good at training her staff.

The therapist then proposes an experiential exercise for her to better recognize the *ugly and fat* core self-image as an idea believed to be true, rather than a fact. She asks Marianne to re-experience her positive self-images and then enact a chairwork where her mother criticizes her for gaining weight. Marianne starts chairwork sitting in her mother's chair. From that stance, she makes a razor-sharp comment: "You suck, no one will want to pick you up."

The therapist now asks her to go to the chair where her *ugly, fat* self is. Marianne experiences the pain of seeing herself humiliated. At this point, the therapist asks her to retrieve her valid self-image and try to use it to respond to her mother. Marianne replies, but still from a position of submission.

M: "Mom, I know I'm ugly, but, you see, at least I'm successfully running Dad's stores, don't you think?"
T: "How do you feel?"
M: "Doctor, why do you want to humiliate me?"
     [*The therapist is surprised, feels guilty, and steps back*]

T: "What's going on?"

M: "My mother thinks what everyone thinks. What's the point of humiliating me again?"

What happens? In this case, the experiential technique is the cause of a major rupture, the interactional pattern 1. Marianne does have a part of herself that she sees as valid, but, as they understand better in later sessions when attachment is activated, she does not have an idea of the other as *benevolent and loving*. She only sees the others as distant and spiteful. Chairwork activates a sense of vulnerability that triggers attachment. At this point, Marianne constructs the therapist exactly like her parents: distant and *sadistic*. The therapist has to repair the rupture. She succeeds because Marianne can read non-verbal signals and recognizes that contempt and disinterest are completely absent. Anyway, the therapist has to give up chairwork and radically reformulate the contract. Marianne, in fact, offers no room for working on her isolation and loneliness. The therapist resorts to the *leaning forward helplessness* position.

T: "Marianne, I've really understood that I have to do everything not to expose you to humiliation. And that if I try and make you figure out that there is something good in the world for you, that you can meet someone who appreciates you and cares for you, I just seem naive. I understand that; I don't insist. But I do ask you: if you feel alone but refuse any form of social encounter, be it even just for making friends, how can therapy help you?"

After several sessions and an exacerbation of loneliness, which has become full-blown depression, Marianne finally agrees to increase social exposure. She is still at a minimum level of differentiation and contact with a positive self-image.

M: "All right, I'm going out. I realize that I have to risk meeting men, maybe I don't suck. Let's be clear, though: I'm not taking them home!

T: "Heaven forbid!"

Fostering shifts between positive and negative self-images so that the patient realizes that these are mental representations

A therapeutic step of great value for differentiation is to bring patients into contact with the positive aspects of the self and then point out how they immediately return to seeing themselves in the light of negative core images (Figure 9.1, Box 12). Therapists, moreover, can promote repeated shifts between negative and positive images, as we will show next. The goal is neither emotion regulation nor challenging negative beliefs. We want to help patients become aware of their own mental processes, how they have multiple, parallel self-images, how they are inhabited by various *characters*, *voices*, or *positions* (Hermans & Dimaggio, 2004), and how their mind is quick to slide toward negative ones. Through these operations, patients come to a metacognitive awareness that sounds like "My mind has difficulty focusing on aspects of me that I like. Instead, it tends to focus on the negative and believes it to be true, and it is pretty good at this job."

We have not yet arrived at: "I can stop believing that negative ideas about myself and others are true," but are at a preliminary awareness: "My mind is populated with various ideas about me; there are various possible *mes*, and the more negative ones tend to prevail because my mind works according to automatisms that I am now discovering."

We describe this step while continuing the story of Laura, the 23-year-old humanities student. During the first part of the imagery, the therapist has her dwell on the moment when she was flirting. Laura feels excited, amused, attracted, and curious, and the therapist points out how these feelings belong to her and are beautiful, and how, on the other hand, self-criticism is absent. The therapist makes Laura identify the core negative self-images and then lets her return to those moments.

T: "Pay attention to that. You don't always believe you are *the Insensitive One*. By the way, do we agree that's how we call it?"

L: [*Smiles*]: "Yes, it sounds very much like a Sicilian love story."

T: "Great. So, we have seen that you can experience moments where you are fully in touch with beautiful, vital feelings, where you know what you want, savor it, feel it is yours and are? ok. At the beginning of the message exchange, you were having fun, and you felt like playing and joking. That's who you are; you're witty, nothing wrong with that. Makes sense?"

Laura looks proud; these parts belong to her, and she is happy about them. She recalls various episodes, both with her previous boyfriend and with friends, where they appreciated her jokes.

T: "Very good. So, we can say that in your mind both the *Insensitive One*, who hurts others, and the ironic, witty, curious Laura dwell. And both are parts of you?"
    [*Laura nods*]

T: "What gives you pain, perhaps one of the reasons you asked for therapy, is that you instinctively give more credit to the negative idea. You would like to spend more time playing, being curious, and following your own path. However, if without any external trigger, but even more so if someone reacts negatively, you freeze, paralyze, and start self-criticizing. At that point, the curious and vital Laura . . . amen! She's evaporated, gone. You look in the mirror and see only the Insensitive One. Then your purpose is no longer to do what you really care about. Instead, you apologize and ask for absolution. Yes, you rebel a little because the vital part is not dead, but it lasts only a short time before fading away for good."

Laura sees herself again in the description. Now it is possible to redraft the contract: "Can we agree that therapy will aim to take away space from the *Insensitive One* and to give more space to your creative and vital aspects?"

Laura finds it a good plan; she is just afraid she cannot put it into action: "When I get into it, I just freeze."

The therapist replies that this is normal and the work will be precisely this. In metacognitive terms, she has paved the way for the two pivotal operations of change: differentiating and empowering the healthy parts. We will describe these in the next chapter, but before moving on to these operations, it is good to consolidate the understanding achieved so far. Patients need to realize that the object of therapy is their own internal functioning and not their way of responding to the behaviors of others to obtain more satisfactory reactions. Experiential techniques are an effective means to achieve this end.

The process begins with raising negative emotional arousal by embodying negative self-aspects. Then, we ask the patient to impersonate a different, positive part, and report what idea of themselves they have now. Finally, we ask them to assume an observer's position (Hermans & Dimaggio, 2004) and note the transitions: at this point, they discover how their own mind is able to move from one state to another, to be one character and then a different one, without either falling prey to the negative state or believing the negative core self-concept to be true.

We explain the procedure by continuing to describe the work with Laura. The therapist proposes another imagery exercise. He asks her to recall the moment when she was flirting and feeling good, to evoke bodily sensations, name them, and communicate them aloud. Laura succeeds and enters a positive state. At this point, the therapist asks her to return to the moment when the boy was offended and to explore the cognitive, emotional, and somatic correlates again. Laura describes the change in mental state and how the *Insensitive One* has now taken over again. The therapist asks her to make various imagery shifts between the two moments. At the end of the exercise, he highlights how she had ideas of herself that changed as the imagery unfolded in her mind.

T: "You see, you have the idea you are insensitive, right? But we agree now that it's not true. That it's not you, it doesn't define you. It just seems true from a certain angle."

Laura realizes with surprise how typical this functioning is.

L: "Wow, that's really me! It's just that sometimes I get fixated and I forget that a lot of times I'm really happy with myself."

T: "Excellent! Did you also notice how the moment you came back to focus on when you were having fun and flirting, you saw yourself in another way? Not only that, you were capable of seeing yourself positively just a few seconds after being very self-critical!"

Laura now truly understands how suffering springs from her idea of herself and not from truly being *the Insensitive One*. She understands this because she notices how differently she sees herself if only she passes to experiencing activity, vitality, playfulness, and being seductive.

The therapist also points out to her how quickly she was able to consciously shift from the negative to the positive state. This means she can anchor herself to positive self-images and let the negative images fade away with a minimum of psychological effort.

The therapist explores the relationship: Laura is grateful to him. At first, she confesses she experienced a brief moment of sorrow and anger because she thought the therapist did not take her pain seriously. She fleetingly perceived the therapist as distant and herself as unlovable and lonely, but then she paid no more attention and became involved in the work.

Pattern 3 thus takes place: a momentary rupture followed by consolidation. The therapist did not even get a chance to notice this. Instead, at the end of the exercise, the interaction is pattern 5: the relationship gets consolidated because the patient has discovered that she has power over the pain and feels the therapist is support-ive, encouraging, and able to guide her energetically toward improvement.

At such times, relational ruptures are possible while performing a technique. We explain this with Catherine, a 45-year-old lawyer who suffers from dependent and obsessive-compulsive PD and is in therapy with a colleague in the early stages of MIT training. She begins therapy for a chronic state of emptiness and sadness and Obsessive Compulsive Disorder. The latter was solved through work on repetitive thinking combined with exposure and response prevention.

Catherine has strict moral standards for herself and others and has difficulty making decisions independently; she constantly asks for advice and becomes para-lyzed. For example, if she goes out with her current partner, she cannot express where she would like to go, whether she prefers sushi or pizza, what dress to buy, and so on. She comes from a strict and punitive family, and this has led her to repress her homosexuality. Only for the past few years has she been in a relation-ship with a woman, but she has not come out. In the past, her dependent function-ing appeared in friendships, in which she compulsively took care of others and self-sacrificed. In this way, she protected herself from loneliness. In addition, she left all decisions to her friends so that she would not risk making mistakes.

Together with the therapist, she reconstructs that emptiness and depression are the consequences of prolonged alexithymia and failure to connect with desires. During dynamic assessment, Catherine has fleeting access to healthy parts related to her love of nature and travel. The therapist helps her recognize how she is driven by a core self-image that she takes to be true: *imperfect and stupid*. Now, the thera-pist would like to help her realize that she contacts the positive aspects but does not keep them in her mind and immediately slips into the negative ones. The therapist proposes an imagery exercise to Catherine: contact the desire to go on a vacation to Puglia and tell her partner. Catherine agrees, but the therapist overlooks non-verbal signs of tension and thus does not explore the therapeutic relationship.

Catherine sees herself at the beach, diving into the water, and likes it. At this point, the therapist asks her to 'wear' this image and keep it as she tries to tell her partner that she would like to spend a weekend together by the sea in June. Catherine immediately becomes tense and freezes. The therapist then asks her to return to the previous moment to better inhabit the positive part of herself. She suggests that she focus on the physical sensations when she dives into the water. Catherine feels good for a moment. But when she tries again to talk to her companion, she fails. They interrupt the imagery.

T: "How was the exercise? What was it that stopped you?"
C: "I did it wrong. I was worried that you thought I was not capable."
T: "No, no, Catherine, you were great. Look, how was the contact with the good part?"

The therapist tries to reassure her, an operation that is actually incorrect! As we have explained, if patients construct therapists in a schema-dependent way, there is no point in refuting the belief; one must work on the rupture in the ways described in chapter 3, which we refer to.

C: "It was a superficial thing; it all sounded silly to me."
      The therapist is puzzled; she did not expect such a reaction.
T: "In what way? I felt like it was going well."
C: "I felt ridiculous, it's a waste of time. Yes, I tell her I want to go to the sea. So what? She says 'no' anyway, and I have just made things worse."

The therapist notices the relational rupture taking place and asks the patient if she feels judged by her. Catherine says no, she does not. At the end of the session, the therapist, who is unclear about what is happening, tells her that they will reflect together in the next session.

In supervision with one of us, the reasons for the problem emerge. The first is that the therapist asked Catherine to enter imagery without having first monitored the relationship. Catherine, in fact, was not driven by curiosity to explore her inner world but by social rank: she wanted to function perfectly in the therapist's eyes and feared her judgment. The therapist thus did not understand that even when Catherine got in touch with the healthy part – which is good anyway – she immediately read her experience in the light of her search for approval: "Am I doing what the therapist is asking me well?"

In this case, the technique-relationship interaction is related to pattern 2: the technique has a negative effect on the relationship. The relational breakdown existed before the imagery, which, however, accentuated the patient's fear of judgment.

The second reason is that the therapist worked inconsistently with the decision-making procedure. This passage ought to make Catherine aware of the shifts between the healthy and schema-dependent core self-images. Instead, the therapist, without realizing it, tried to empower the healthy part to refute the negative belief, which is a more advanced change-promoting operation. Had she realized this, even with all the relational breakdown, the exercise would have been a success! That is, the therapist could have said

How wonderful, Catherine, you really contacted how much you like the sea, the sensation of the sand under your feet, the water, the sense of freshness and freedom. Yet, look how quickly you switch to self-criticism. 'I thought I was being frivolous, plus the important thing was to do the therapeutic exercise well!' Do you see that even with me, you worry about being good? It's hard for you to allow yourself to use therapy for what it is, something that allows you to feel better, overcoming emptiness and sadness.

With such an intervention, the therapist would have handled the relational rupture correctly and increased the patient's awareness of having healthy parts that are, however, immediately obscured by schema-dependent ones. How come she did not formulate it? Partly because of inexperience; it was her first MIT supervision. However, the rupture also depended on a second reason: the activation of a schema in the therapist, in the social rank domain. By the time Catherine got in touch with the healthy part, the therapist was satisfied and relieved; she thought she was being effective. But when Laura returned to seeing herself as stupid and frivolous, the therapist worried, "What am I doing wrong?" She saw herself as incapable and, under pressure, could only postpone problem-solving until the next session.

We have just described one of the most frequent mistakes: using patients' access to positive states as a marker for therapeutic success. But when schemas take over again, therapists get worried, scared, and tormented. Instead, it is a physiological process they must anticipate. We will also see this in chapters 10 and 11.

We return to the question: how to get patients to discover that their mind, after contacting the positive parts, quickly returns to reading themselves and the world in light of the schema? Body work is particularly useful for this purpose: we make patients swing between schema-related somatic states and healthy or positive somatic states and vice versa. In this way, they discover how cognitions and emotions depend in part on posture and movements and that negative ideas do not describe an objective reality but are just a point of view that changes as the body moves.

Identify what coping is activated as part of the self-response and strategies for dealing with it

In reconstructing functioning, it is important to note that patients procedurally resort to cognitive and behavioral coping to alleviate the suffering that emerges when the response of the self is activated in response to the other. Simply said, using the example of a young man with avoidant PD, this is how it works:

I hope to be appreciated. The other criticizes me (*response of the other*). I think she is right and that I am unworthy and I feel ashamed (*response of the self with the associated pain*). To soothe the pain I avoid further relational contact with worrying about what could I do next time to prevent further criticism (*behavioral copings and repetitive thinking*).

These copings are automatic protective procedures that increase suffering and relational problems. In the case of the former example, the patient finds himself incapable, ashamed, and to protect himself from pain, isolates himself. What is the result? The increased sense of painful exclusion, and then repetitive thinking increases anxiety and leads to depression.

In Chapter 8, we have already described the procedures for reconstructing coping mechanisms and their interactions, for example, how repetitive thinking can trigger maladaptive behaviors. In this step, we focus on the operations to make patients aware of how, when they conclude that the others' response is negative, the negative self-image and related emotions emerge; they believe it to be true without even questioning their truth-like value, and at that point, they resort to coping to protect themselves from suffering.

This is often a very rapid mechanism, mediated by fast, embodied, sometimes preconscious cognitive-affective processes. The sequence goes something like this: "He criticized me. He is right. I am ashamed. I avoid." At other times, the coping reaction is mediated by conscious reflection and repetitive thinking.

As long as patients rapidly enact coping mechanisms like binge eating, perfectionism, aggression, or substance use, they come to a point in their life where they are unable to tell the reasons underlying these behaviors. To discover the cognitive-affective processes underlying the reasons for using coping in response to others' negative reactions, therapists have to invite patients to attempt abstaining from these protective processes because, as long as they are active, it is difficult to make them aware of the cognitions and emotions that define the core self-image.

Remember that the other's response activates the self's response, but the latter is not a simple reaction of the kind: "She criticizes me, I feel criticized." The real driver is what patients think about themselves, and making them aware of this allows them to get to the core of personality pathology. So the process we want to reveal sounds like: "When she criticized, I think she is right; I am a failure. This is the reason why I feel ashamed and then avoid." Changing nuclear images such as "I am a failure" is the main goal of treatment (Figure 9.1, Box 13b).

Patients like Alina, when they reach the levels now described, are at the threshold of true change promotion, as we have already shown for Marianne. We have thus arrived at the most important juncture in therapy. Patients have achieved full awareness of their own functioning; the formulation is shared. They have assumed a beginning of critical distance and have some regulatory abilities. Therapy must now lead them to break the maladaptive interpersonal patterns and form new ones, and then take different, healthier paths. The next chapter is devoted to the first steps necessary for this to happen.

Chapter 10

Differentiate and strengthen the healthy parts, recognizing the shifts back to the schema

We now start promoting change; here lies perhaps the most technically complex step. We have led patients to understand they are guided by schemas and to reconstruct their structures with us. We have helped them discover that they are inhabited by healthy and vital self-aspects. The time is ripe for these understandings to become solid and stable, and take over schema-dependent ideas, emotions, and behaviors.

Strictly speaking, MIT therapists begin to move toward change from two parallel operations: promoting differentiation (Figure 10.1, Box 1) and consolidating and strengthening the healthy parts (Figure 10.1, Box 2). As explained in Chapter 5, some operations are forbidden at this stage; we consider them serious technical errors: therapists should not attempt to bring patients to change their social behavior to act more appropriately, or to better understand others, or to become aware of their contribution to creating or sustaining the very dynamics that cause them to suffer. These are operations to be carried out after differentiation and empowerment of the healthy parts have become established. We will describe them in later chapters.

At the end of the shared formulation, patients begin to realize that the reasons for chronic suffering are internal and schema-dependent. It is a passage with great instability; patients' awareness fades easily or does not hold up to the lashing waves of reality.

How, then, can we bring patients to believe less in schema-dependent ideas, to feel them less true, and conversely learn how to embrace positive, benevolent core self-images capable of motivating exploration and restoring agency? In this fundamental and unstable transition, techniques are very good at changing, provided they are used correctly.

Before describing the procedures, we summarize what forms of awareness differentiation can be achieved.

(a) *Move from "true" to "historically learned."* From "I would like to be liked, but I am worthless, and others criticize me" to "I would like to be liked, but I tend to think I am worthless, and others criticize me because that is what I learned in childhood." When patients do not remember core episodes (Dimaggio et al.,

DOI: 10.4324/9781003570967-10

Differentiating
Box 1

Consolidating and empowering
healthy self aspects
Box 2

Discovering how after having accessed the
healthy self, the mind returns to read the
world through the lenses of the schemas
Box 3

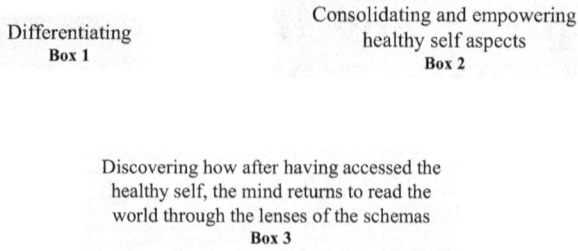

Figure 10.1 Changing inner representations of self and others

2013), we always work by promoting associations but moving toward the future. We ask them to pay attention to relational narrative episodes in the days following the session. Through this and noticing recurrences together, patients move from "*true*" to "my usual way of reading events that is not necessarily true."

In both cases, the driver of differentiation is the discovery of recurrences in one's way of reading social relations. Patients understand that even if the world hurts them, structural suffering depends on the perspective from which they view it and the lenses they wear.

(b) *Move from "Always true" to "Sometimes I think it is true, but at other times I have a positive view." Patients pass f*rom "Others always criticize me because I am a joke and they see it" to "At times, I see myself as capable, and have a sense that others can appreciate me." It is thus differentiation through access to healthy parts.

(c) *Assess the degree of certainty in the negative belief.* If therapists ask patients what percentage they believe their ideas about self and others, and they answer "100%," they are not differentiating. If they answer "80%," they have reached a minimum of critical distance; their idea is a hypothesis, believed to be mostly true, yes, but not certain. Of note, this type of differentiation corresponds to Beck's concept of cognitive insight (Beck et al., 2004).

(d) *Promoting agency over mental states.* This is a fundamental modality in MIT; many patients are deeply convinced that their pain is caused by others: "I'm suffering because the other person makes me . . ." or that they are at their core defective, unlovable, and inferior. They focus, therefore, on the other causing the harm or on the impossibility of change. They believe these ideas are true and often ruminate. The associated memories only confirm the idea: "You see, it has always been this way; it's the story of my life!" Healthy parts lie in the shadow, hardly ever surfacing.

What do we therapists do, then? In a calm but unflinching way, we point out that, yes, others may hurt them and that, yes, the idea of being worthless is painful, and we do not expect them to change their mind. But we highlight that the pain they feel is largely due to their tendencies to remain attached to those ideas and not do anything to change their state of mind: "The other person made you suffer, but staying in a state of suffering is up to you. Remaining sad, angry, guilty is an active mental operation, which we can either go along with or interrupt."

This is a differentiation based on changing agency beliefs with respect to mental states. Patients must move from "The other makes me . . ., and I react passively to the stimuli," or from "I am defective and can only suffer in thinking about it" to "I have agency over my mental state, and if I use it I will be better off." MIT therapists must constantly have before their eyes such an operation leading to renegotiating the therapeutic contract:

Would you rather stay ruminating about your defects, whether real or false? Would you rather stay talking about how much the other has hurt you in the past or hurt you today? Or do we choose to act to ease the pain and move toward health?

(e) *Revise the belief, recognizing that one's negative ideas were unrealistic.* MIT adopts this tool practically only when therapy is in its advanced stages. For two reasons, the first is that the ideas expressed by those suffering from PD or PTSD are almost never false. They are attributional biases, tendencies to read the world from the same angle, and a constant veering to the negative. But they can be true and often are. Is the world a safe place? No. Are people benevolent and well-disposed? Maybe. Did bad things happen in the past? Sure. To consider such beliefs "irrational" or "wrong" would be a real mistake. The second reason is that if therapists refute the belief, they force patients to expose themselves to situations that evoke dangerous scenarios. If we try to convince a young avoidant man that he is wrong to see himself as fat, ugly, stupid, or inferior, he will immediately see himself exposed to the other's gaze and experience anxiety, fear, and shame. He is likely to erect protective barriers. Consequently, in this volume, this is not the kind of differentiation we suggest promoting; we consider it may be more useful in some symptom disorders treated with CBT.

We promote differentiation and access to healthy parts simultaneously. The most obvious example is fostering critical distance by moving from "I have negative ideas about myself and others that are always true" to "At certain times, I realize I read myself and the world from a more benevolent angle."

In the other manuals, we covered the operations of differentiating and accessing the healthy parts separately for the sake of clarity (Dimaggio et al., 2015, 2020). Since we focus here on what happens as we adopt experiential techniques to take these steps and what impact they have on the therapeutic relationship, we treat them together. We then use illustrative examples where the therapist, at the same time, promotes both differentiation and access to healthy parts.

The risk of new relational ruptures here is high. Patients' patterns are still active and quick to take over, and therapists' schemas do play a role. But often, ruptures come from technical mistakes, as we see in the next section.

Before differentiating and accessing healthy parts, avoid mistakes

We have learned from supervision experience that this is the time when therapists most easily make mistakes and persist in them. What mistakes do they make? They note that patients have achieved a good awareness of their internal world, a high level of metacognitive monitoring that includes some capacity for integration:

> I think I am incapable and others will judge me. I have this idea almost all the time and it makes me anxious when I have to expose myself or ashamed when I am inside situations. But it's not always like that. With friends having drinks, I'm fine, huh!

At this point, therapists become convinced that patients are aware of the pattern and move to help them change their minds. They propose guided imagery exercises, bodywork, and behavioral experiments. However, patients do not respond, and relational ruptures occur. Therapists become impatient, worried, or judgmental, and patients feel pressured, controlled, disappointed, or neglected. What has happened? Patients have not differentiated at all! They are only aware of their own ways of thinking and feeling in a metacognitively advanced way, but they still believe their ideas are true!

Therapists can make a mistake at any moment, but here we are talking about an inherently technical one. Then, as always, it can be aggravated because therapists enter negative states of mind, mostly characterized by shame, guilt at the idea of harming patients, sorrow for their suffering, or fear of the professional consequences of an error. Driven by core images of themselves as undeserving, harmful, and doomed to failure and poverty, therapists insist on promoting change. In doing so, however, they exacerbate problems. They propose other techniques and behavioral experiments and press for patients to rescript narratives successfully. Alternatively, they experience frustration and swing between helplessness and frustration, criticizing patients: "Why doesn't he engage?" "Why doesn't she understand that if she doesn't do something, it makes me feel bad?" Driven by this range of thoughts and emotions, they do not act in line with the formulation, which would instead require them to take steps back and understand what is going on in the patients' minds. On the other hand, they contribute to dysfunctional interpersonal cycles in session.

How do we remedy these errors? Therapists must become aware they have entered a problematic mental state that contributes to the interpersonal cycle and work to get out of it and repair the relationship (Chapter 3). They must then rethink the formulation and remember what psychotherapy is at the core.

The essence of psychotherapy

Psychotherapists' job is not to push patients toward health. For them to improve and heal, three steps are essential:

1) that patients form a mental model of their own functioning;
2) that they know that it is just a map of the world and not the world itself;
3) that they intend to use this map, together with the therapist, to change by acting differently.

Where do therapists go wrong, and in what ways do they disregard these steps? The mistake is that they confuse their own understanding of the schema with the idea that patients know they have a schema. This is almost always not the case. The therapists' skill is not to understand and intuit but to hypothesize and ask for feedback. Therapists must therefore always summarize patients' functioning and then ask them: "How true do you believe what we just described: that you are worth little and that others criticize you for good reasons?"

Therapists must purposefully investigate patients' cognition about themselves: "Others criticize you, but observe yourself in the scene where it happened. What do you think of yourself?" Getting an answer to this question is crucial for therapy to work.

There is only one reliable signal to really access change operations, an explicit and unequivocal response: "I realize that I tend to think I am worthless, that I cannot affect events, that I am unlovable. But now I am beginning to realize that this is not necessarily the case. Of course, it is difficult to change perspective." These are the statements that indicate nascent differentiation. It needs to be consolidated, but patients are ready to change.

Let us be honest, we do not believe much in implicit change. That is, that patients automatically, through corrective emotional experiences (Alexander & French, 1946) in the therapeutic relationship, internalize new interpersonal patterns and apply them in real life. The embodied, procedural component of maladaptive interpersonal patterns makes them little permeable to change.

Our work therefore consists, first of all, of subtracting land from the realms of the implicit. We want patients to say out loud what they are suffering from and if they are starting to detach themselves from their negative ideas. We want them, on this basis, to formulate with us a contract aimed at changing their meaning-making system and, more importantly, their in-between session behaviors.

Yes, a good therapeutic relationship helps. Having passed tests (Weiss, 1993) helps. Having dealt with relational ruptures and having repaired them (Muran & Eubanks, 2020; Safran & Muran, 2000) helps. But changing personality structures comes through conscious work and training in new perspectives and actions. When patients start practicing any new activity, they have to know they are going to engage themselves in numerous repetitions before they see results. We need to be aware of this, both for the sake of the patient and to spare therapists' frustration and stop them from banging their heads against the wall.

Differentiating and accessing healthy parts: the role of techniques and the impact on the relationship

The starting point for accomplishing these two operations, as just noted, is for patients to have an emerging awareness that their reading of relationships is not necessarily true. They begin to realize that they suffer partly because reality is not always loving and cheerful, but mostly because of their own worldview. They would now like to climb another hill, look at the sea from a different shore, but they do not know how to get there. This is where the attempt to change starts.

Experiential techniques in this transition can be decisive, and we know that, in general, they are safe and effective (Hoppen et al., 2022). However, cognitive therapies and other experiential approaches are known to have dropouts and treatment failures. It is likely that these problems do not depend on the techniques themselves but on having applied them without following a set of principles.

Our working hypothesis is that to make experiential techniques safe and effective and to avoid relational ruptures, a series of steps are necessary, which we describe. We illustrate them here because we are at the beginning of change promoting, which is when the techniques work full steam. We focus on how to apply guided imagery and rescripting, but with minor modifications, the steps are the same as for role-play and chairwork. Of note, MIT applies guided imagery and rescripting in a largely different way from the *Imagery Rescripting* protocol adopted by Schema Therapy (Arntz, 2012), though we do not get into the details of the many differences between the two procedures for the sake of space.

We repeat: the procedures we now outline are aimed at maximizing the effectiveness of the techniques and preventing ruptures, especially those resulting from erroneous interventions that are inconsistent with the shared formulation.

1.   Have in mind the maladaptive interpersonal schema and a plan for the rewriting

Therapists should organize imagery only if they have a clear idea of the structure of schemas and a plan for rewriting them. They must know which wish to support and have already programmed actions and phrases that support them and interrupt coping. It is not good to go into imagery improvising or letting patients decide what they would like to say or do differently. The latter seems to give agency and freedom, but the result is usually negative. Left to themselves, patients very easily adopt coping procedures and compromise solutions. Let us imagine that the goal is autonomy and that, to achieve it, it is necessary to abandon compulsive care of the suffering of others. What if we say "You are facing your mother who is sick. What can you do now to move toward your own autonomy?"

We have collected many similar examples: imagine a woman who tries to convince her mother to let her go, explaining that she loves her still, even if she is leaving her on her own. She promises her mother that after a while she will be available. What is this patient doing? She is trying to be autonomous but at the same time, to be forgiven by her mother and shield herself from guilt; she hopes her mother will not feel abandoned. In this way, she does not break the pattern!

Instead, the intervention should sound like this: "Try telling your mother that you are going on vacation with your boyfriend, that you are sorry she is suffering, but you are going anyway." The patient, at this point, hesitates, and only if the therapist supports her will she not succumb to guilt. If the therapist does not intervene in this way, it is easy for the patient to perform the exercise in imagery, but then, in daily life, instead of pursuing her own desires, she continues trying to convince her mother to let her go and is possibly not feeling abandoned!

2. Summon the healthy parts first

Entering guided imagery requires exposing oneself to painful images and emotions, governing them, and acting in new ways. Patients face others who are critical, threatening, distant, cold, or suffering. Nothing is easy. To succeed, they have to anchor themselves in a valid, competent, energetic, motivated, and curious sense of self. It is difficult to evoke this while painful emotions and cognitions surface.

It is good practice to invite patients, before guided imagery and rescripting begin, to evoke, both in their mind and in their body, a healthy part they might recall when in the heat of the episode they are re-experiencing: "Think of a time when you were capable and competent, experience the emotional and somatic correlates, and keep the sensations in mind." In this way, when moving to rewriting, the therapist can say "Recall that part of yourself we contacted earlier."

3. Patients must understand and agree that they are working on their internal space; that is, they must have begun to differentiate

Many therapists bring patients into guided imagery, making the aforementioned mistake of thinking patients know they are working on their schemas when they are not. They are still reasoning on a reality basis. They are in the "I have no power to correct my faults" or "The others should treat me better" position. Therapists try to change the scene, but patients either do not respond or follow their suggestions but do not change their inner world one iota.

This is the pattern 2 technique-relationship interaction: the technique creates a rupture that needs attention. But the very reason for the alliance rupture is the therapeutic error. Before entering imagery, therapists must be crystal clear that patients know that the goal is to change internal structures. That is, patients need to be already aware they are guided by schemas, but taking another perspective is difficult for them. That is what imagery and other experiential techniques are for: to discover in an embodied way, by adopting it, that there is another angle from which to view the world. Again, patients must be aware that a different angle is indispensable before entering imagery.

4. Guided imagery is not aimed at changing behavior in reality

We are at the stage where we want to change interpersonal schemas. We explain to patients that we are not asking them to prepare to act differently in reality; this may induce ungrounded hopes, fears, and protective mechanisms. They need to know that they are going to try new ways of feeling and acting, of embodying healthy aspects of themselves and giving them a voice, and of disrupting habitual coping. Only when these new perspectives are subjectively true and plausible do we agree on the behavioral experiments that we describe in Chapters 11 and 13.

5. Breaking the link with reality and fostering emotional regulation before imagery: the preparation step

To clarify that we will be working on internal space, we begin imagery with an introductory phase. We usually ask patients to close their eyes and breathe steadily, paying attention to the contact points of the body with the world. We can alternatively, preferably with eyes closed, have them adopt a grounding position in which they feel their body anchored to the floor. This stage usually lasts about a minute and helps patients detach their minds from reality, to deflect attention away from the therapist, so as to explore their inner space, knowing that they will be working on that.

If the scenes are very painful or frankly traumatic, emotions are likely to rise intensely. It is good, then, that the preparation phase has a true pre-regulatory component. The therapist should prolong it until patients have optimal emotion regulation. In this way, when emotions mount and are on the verge of spiraling out of control, it is easier to resume the exercises already begun before imagery and calm down. This operation prevents pattern 2 ruptures: if patients know they will experience intense painful emotions but can regulate them, they are unlikely to view their therapist negatively when it happens.

6. Remove the filter of the narrating ego and speak in the present tense

Experiential techniques serve to access the sources of emotions and cognitions, to identify those thoughts that generate action and control it. They aim to remove the interference of semantic reasoning and turn off the protective coping mechanisms, such as experiential avoidance, that patients use unconsciously. At the same time, these techniques promote self-reflexivity. We bring patients into the scene, activate arousal, and ask: "What are you thinking and feeling at this exact moment? You are looking at the face of your father, who is scolding you, observing him. How does it affect you? What are you thinking and feeling?"

For patients to unfold their full capacity to increase self-reflexivity, two operations are necessary: first, they should not put themselves in the position of the storyteller, which in itself grants emotional distance from the scene; second, they should not speak in the past tense, because it would mean not remembering and reliving the scene in the present *as if* it were really happening now. So we say "Speak in the present tense and report to me what you are thinking and feeling as you experience the episode." Whenever patients use the past tense, the therapist gently invites them to return to speaking in the present tense.

7. Avoid questions that evoke reflection and prevent associations to other memories

Once imagery has begun, we aim to intensify arousal and increase self-awareness. If patients begin to reason abstractly – "What happens means that . . ." or associate other memories – therapists immediately intervene: "Reflections, associations, are important, but not now. Please tell me what you are thinking and feeling as you face your sister, who is blackmailing you."

Therapists need to evoke only cognitions, emotions, and action tendencies related to the scene. They ask questions moment by moment. If the scene changes, they ask, "Well, and now that your sister has called you selfish, what are you thinking and feeling? What would you tend to do?" In summary, we consider any higher-level cognition an obstacle or avoidance. Valid questions are those that explore the internal world in the scene. Instead, questions such as "Why do you think . . .? What would happen if you . . .?" are forbidden, as this would be therapy as usual but with eyes closed! It makes little sense.

8. Acting in imagery to improve monitoring and explore alternative scenarios

We have forbidden the exploration of alternative cognitions and the stimulation of semantic-abstract reasoning. However, therapists need to know what would happen if a patient did something different. How do they find out? Simple: by exploiting imagery. They ask patients to act differently in a scene and report how cognitions and emotions change. Do we want to find out what would happen if a patient moves away from his depressed and complaining mother? We invite him to move away and tell us what happens. We want to know what a patient fears if she tries talking back to her screaming father. We ask her to talk back. Then, we stimulate action tendencies and new actions and investigate the cognitions and emotions that surface. No problem if patients have difficulties or a relational micro-rupture arises. We ask how they feel at that moment and whether they need to stop the exercise. Based on the response, we can encourage them to continue or agree to stop the imagery and reason together about what happened.

9. If patients insist on associating and thinking, open their eyes and speak in the past tense despite the therapists' interventions, discontinue imagery

Therapists have tried to make the most of the imagery's power to improve self-reflexivity and increase emotional arousal. However, some patients persist in reasoning and assuming the position of the storyteller of events distant in time. The scene loses the quality of immanence that we seek. At this point, it is unnecessary to insist because the working alliance is broken and patients do not accept the task. To persist would sustain the rupture and be unproductive. Therapists should, therefore, interrupt the imagery and, in a non-judgmental way, point out to patients that they have not really entered the experience. They highlight markers, for example, "You opened your eyes often, kept talking in the past tense," and invite them to reason about what happened. The goal is to find out how imagery activates negative schemas and how patients construct the therapist.

A relational rupture is almost always present in these cases. If, for example, a woman with borderline PD says: "I'm afraid that if I go on, I won't be able to handle the emotions that come up but it's my problem," she has an emotion regulation problem, sure. But in fact, faced with an emotional difficulty, she does not think the therapist can help her. She implicitly configures the latter as absent, distant, and unable to help. A negative interpersonal schema is thus active in the therapeutic relationship. At this point, therapists need to work to repair the rupture before moving on with the technique.

10. The search for the core negative belief: The heart of therapy

Personality disorders revolve around core ideas about oneself that are believed to be true. Bringing patients to realize how true they believe these ideas to be and to detach from them is the cornerstone of psychotherapy. Many therapists forget to ask the central question, and as a result, therapy is ineffective, and alliance ruptures appear. When we bring patients to narrate an episode and then relive it experientially – in this case, in imagery – a patient like the 25-year-old Jade, suffering from dependent PD, is able to tell us "My boyfriend told me he didn't give a damn that I was sick and locked himself in his room. I felt lonely, abandoned, shitty." Jade's therapist is convinced he has the necessary material to move toward change and that Jade knows that the core idea underlying her attachment wish is *lonely and abandoned*. This is not the case, as it almost never is. Patients' minds remain in the "The other makes me . . ." mode: "When my boyfriend treats me like this, I feel lonely." As a result, they are not predisposed to changing internal structures. They are outwardly oriented: "If he treats me differently, I will feel less lonely. How can I make him treat me better?"

How do we overcome this problem? Remember that the experiential attitude to psychotherapy remains consistent with transparent cognitive inquiry! We simply investigate cognitions during experiential exercises. We have brought patients, like Jade in this case, to the moment where the other has stopped responding to messages and so she feels lonely and abandoned. Now, we investigate the cognitions about the self with direct questions (Chapter 9). The therapist asked Jade during imagery to step outside herself and become an observer: "Look at yourself and tell me what you think of Jade, who is now alone in the room after her boyfriend has just locked himself in his room?"

What happens if the therapist neglects this step? The rewriting gets stuck, and often the alliance is broken, unless Jade becomes able to answer: "I think she deserves it, she is whiny, insufferable." So the therapist can ask if she realizes the problem is not her boyfriend's reaction, but the idea she has about herself. Once patients like Jade agree the therapy target is the negative core idea and not the others' reactions, the time is ripe for promoting change through imagery or other experiential techniques.

Scarlett is 28 years old; she works as a social media manager and is a very beautiful woman. She is treated by one of our colleagues, who tells the supervisor about the case. Scarlett suffers from borderline PD with histrionic and narcissistic traits and is depressed. She knows that the trigger for her depression is relational and asks for help because she fears rejection and abandonment. She cyclically finds herself in situations where she needs to receive constant appreciation, and when it does not come, she imagines her boyfriend will leave her because he does not value her much.

When she sees the impending abandonment, she reacts either by trying to please and submit, by seducing, or by getting angry if she considers the abandonment unfair. She has verbally and physically assaulted her exes – she hit one with her car, with no consequences, luckily –. At other times, she throws herself desperately at her partner's feet, holding him and begging him not to leave.

In other relationships, she uses the same attention-seeking mechanisms: physical appearance, clothing, and seductive gestures to attract, place herself as the center of attention, and counter the creeping idea of being unappreciated. She is frequently driven by social rank: at work, she is a perfectionist, and sexually, she competes with other women, something she will realize only later in therapy. When she sees a man looking at her with interest, for a moment, she feels fluttered and pleased: "If he realizes I'm hot, he can't leave me!" However, the positive image is unstable and context-dependent.

Seductiveness has caused her problems: she once found herself in an isolated parking lot with a friend with whom only in retrospect did she realize she had flirted. The boy did not harass her, but Scarlett was afraid. She also tended to unknowingly flirt with her friends' boyfriends and lost a longstanding friend for this reason.

The therapist and Scarlett jointly reconstruct her functioning. The therapist begins with a structured summary of events. Here, she makes a first mistake: she does not explore what it means for Scarlett to be abandoned. What does she fear? Remember that the therapist, consistent with the basic assumptions of all cognitive therapies, must always investigate the feared scenarios. The correct question would have been: "If you are abandoned, what do you fear? What is so terrible about it?" Instead, the intervention was as follows:

T: "We have seen that, in the episodes that made you suffer, there is a pattern that repeats itself. You stand in front of the other and feel the desire to be appreciated, which is ok, it is human! A moment later, however, you are afraid to see the other as critical and dismissive. At that point, you believe you are worthless, 'He doesn't appreciate me because I suck'. You are convinced that precisely because you are worthless, the other will abandon you. To avoid finding yourself experiencing this, on the one hand, you continuously strive to be perfect and flawless, and on the other hand you become seductive, more or less consciously: 'If I'm beautiful and I attract him, how could he reject me and leave?"

Scarlett recognizes herself in the description, and the therapist asks her for associated memories. After collecting them, she makes a second mistake. When Scarlett notices that there are indeed regularities that connect remote and recent episodes, the therapist becomes convinced that she has realized she is driven by a schema. Instead, Scarlett has only become more aware of her own functioning.

What happens is that Scarlett recalls a memory in which her father criticized her. The therapist proposes that she process the episode in guided imagery, still convinced that Scarlett knows she is working to change a schema. In the first part, Scarlett relives the scene: she is 6 years old, in the company of her father, whom she adores. She shows him her drawing, wishing very much that he would say 'good girl'. Instead, her father, with a stern expression, grabs the drawing and, without even looking at her face, tells her: 'Forget it, you can't draw, this really sucks'. Scarlett is ashamed before her father's scornful eyes; she thinks she is worthless. The father turns his back on her and leaves the room, leaving her alone and sad.

Emotions are intense; conditions for rescripting seem to be present. The therapist suggests responding consistently with the wish to be appreciated. Scarlett tries.

S: "Daddy, you're hurting me like this. I'm a child, I need you to appreciate me [*suddenly opens her eyes and bursts into angry, helpless crying, and then speaks to the therapist*]. It's useless! I can't do anything to change that look; he has never appreciated me, and he never will."

T: "What's going on, Scarlett?"

S: "Should I try telling my father: say I'm good? Then what? He'd answer I'm fucking useless, as usual. What's the point in making me feel like crap again?"

T: "I'm sorry, Scarlett. Can you help me understand what's going on with you? Does feeling lousy mean you think you're worthless? Are you sad, angry? Even toward me, maybe?"

S: "Yes, angry at you as well."

A pattern 2 technique-relationship interaction emerges here: the imagery generates negative emotions that provoke a rupture.

T: "All right. How did I upset you? How do you see me now?"

S: "You seemed annoyed because I couldn't do the exercise."

T: "Which makes you think that . . .?"

S: "That I am a moron!"

T: "In my eyes?"
S: "Mine as well."

At this moment, Scarlett constructs the therapist in a schema-dependent way. The therapist moves on to repair the rupture until Scarlett realizes that the former was not criticizing her and was not disappointed; on the contrary, she was sorry and concerned that the therapy was hurting her. For a brief moment, Scarlett differentiates, not through the exercise but through working on the therapeutic relationship (Dimaggio et al., 2015): first, she applies the schema to the therapist and then, through repair, she realizes that her idea was not true, that the therapist was not really criticizing her.

But why does the imagery not work? Part of the answer is that Scarlett reads the therapist in a schema-dependent way. The other part is caused by a technical mistake. The therapist does not explore in detail the core self-image surfacing in Scarlett after the other's feared response. Then, the therapist does not investigate the feared scenarios by asking: "What happens to you if the other leaves? You are left alone and . . .?" Nor does she include the healthy part in the structured summary of the episodes. In fact, she should say:

At some moments, you manage to think that you're worth something, regardless of whether the other's look acknowledges it or not, but then, as soon as you think the other does not give you attention or notice signs of criticism or disinterest.

Again, the therapist does not ask the patient for feedback after expounding the summary of the structure underlying the episodes. She takes for granted that Scarlett understands she is schema-driven without explicitly asking if that is the case.

Finally, and this is the most important mistake, she does not already ask questions about core self-cognitions when expounding the structured summary of the stories with boyfriends, and even more so when inquiring about the episode with Scarlett's father. The correct intervention would be: "Okay, Scarlett, now that your father has treated you like this, you are suffering, but look at yourself from the outside, look at little Scarlett: what do you think of that little girl?" At this point, Scarlett could respond "That she is stupid," and an opening would open up for her to point out how the pain arises from a core belief about herself and not from how real others treat her.

Because of these mistakes, Scarlett enters imagery with the implicit expectation that her purpose is to convince her 'real' father that she is not stupid. The therapist wants to help Scarlett contact, when under stress, an alternative benevolent self-image and support her even in the face of criticism. But the aim is only in her mind.

When done correctly, experiential techniques are a powerful tool for getting an answer to the crucial question: "Yes, okay, the other person made you suffer. But what are you thinking about yourself right now?" Let's show what happens when therapists correctly follow the procedures.

We go back to Jade and see what the therapist asks her about the moment the boy locked himself in the room.

T: "Close your eyes and go back to the moment when you are alone on the couch. Your boyfriend has just closed the door . . . Observe yourself; look at yourself when you call him and silence is the only answer. Observe Jade alone and forlorn. Look at her from the outside, and tell me, what do you think of that Jade? Okay, the boyfriend told her that he doesn't care that she is sick. But in your own eyes, who is that Jade?"

J: "I don't know, she feels bad."

T: "The boy walked away and left her alone. But what do you think? That the boy is right that Jade deserves abandonment?"

J: "Yes, she deserves it. It's her destiny."

A core self-image has emerged. There is a real trigger, but it is Jade who harbors a negative idea of herself. That idea will be the target of therapy. Once finished with the imagery, the therapist summarizes.

T: "Very good Jade, so do we agree that this is our real problem? Your boyfriend is distant and this, understandably, gives you pain. But the problem is that you think of yourself as unlovable and lonely, and you believe it to be true. Can we agree that the goal of therapy is to make this idea less true, to bring you into contact with a Jade that you see as lovable, deserving?"

In this way, patients make the step that transforms therapy: understanding that the heart of suffering does not arise from "I am unloved, criticized, hindered, threatened," thoughts that are only the source of contingent pain. Structural pain arises from ideas such as "I believe myself unlovable, inferior, crippled, vulnerable." Once such ideas have emerged, and patients know that these are ideas and not necessarily what others think of them, work is done to differentiate and access alternative images of self.

11.   *During imagery (and other experiential techniques), arousal must rise*

To rewrite a pattern, it is necessary to reactivate it. The principles of behavioral therapies have already argued this (Wolpe, 1973): to extinguish a behavior, the associated emotions must be evoked. In recent years, memory reconsolidation theory has clarified this (Nader & Einarsson, 2010; Solms, 2021; see Chapter 1). When memory is reactivated, laden with emotions that make it seem "true," it enters a phase of instability. If one works to modify the narrative at this time, at the end of the work the mind stores a modified version. It becomes a new memory that functions as an updated world map. So, if we want to rewrite the way patients see their relational world, arousal must rise. If it does not, therapists can use one of the following strategies: a) activating interventions, for example, they give voice to the 'negative others' almost as if they shared their ideas, addressing patients with "You let me down"; "Because of you I am alone and desperate" and so on, and observing whether emotions emerge; b) push patients toward behaviors that interrupt coping. This is a rescripting operation that we describe later. Here we only show its activating power: "Your father was offended because you talked back to him. Try not going to him to make peace"; c) if the emotions still do not get activated, therapists stop any intervention and monitor the therapeutic relationship: if the relationship is good, they revise the purposes of imagery because it is likely that patients are performing it guided by schemas active at that moment that therapists did not notice.

12.   The forms of rescripting: promoting the wish

Once the scene has led to reading emotions, cognitions, and action tendencies or adopting coping, it is time for rewriting. This has two goals, usually simultaneously: 1) moving toward the primary wish by anchoring in the healthy parts and 2) abandoning coping. In both cases, we promote differentiation and access to healthy parts.

How is this rewriting differentiation? When the patient tries to act differently, it means that he is giving a chance to the possibility that his positive representations are true, become embodied, and have power. Put more simply with an example: the patient, before imagery, knows that he is guided by the idea that if he explores the world independently, his mother will suffer and criticize him, and consequently, he sees himself as bad and guilty. He realizes that it is his way of thinking and that he is not really bad or guilty, but in reality, he is immobile. The moment when, during imagery, we ask him to say goodbye to his mother and leave, and he tries, he is, in fact, differentiating! He is acting as if the pattern is no longer true, and an alternative reality becomes possible and takes control of the mind and body.

In some cases, we ask a patient to act according to the wish; disrupting coping will be an indispensable step but not the primary goal. In others, the figure-background relationship is reversed; the primary goal is to stop coping, and moving toward the wish is a beneficial but secondary effect. The following is an example of a rewriting aimed at sustaining the wish and, as is always the case, in pursuing it, the patient has to give up coping.

In Chapter 4, we described Daniel, a 40-year-old painter and architect. He has entered treatment for alcohol and substance dependence along with narcissistic and borderline PD. We have had initial difficulties, which were soon overcome, in formulating the contract. After a year and a half of therapy and several relapses, the addiction regresses to the point that it is no longer a problem. Daniel, however, is exhausted from overwork. He is successful, receives important architectural commissions, and his paintings are appreciated. He has difficulty saying no, but his days have an unsustainable pace. Together with the therapist, he has realized that for him to say "no" means exposing himself to the idea of being a "total loser." This is backed up by family memories in which his mother was anxious and afraid that he would fail at anything and in which his father distrusted his qualities. A closeted teenager, he has memories of exclusion from the group: boys teased him, and girls ignored him. Over the years, he has overcome them, has had many romantic relationships, and is fully integrated into groups, but he still harbors the idea that it is all due to his professional success: "If I quit for a moment, they'll think I'm nothing, and it takes me a moment to get back to where I was." This is narcissistic coping, in an obvious way, and the price Daniel pays is his inability to relax and, often, to choose only in line with his preferences and not with the coping wish of being liked, and considered top (Dimaggio, 2022). The therapist points out that his pace of work is unsustainable, or rather, he can maintain it but pay the price of fatigue and the sense of alienation that pervades him. Daniel realizes that the therapist's words make sense. He knows that he should refuse assignments, but the price for him is very high.

D: [*Laughing and feeling ashamed at the same time*]: "Doctor, it's terrible what you're asking me! You're telling me that I should feel like a loser!"
T: [*Smiling*]: "I admit it, yes! Of course, you can also spend the rest of your life killing yourself with work, be wildly successful, and then kill yourself with work . . ."
D: [*Smiling*]: "But this is not therapy; this is torture!"
T: "Actually, when you say it like that, I think you're right."
D: "OKAY, SO WHAT DO I HAVE TO DO? I ARRIVE THERE NAIVELY AND SAY: 'SORRY, I'VE PRESENTED THIS GREAT PROJECT WITH MY COLLEAGUES; HOWEVER, DO YOU KNOW WHAT'S NEW? YOU GUYS CLING TO HEAVEN KNOWS WHAT AND I'M PULLING OUT; THEY'RE DOING IT."
T: "No, no, it's okay if therapy is a torture – but in moderation. It would be too much today! What we need is for you to have the experience of saying no and facing disappointed responses."

This is a typical dialogue in therapy with patients with narcissistic PD and a good alliance; the tones are ironic and playful. Daniel agrees and asks what exercise the therapist is thinking about. They draw up a guided imagery together. Daniel focuses on the moment he accepts the assignment. They pinpoint the desire he felt at that time. He wanted to travel to Scotland to visit his friends Luke and Patty, who live on the edge of a hilly forest. It was going to be a nature vacation, and he really cared about it. He had to cancel it because of the deadlines piling up.

There are two steps to imagery. In the first, the therapist takes Daniel back to the moment when he is talking on the phone with his friend. A sense of brotherhood emerges; Luke has good memories even during difficult times, and when he is with him and his wife, Daniel always experiences a sense of belonging. They are almost a kind of foster family compared to the distressed, controlling, and pessimistic family he comes from. Daniel now has a forward-looking, open face and feels a sense of warmth.

The second step is to stand in front of his colleagues, who have asked him to be the frontman of a project, and say no. The goal is to pursue the wishes of autonomy/exploration, feeling the pleasure of the nature in which he is going to immerse himself and belonging to the group. The scene shifts to the office: they are all standing around the meeting room table. In imagery, at the moment of saying, "Guys, I'd rather not," Daniel's face twitches. He moves back and forth, gesticulates, bends his shoulders, and rotates his neck as if trying to loosen his muscle contractions.

D: "It is too difficult."
T: "What makes it difficult?"
D: "It is not done."
T: "Try telling your friends. You don't because now I say it and they . . .?"
D: "They think I'm worthless."
T: "A loser?"
D: "Oh, how awful!"
T: "Do you think so yourself?"
D: "Sure."
T: "Good. Now go back to the times when you felt fine with Luke and Patty . . ."

Daniel returns to those moments and experiences the positive feelings again. The therapist asks him to visualize moments when he has been before in that house and the woods around it. Daniel recovers the feelings of warmth, beauty, and surprise at seeing the animals around the house in the morning.

T: "Keep these feelings and come back around the table. Now, try to tell your colleagues that you will not take the lead on the project."
D: "Guys, I know you'll be pissed off, and you're right too. But I just can't do it. I've had enough, I need to go to see Luke and Patty."
T: "How are they responding?"
D: "They object . . ."
T: "And what expression do they have?"
D: "Hm . . . not worried, more . . . he's sorry."
T: "Are there any signs that they are thinking: 'See this poor loser'?"
D: "No, no, it's just that it's a challenging project . . . They really need me."
T: "How do you feel now?"
D: "A little bit guilty . . ."

This emotion has already surfaced, particularly when Daniel dealt with a moment in his father's depression: then he said he would enroll in a college in London, far from his hometown. The therapist works to regulate his guilt and let him return to being driven by wishes to explore and to belong. Eventually, Daniel is able to freely express his wishes.

D: "Guys, I swear I'll help you. Really, but I just can't sign it, it's too much; I can't take do it. If I don't leave, in a little while, forget about projects . . . I'll fall on the ground, dead! And what you'll draw is my silhouette! With chalk. On behalf of the police!"

T: "How do you feel about saying that?"

D: "I tremble."

T: "Observe your colleagues; how are they reacting? Is there any face that strikes you?"

D: "There is Gennaro spreading his arms wide."

T: "And it means that . . .?"

D: "If you have to do it, Daniel, do it."

T: "And how do you feel?"

D: "A bastard . . . Wait, no, a little better."

T: "Still guilty?"

D: "Less than before."

T: "Try saying out loud, 'I feel bad. I feel sorry for my colleagues. I care about them. But I need this trip, it's important to me.'"

The therapist invites him to repeat this several times. Daniel gradually says it with more conviction and confidence, and he notices that the sorrow in his colleagues' faces no longer makes him relent. His guilt fades and gives way to a desire to travel.

T: "Say it out loud, 'I feel like leaving,' say it in your own words."

D: "I want to leave. I want to have dinner with Luke and Patty and joke with them. I want to wake up and see the hares outside the window and walk in the woods."

Daniel now has full contact with his wishes for exploration and group inclusion. Guided imagery has enabled him to sustain them and, in parallel, not to give in to copings generated by negative self-images. We note one element: Daniel entered imagery with the idea that if he takes time for himself, the other will judge him, and he sees himself as a 'loser'. In the course of the experience, however, the dominant other's image was *downcast, sad*. Noticing this, the therapist leads him to explore developmental memories again. The importance of his father's depression emerges, and how Daniel, despite always reacting with anger and defiance, harbored a sense of pity and guilt, as if making his father happy was his responsibility.

13.   The forms of rescripting: interrupting coping

What happens, however, when patients are paralyzed by either behavioral or IRT coping? These are stubborn mechanisms, supported by positive meta-cognitions such as "I must behave that way or else I will suffer," or negative ones such as "I am impulsive, I am unable to resist from acting that way," "I can't decide what to think." In these cases, rescripting focuses on interrupting coping. What, then, does differentiation consist of? Mainly in moving from "I respond automatically and passively, and it is a fact" to "I have agency over my mental state and behavior." Let us illustrate these operations through an example.

Thomas, 28, suffers from narcissistic PD. When not working, he is motionless, dull; there is no inner drive moving him. He shields himself from emptiness by filling himself with commitments. Sometimes, however, it is impossible, for example, during Christmas or summer vacation. Then he becomes apathetic and abulic and begins an unapologetic internal dialogue: "You're a joke, inept, a clown." He foresees catastrophes and worries: "I'll get everything wrong, I'll never find a place in life." The only active desire that brings him out of the state of emptiness is looking for girls on dating apps. He fantasizes about a special one: if he finds her, his pains will vanish.

Thanks to a dating app, he meets Julia: she seems the embodiment of the woman he dreams of. He dates her a couple of times, they have sex, and he idealizes her even more. He wants to be sure Julia will be his forever, pushes on the accelerator, and suggests they stick together. They have only known each other for a very short time; she refuses, and Thomas suffers. Passivity and devitalization resurface.

The therapist first reconstructs the time sequence of events: first comes boredom, and then the core undeserving self-image is activated. Now coping begins: first worry ("I'll fail at everything") and rumination ("I made a mistake that time . . . I should have instead . . ."), which accentuate the emptiness and make him anxious and then depressed. The solution he adopts crystallizes the problems: he switches to desire thinking to retrieve the grandiose, typically narcissistic self-image. This is where behavioral coping starts: he searches for partners on dating apps, and when he has found "the one," the perfect woman, he becomes dependent, as frequently happens in many PDs, narcissism included. Driven by dependence, he becomes impulsive.

Through this reconstruction, Thomas understands that this is his typical way of functioning and that Julia is not the solution to his problems. He understands that he needs to regulate emptiness without resorting to coping. The therapist and patient plan how to cope adaptively with this state. It is necessary to start with an attempt to refrain from coping, both the behavioral type, that is, compulsive seduction and avoiding making appointments, and IRT. Thomas knows that the moment he does not look for a girl, he will feel empty, and then he will probably start worrying about a catastrophic future.

He manages to refrain from behavioral coping and, as expected, feels useless and worries, a process he cannot interrupt. In the next session, the therapist takes him into imagery to return to a moment of emptiness and find out how to get out of it without worrying. Before imagery, she asks him to recall a memory where he is active, vital, and confident in his abilities. Thomas succeeds, notices the positive feelings, and keeps them in mind for a while. At this point, they select a moment of emptiness from the previous week, and imagery begins.

Thomas is on the couch, turned off, and doesn't even feel like watching his favorite series on TV. He opens the dating app, goes from one profile to another, and is almost obsessed. He has no sexual desire, yet he can neither turn off his phone nor close the app. He refrains, however, from sending a message to a girl with whom he has a match. The emptiness rises, and the worried brooding begins. The therapist asks him to recall the healthy part and to assume the posture and facial expression of the *effective Thomas*, as they call him. Then she invites him to voice the qualities he perceives at that moment, and he says, "I am solid, reflective. I don't react. I can find solutions without haste. I have control over myself." His body is consistent with his words: his legs are firmly planted on the ground, shoulders and chest are open, and breathing flows calmly. In imagery, Thomas refrains from shifting from scrolling and especially does not worry. The therapist asks him to do something concrete and useful now. Thomas decides to set up his desk and make tea.

Having completed the exercise, Thomas is motivated to try to react to emptiness once home but without resorting to dating apps. He knows that worry will be more difficult to counteract, which will be the target of the coming sessions.

Thomas has now achieved two types of differentiation. The first is the awareness that, at certain times, he has positive self-images, in alternative to schema-dependent ones. The second concerns agency beliefs about his own behavior. He went into imagery thinking: "I have no power over my behavior and thinking when I start to worry." After the exercise, he discovers that

> There are different Thomases. I know that at certain times, I think I am good; it's just that I forget! When I get into a state of passivity, it's not true that the only thing I can do is try nonsense dating. I have the power to get out of it, to become active and vital again. Giving up tormenting myself about the future is more difficult, but I want to work at it.

Therapists are pleased when patients make these steps. They are bewildered when, a few seconds later, or in the next session, they return to reading the world through the maladaptive schema lens: "But he did improve! What happened, where did I go wrong?" This continuous returning to schemas is, instead, physiological, and has to be approached calmly by relying on procedures.

Schemas take back control: promoting differentiation and access to healthy parts again!

We repeat that this chapter contains the keystone of psychotherapeutic change: recognizing schemas as such, taking away their power, and making room for alternative, benevolent views of self and others. This is not easy, especially since schemas are embodied structures built and established over a lifetime. They tend, therefore, to take back control even when new structures have emerged. Consequently, change is by nature unstable.

If clinicians expect differentiation and access to newly achieved healthy parts to be consolidated, they make a naïve mistake. They should instead assume that schemas will regain power. How should they act, based on this knowledge? Not only do they watch schemas get back in the saddle, but they themselves give them power and control! With an instrumental purpose, by the way.

Schemas can take back control: a) after the session, often because of relational triggers; b) suddenly, in session, and in the form most unexpected by therapists, which causes most technical errors; c) as a result of intentional action by therapists; we will show how to let schemas take the lead during experiential techniques.

As regards the first eventuality, the pattern is often reactivated after a session in which it has been overcome. New relational events – obstacles, accusations, criticism, aggression, and abandonment – are typical triggers. In response, patients lose the awareness achieved and suffer on two levels. The first is normal, human, and reality-based. The second is schema-dependent: "He rejected me, and he is right, because I am not lovable." One must, in these cases, simply take a few steps back in the decision-making procedures and work knowing that, at that moment, the patient does not differentiate.

Often, however, the mental state shift occurs in session, automatically. Patients have entered the new world and have tasted it, but this means exposing themselves further to the negative consequences from which they previously protected themselves with coping. So they suddenly go back to reading themselves in schema-dependent ways or activating various forms of IRT: "What if I make a mistake? Then what if the other person leaves me? What do I do? But on the other hand, I can't keep submitting. Yes, and then who helps me when I'm alone?"

What do therapists do when patients, even seconds after differentiating and contacting healthy parts, go back to reading the world through the lens of schemas and, at that point, return to repetitive thinking? We illustrate the next step in the procedures by continuing with the example of Thomas's therapy.

Thomas benefited from guided imagery in which he activated a healthy part characterized by vitality, reflexivity, agency, and good self-regulation. He was able to stop being seductive but not worrying. The working alliance at that moment was solid, and the case formulation was shared. So, in the next session, the therapist puts him through a kind of "stress test," explaining the rationale: to evoke states of boredom and monitor the internal world. Thomas is curious and determined to reduce worrying.

The therapist asks him to close his eyes and focus on his stream of consciousness, with the aim of observing when desire thinking starts and how his mind reacts from that moment on. She then invites him to pay attention to various parts of his body and intersperses her instructions with prolonged silences. From time to time, she asks him, "Thomas, where is your mind now?" Thomas regularly finds himself rambling on about desirable scenarios, girls to contact, friends to see, and himself walking the streets of London or scuba diving in the Red Sea.

T: "Well, now try to let go of these beautiful, desirable scenarios. You go home, you're there, alone. What are you thinking? How do you see yourself right now? What is your self-image? What body signals do you notice? What emotions do you feel?"

THOMAS: "Hollowness in the pit of my stomach. My upper body is heavy . . . weak . . . my head . . . you know, when you get sleepy on a train and fall forward? My feet feel nervous . . ."

The therapist suggests that he should indulge the tendency to bow his head. Thomas bends it forward. Emptiness at the entrance to his stomach and a tendency to tap his feet increase. He struggles to remain in this state without opening his eyes and stopping the exercise. He scratches and rotates his neck.

T: "Conjure up the calm and effective Thomas. Can you?"
THOMAS: "Yes . . ."
T: "Try and wear that posture and facial expression as if you were wearing that vital Thomas."
THOMAS: "Yes, I am."
T: "How are you now?"
THOMAS: "I'm breathing better. My foot has stopped [*stopped tapping*]. I feel alive, alive again . . ."
T: "Good, you did it easily. Would you like to go back to bringing attention to your body and see if the calmness is lingering? Or has the calmness disappeared and you've turned yourself off again? Let me know when you notice that something is changing."

After a while, Thomas feels concerned but identifies the moment when worrying starts. The therapist invites him to impersonate the *effective Thomas* again.

THOMAS: "I feel my head falling again, but less. Above all, there is no more agitation . . . I don't like it, but it doesn't scare me anymore. Maybe I don't even need to become effective. In the end, it's just a tinge of boredom. There, as I say it, I'm breathing better."
T: "Do you want to give voice to this state? Like: I,   Thomas,   now that I'm like this . . . I'm . . .?"
THOMAS: "Hm . . . I can be on my own. Emptiness doesn't scare me."
T: "How does it feel saying it?"
THOMAS: "True, it calms me down. I don't need to raise hell, don't need to run away."

Once the exercise is finished, Thomas adds, "I realized something. I get bored, I feel empty, and of course, it happens, that's normal. But if I notice it as soon as it starts, I can deflate my negative thoughts."

When the therapist asks him how he felt her presence and their relationship during and after the exercise, Thomas replies that it was important to feel her confidence even when he was experiencing some difficulties. Now he is surprised at the power of the exercise, which makes him even more optimistic about the usefulness of therapy. Pattern 4 was thus triggered first: thanks to the technique, the patient already felt the therapist to be solid while carrying it out. Then pattern 5: the beneficial effects of experiential work strengthened the relationship.

It is helpful for therapists to voluntarily reactivate schemas during experiential work, even several times. When patients have successfully rescripted an episode, therapists intervene by embodying the negative characters and encouraging a return to schema-dependent reading. The painful emotions resurface.

The purpose is to train patients to resist the schema at increasing levels of intensity. It is an exercise that will help patients resist when schema-driven thoughts, feelings, and actions resurge in everyday life and consolidate the capacity to free themselves from schemas through behavioral experiments. If therapists did not increase the level of exposure, it would be difficult for patients to resist the schemas when necessary; that is, when they are under the pressure of the many forms in which reality manifests its harshness.

This is not easy for many therapists, as they must go against their tendencies to embody the position of the helper, the savior, and the wise. We have instead to play the villain for some moments and be credible while we say nasty words to our patients. We need to be in full control of our own emotions and ideas to remain in the role as long as necessary, which means until negative arousal mounts again. Once patients experience schema-related thoughts and emotions again, we suddenly turn back to our helper/supporter position and invite them to retort, react, and embody the vital, healthy, strong, free self they achieved a few seconds before. But this time they have learned they are capable of being in control even under pressure. They are now ready to face the challenges of everyday life.

Embracing coping as a form of differentiation

We assume that we have correctly formulated the case. Patients agree on the formulation. We have also investigated negative core cognitions; the patients have identified them and acknowledged these are ideas, not necessarily true. Everything looks okay; the conditions for rescripting during imagery or through any other experiential work are set. Yet, patients do not move a step. A therapist's insistence is, as always, counterproductive; it would only trigger maladaptive interpersonal cycles.

At these moments, it is almost a must to return to negotiating the therapeutic contract. We tell patients it is not a problem for us if they give up exposure, exploration, reducing perfectionism, abstaining from binge eating, compulsive caregiving so as not to feel guilty, and so on. We simply need to redefine therapy goals.

Even in these difficult situations, experiential techniques offer an opportunity for differentiation that promotes progress, makes contract renegotiation easier, and reduces the risk of relational ruptures.

What kind of differentiation are we promoting here? It is a matter of moving from an idea such as "Bad things happen, others treat me a certain way, and I can't do anything about it," to "I have the power to behave differently, but I decide not to act." Beliefs about agency change from "I thought I had no power" to "I know I have power, but I decide not to use it"; from "I act because I can't do anything else" to "I decide to act this way because I don't want to expose myself to the negative image of myself and to the resulting emotions."

Simultaneously, patients move from "Therapy is not helping me, and the therapist is doing something wrong" to "I am making a conscious decision to stay within a safe zone, knowing that this will not help me solve my problems."

How do we promote this transition experientially, in this case through imagery? We bring patients into the scene and ask them, metaphorically, to "embrace coping." That is, we invite them to say out loud that they are consciously, intentionally, deliberately choosing to act or not to act in a particular way. By enhancing the sense of intentionality, of deliberate choice, the patient will thus not be in a position to protest that therapy is useless!

This is an extremely difficult step, especially emotionally. Indeed, therapists have to deal with patients who decide not to take steps that appear reasonable, necessary, and healthy. At times the problem is that therapists moralistically blame patients for their coping behaviors, especially when they cause emotional harm to others. Supervision is therefore often necessary to accomplish this step. It requires adopting the position of *leaning forward helplessness* (Chapter 3) and, to reach it, therapists need to pass through their own inner dark places.

We see this in the therapy of Amanda, a 37-year-old vice principal of a prestigious high school. She has two daughters, ages 5 and 3. She sought therapy for depression, supported by what appeared to be dependent PD. She has difficulty making her own choices and systematically tries to please her mother and husband. Both are dysfunctional relationships: her mother is tyrannical and intrusive, while her husband lives out of town most of the time, is distant, dismissive, and spiteful, and blatantly cheats on her. Yet Amanda is not detached from either of them and has become dull and devitalized; nothing turns her on.

She believes herself to be a good mother, but it is evident from her narratives that she neither spends time with her daughters, entrusted to a full-time nanny, nor gives them any emotional attention. The main diagnosis becomes clear: covert narcissism. Amanda, in fact, derives economic and practical benefits from depending on her mother and husband and considers them vested rights. Her main motivation is status. The therapist is at the beginning of her MIT training and has difficulties. Amanda is depressed but does not agree to take any steps to get better; the therapist therefore feels frustrated and inadequate. She also judges Amanda morally: she herself recently had a child, and seeing Amanda so disinterested in her daughters makes her angry. Thanks to supervision, the therapist realizes that Amanda reminds her of her own mother, who was incapable and "childish" and neglected her. The therapist realizes that it is like coming to terms again with the sense of abandonment she experienced in childhood. In her eyes, Amanda, at certain times, is not a patient to be treated but a mother to protest with.

Once this became clear, the therapist and her supervisor agree on *deliberate practice* exercises (Chapter 3). Immediately before the next sessions, the therapist evokes images in which her mother neglected her, lets the arousal surface, and then enters an internal dialogue in which she says to her inner child: "You weren't neglected because of your flaws. Mom was like that, so weak. You felt lonely, and it was normal, but you didn't deserve to be left alone, you are lovable." Through this work, the therapist enters the following sessions in a well-regulated state.

Technically speaking, the formulation is agreed. Amanda's core wishes are attachment and exploration: she desires both to have someone take care of her and to act guided by something of her own. She faces a distant, controlling, spiteful, and unreliable other. The initial reaction is shutdown, supported by core self-images such as *unlovable* and *powerless*. She understands that this is at the heart of her depression and passivity. The therapist carefully explores her core cognitions, and Amanda confirms that, yes, the other treats her with distance and contempt, hinders her autonomy (her mother), and betrays her (her husband), but she is the first to think: "I am unlovable" and "Left on my own, I am unable to do anything."

There seems to be what is needed to try and change, but Amanda remains immobile. She also protests that the therapy is not helping her. The therapist, together with the supervisor, manages to let the criticism slip away without reacting. Then, through supervision and deliberate practice, in a modulated emotional state, the therapist calmly returns to negotiating the contract. She repeats the formulation and explains to Amanda the importance of behavioral tasks to overcome ideas such as "helpless and deserving abandonment." Amanda stops protesting and seems to agree to implement autonomous behaviors, such as going out with friends while leaving her husband at home the few times he is there, and refusing some of her parents' dinner invitations. But in reality, she does not implement them and continues to be depressed, so the therapist again experiences frustration, which she can easily self-regulate now.

The therapist also realizes that Amanda quickly veers toward the social rank motive: she expects the other to care for her almost like a servant and to guarantee her the standards she is entitled to. As a result, she does not act independently because she would feel she was giving up receiving what she deserves. This part of the formulation is still not agreed. When the therapist points it out to her, Amanda does not reject it but is confused. The therapist asks her if she can evoke an episode in which she lost status. A key memory emerges. Amanda takes her eldest daughter to horseback riding, but the girl shows clear signs she dislikes it. She is also afraid, cries in despair, and vomits. Still, Amanda cannot let her daughter decide to stop riding. Amanda suffers from seeing her sick, but each week, she renews the agony. The therapist tries to agree on behavioral experiments, but nothing changes. Amanda takes the child riding, sees her suffer, and complains about the situation, but the next lesson she takes her again. A first reason emerges: "My mother has paid for everything; if I take her off the course, she will be offended." The episode is the latest in a series of scenes in which Amanda gives up her autonomy, self-love, and personal worth either to not make others criticize her or to keep them from suffering.

This is a difficult passage for the therapist; she is a young mother herself. Leaving schemas apart, Amanda's behavior is one of real neglect, and in her soul, the therapist criticizes her and gets angry: "How can she treat her daughters like that! I would feel so lousy!" Through further supervision, she realizes that following ethical principles would be useless; Amanda would not change her behavior and would only feel judged. She then agrees with the supervisor to conduct imagery to lead Amanda to embrace coping. The goal is for her to become aware that her behavior is not ordered by anyone; it is intentional, and she therefore needs to accept paying the consequences.

They agree to return to the moment when the daughter is riding, crying desperately and about to vomit. The rescripting apparently aims to get Amanda to care for her daughter. Warning: the purpose of this first step is only instrumental means to an end. It is, in fact, necessary for Amanda to try to act in a healthy way and fail. Only then does the real exercise begin: rescripting by embracing coping.

In imagery, Amanda, as expected, fails to tell her daughter that she can get off the horse. The therapist asks her to dwell on that moment and observe where she feels the pain in her body. Amanda does not recognize body signals; it is more of a thought, something in the head.

T: "Try saying: 'I'm sorry my daughter is sick, but it's more important for me to do what my mother wants. I am choosing to make my mother happy even if the consequence is painful for me and my daughter."

After several rehearsals, Amanda speaks her own words.

A: "For me it is essential that my mother is happy; I don't want to contradict her."

After finishing the imagery, Amanda is thoughtful. She feels guilty about her daughter but is aware that it is more important for her not to displease her mother, although it is not clear what consequences she fears. She agrees with the therapist that, on this basis, it does not make sense to ask her to soothe her sorrow for her daughter or to achieve other goals. Amanda now knows that most of her dependent behavior is her choice, not imposed by anyone.

In subsequent sessions, Amanda understands better why she enacts submissive coping behaviors and why: to protect herself from her feared scenarios.

A: "You see, my mother pays for everything, and my husband also provides me with a high standard of living, so I don't want to give that up. If I take my daughter away from horseback riding, my mother gets hurt, takes revenge and stops giving me money for a lot of other things . . . Then, for me, it's important my daughter goes horseback riding in that club. There are girls from all over high society, and if she stops going there, I feel left out. It's the same with my husband, I know he's cheating on me, but what can I do? Leave him?"

Amanda is now fully aware she is driven above all else by the social rank motive, narcissistically, and that paralysis and suffering – her own and her daughter's – are the price she chooses to pay.

A: "I live in a gilded cage, and I'm not sure I want to leave it."

The therapist is relieved. She felt responsible for the well-being of the patient and her daughters. Frustration and sorrow for Amanda's children remain, but she knows she cannot help her. She can adopt the position of *leaning forward helplessness* and asks Amanda what goals therapy can serve. Over the course of the next few months, the patient discovers that the gilded cage comes at an unbearable cost to her. She curbs her mother's intrusions and tells her husband she wants a divorce. She realizes that motherhood necessarily involves hard work and stops avoiding it: she spends more time with her daughters and discovers their emotions, sorrows, and preferences. Upon returning from summer vacation, she informs her mother that her daughter will no longer go horseback riding.

In rare cases, it is possible that after contract renegotiation or through experiential exercises aimed at embracing coping, patients realize that they have achieved realistic treatment goals, that the life they live is no longer imposed but chosen. They consequently decide to discontinue treatment. Aware of this, therapists can accept the decision more calmly.

The work on differentiation and access to healthy parts, of course, is not conducted through imagery alone. It can be accomplished through dialogue or with other experiential techniques (Dimaggio et al., 2015, 2020). Here we wanted to highlight three new aspects of MIT: 1) redefining the procedures, specifically the part about returning to the schema after initial progress, which deserves attention; 2) describing more precisely the steps to be followed to use the techniques, in this case guided imagery; and 3) describing the interaction between relationship and techniques.

The therapist can use the same conceptual scaffolding, but instead of imagery, engage the patient in role-play, chairwork, bodily exercises, attentional techniques, or combinations of these.

Having reached this point, patients have really begun to change. They manage to differentiate and make room in their inner world for healthy parts. They take steps backward – therapy is a bit like a Game of the Goose – but therapists intercept them, and immediately patients realize that these are just mechanisms that are trying to regain control. What is the next step?

Beginning to come to terms with reality. We will see this in the next chapter.

Chapter 11

Pursuing wishes by exploring the environment and interrupting avoidance

Counteracting tendencies to return to schemas after successful experiments

Here is the element of treatment focused on changing interpersonal structures. The time is ripe to face reality. Patients attempt to act guided by primary and adaptive wishes and healthy self-parts. We have seen they have already accessed these wishes and positive, benevolent self-images. Now therapy is about letting them flourish in the world. It is a transition that requires, on the one hand, a combination of confidence and risk-taking in seeking the new (Figure 11.1, Box 4) and, on the other hand, facing fears and abandoning the usual coping strategies (Figure 11.1, Box 5).

Patients' differentiation has improved; they know their internal world is populated with negative ideas about themselves and others, but they also know that these ideas were learned and generated in the past or, in any case, are not necessarily true. Above all, they come to recognize that they harbor more benevolent images, ideas, emotions, and somatic sensations to guide them while they hope their core wishes can be fulfilled. This is the time for patients to experiment, on the one hand, going in the direction of the wish (Figure 11.1, Box 4); and on the other hand, counteracting fears, avoidance, and any coping still being adopted (Figure 11.1, Box 5). These operations are usually intertwined. For clarity, we first illustrate them separately and then describe a case in which the therapist performs them together.

To follow new paths and discover new parts of themselves, patients need to have experiences and learn through repetition. Therapists have a very active role: supporting, spurring, inciting, and correcting. In this transition, the risk that patients find themselves wrapped in the web of their schemas again is high.

In reviewing decision-making procedures in this volume, we have designed an additional step (Figure 11.1, Box 6), born out of the realization that behavioral change is by no means linear. Often the mind falls prey again to the negative self-image, viewing the world of relationships anew from the initial, schema-dependent perspective.

The techniques help patients read the swings between positive and negative self-images, govern them, and reconnect with the healthy self. Despite the return of schemas to the cockpit, ruptures in the therapy relationship at this stage are less severe. Patients have reached this point because they know that their schemas do not necessarily correspond to reality, even if this awareness waxes and wanes. At the same time, the steps taken so far are a sign that the therapy relationship is solid.

DOI: 10.4324/9781003570967-11

Tackling avoided or feared relational situations **Box 4**	Exploring the environment and pursuing healthy wishes **Box 5**

Discovering how after behavioral homework the mind returns to read the world through the lenses of the schemas
Box 6

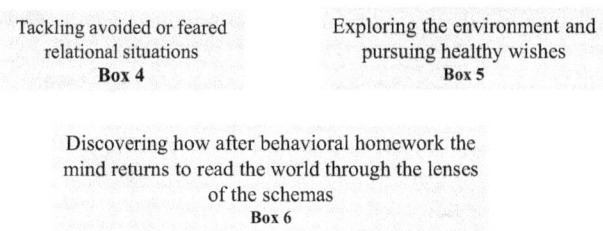

Figure 11.1 Acting to break maladaptive interpersonal schemas

However, precisely because of the mind's tendency to swing, at times when schemas command, between healthy and problematic aspects of self, relational ruptures occur. The reasons are two: the first is that patients may apply the schema, now reactivated, to the relationship and return to experiencing the therapists as dominant, devaluing, disinterested, and so on. Therapists are often bewildered by these ruptures: "What is happening? Until just now, everything was going well, the patient had made progress, and now she has taken steps backwards and views me negatively?"

The second reason is that therapists are anchored in the success they have just achieved and tend to consider patients fully recovered, and thus, as they would with a friend with whom they have an argument over dinner, to refute as being real the schema-dependent ideas that have resurfaced. As a result, patients feel misunderstood, devalued, dominated, and a new rupture is triggered.

These operations are not without difficulties. Patients may get stuck at the threshold of the new path because of fears: "What happens if I leave my partner? Will I remain alone forever?"; "What do I risk if I shun my tyrannical boss who undervalues me? If I send my cv around and only poor quality firms call me?"; "If I move out of my parents' home, will I be able to take care of myself?"; "I can try to talk to my friend and tell her that, even if she was offended, she shouldn't treat me that way. But what if she then insults me?"

When patients hesitate to take a new path, knowing that there will inevitably be emotional costs to be paid, reformulating the contract is essential. Even if the therapeutic relationship is good, we are preparing for transitions that will activate intense emotions. To get better or heal, patients have to give up forms of coping that shield them from negative ideas and emotions and try to fulfill their wishes while challenging their fears. They may not necessarily do this willingly, or with enthusiasm and gratitude toward the therapist!

Contract review involves bringing patients to weigh the costs and benefits of both actions and omissions and state their preference. Do they decide to act for their well-being because the price to be paid is worth it? Or do they consider that costs outweigh benefits, or is it simply too emotionally painful and so, at this moment, they do not want to pay them?

Note that it is not that an MIT therapist is not happy if patients act and disappointed if they remain motionless. Of course, every therapist will experience positive and negative emotions; this is natural. Patients moving toward health give us relief and satisfaction, while those standing still and maintaining their disorder evoke frustration, powerlessness, and other negative feelings. We are entitled to feel the whole spectrum of emotions. But to patients who choose not to act, we must learn to convey the state we have called *leaning forward helplessness*:

> I am willing to stay here and listen to you as long as you want; I am near you and listening to your pain, I embrace it. But we both know that if you do not commit yourself to acting in a new way, you are unlikely to get better. You have a new awareness, and that is a good thing. But if you have awareness and do not act on the basis of it, this will prevent you from achieving relief, well-being, and fulfillment. Really, I am here for you; I remain your therapist for as long as you want. We just need to know that mine will be just a human presence; it will give you transient relief, but I do not promise change and, even less so, healing.

We now describe an example of such a contract renegotiation.

Julius, a 54-year-old musician, suffers from overt narcissistic PD. He knows that the schemas driving him are related to the frustration of attachment. He harbors the idea that, when he is afraid, his fate is to be alone because no one will rescue him. In his narrative, those who neglect do so because of their own suffering, a pattern typical of those with pathological narcissism (Dimaggio, 2022; Dimaggio & Valentino, 2024): in their narrative, when they ask for help, they encounter a weak, sick other, and this leads them to believe they are bad and selfish. This evokes guilt and paralysis and, in Julius' case, frustrates attachment: *if I ask for care, someone suffers*. His mother has been in a wheelchair because of a car accident since he was a child. His father loves him but is tired by the situation and emotionally distant.

Julius has not been in a stable romantic relationship for years because he cannot emotionally separate himself from his sick ex-wife. He does not live with her, but he takes care of her. Abandoning her would make him feel guilty; his wife is grateful, and this keeps the bond alive. Sexuality is also frustrated: he has casual affairs with women whom he leaves when the relationship gets serious because he would risk falling in love. He would then have to consider leaving his wife, but he is afraid to choose a woman who might abandon him. Repetitive thinking worsens things: "I have lots of women, but in the end, I am alone. I would like to separate for good and have a relationship with a new partner, but if I do . . ." and he starts repetitive thinking again.

Julius now differentiates: when he needs care, he knows he deserves it, and at the same time, he can handle loneliness. He is guided by the idea of himself as *lovable and able to stand on my own feet*. At one point, he really falls in love and would like to have a real love story; fear of loneliness no longer disturbs him, and he likes the qualities of his potential partner. He remains guilty at the idea of leaving his wife, but he seems to want to overcome the guilt feeling. The therapist assesses that there are the conditions to help him act in line with his own wishes. Together they plan how to express his intentions to his ex-wife. They plan a behavioral experiment: Julius will refrain from the usual Sunday visit to his ex-wife and be with his new girlfriend, which he would love to do.

In the next session, he is elusive and, when asked by the therapist to talk about the experiment, laughs bitterly and sarcastically.

J: "Doctor, I didn't do it. As usual. What are you going to do? Are you going to cane me, then? I can understand if you want to end the therapy."

The therapist notes the rupture marker and explores with Julius what emotions are guiding him.

J: "I feel weak, I thought you'd say 'Then let's interrupt therapy,' and it would make me feel awful."
T: "You see, Julius, it is interesting that you imagined that I would abandon you."
J: "It's true, but I know you won't, I feel it . . . I just can't stand to leave my ex. Without me, she won't make it alone; I can't stand her being sick because of me. The guilt would eat me up . . . I still love her. I just can't."

What to do at this point? As we have repeatedly underscored, MIT therapists welcome patients' positions by validating their decisions but at the same time emphasize that patients are moving from automatic coping to a conscious decision. This is what guides Julius' therapist.

T: "Julius, I am with you. You are fully aware of what you are giving up. You are deciding not to give yourself a chance at romance. We know it has a cost, but it is a choice; no one is forcing you. And [*smiling*] rest assured that I am not going to end therapy because of that."
J: "Of course, you won't! I'm a coward, but where do you find another nice buffoon like me?"

What happens? Julius agreed to the behavioral experiment, but in attempting the task, he experienced negative affects that led him to give up. Schemas take control of the therapeutic relationship as well. This is pattern 2 of technique-relationship interaction: the very proposal of doing something active triggers a rupture.

At this point, the therapist works on repairing the relationship until the rupture is repaired. The next step is to renegotiate the contract: the goal is no longer to leave the wife and build a new relationship. Julius can certainly talk about his chaotic love situation, but as soon as he complains about indecision, the therapist immediately points out that he is just *worrying* since he has decided to maintain the status quo.

They agree, then, to approach guilt from a different perspective: reducing worries related to either guilt toward his wife: "I am having a good time while she is sick" or toward his lover: "I'm gonna make her suffer through my indecision." He knows that in both cases, worrying starts from the core idea *I am bad and selfish.* But here again, thanks to the work on interrupting IRT (Chapters 8, 9, and 13), he understands that it is not necessary to continually torment himself with useless chains of thoughts. He finally manages to say: "Doctor, I may be a polygamous buffoon, but at least I will ruminate less."

We now go into the specifics of the three steps (Figure 11.1, Boxes 4, 5, and 6) with examples where the techniques accelerate change consistently with any step in the procedures but trigger ruptures in the therapeutic relationship. We show how therapists deal with them.

Exploring the environment and pursuing healthy desires

Patients clearly see wishes that, until recently, they felt were unattainable because of their schemas. We help them recognize them, value them, and attempt to pursue them: ultimately deciding to apply for that job they always avoided for fear of failure, taking up a hobby that requires changes in routine, engaging in creative and leisure activities avoided for fear of judgment, shame, or guilt at the idea of being selfish. New goals surface: "I would like to invite that girl, I didn't so far because fear of rejection paralyzed me"; "I finally feel entitled to travel and study in another city without letting the idea of someone suffering because of me hold me back"; "I can play competitive sports without being crushed by the idea that only winning matters." It is about empowering patients to fulfill frustrated wishes and, in general, to reactivate the exploratory system. Therapy at these moments is creative, vital, and often fun, but full of pitfalls and relapses.

Patients need to be supported in discovering what they like, and therapeutic interventions become very active: during guided imagery, we ask patients to figure out a future scenario in which, for example, they finally play rock guitar or sail a sailboat. We can ask them to actually paint in session, bringing canvas and colors. If we have gone through the decision-making procedures correctly, patients have already contacted, and sustained, healthy self-parts and positive emotions.

What changes from the work on healthy parts, done preliminarily at the beginning of therapy? Now the focus is on concrete actions: it is time to move into the world. We invite patients to act concretely, taking initiatives that bring them closer to fulfilling their desires. Therapists work to empower agency, helping patients intercept desires and goals that they feel authentic and, most importantly, pursue them concretely.

Therapists' interventions are active and supportive, like a sports coach or mentor: they help build action plans and weigh advantages and disadvantages, and propose behavioral experiments to train patients in finally moving along the paths they have avoided because they saw them as full of risks and dangers. In session, therapists initiate role-plays or guided imagery to help patients communicate an intention to someone or to help them better visualize the details of desired scenarios.

The techniques here may consolidate results or allow exploration of why experiments are not working. Experiments often enhance confidence in oneself and in the therapist. It may happen, however, that they generate a micro-fracture: a frightened patient may refuse the exercise. Conversely, the experiment may consolidate the relationship: patients try a new course of action which makes them feel better, and they trust the therapist more.

Problems may surface: during these advanced steps, therapists have gone through painful memories with patients who are now actively involved in attempts at changing with confidence. The risk of being caught off-guard is high: therapists tend to enthusiastically push patients down new paths but risk overlooking signs of returning to old functioning. Schemas are embodied structures, and their procedural component is more change-resistant. They therefore lurk for long, ready to regain control. What happens when therapists insist on engaging in a behavioral experiment, neglecting the emergence of signs of fear?

Sara is a 27-year-old mathematician, suffering from covert narcissistic PD. She asks for help for anxiety that assails her on every working and social occasion; she fears being judged incapable and "strange." She considers herself inferior and others superior and judgmental. She desires to belong to groups but sees others as close to each other, sharing something she is left out from, which further fuels her self-image of being strange, defective, and marginalized.

Simultaneously, when she sees herself excluded, she gets angry because part of her believes that the exclusion is unfair. She describes others as snobs, becomes motivated by competitiveness, and on the one hand, sees herself as inferior, which makes her ashamed, but on the other hand, thinks she is morally superior and the others are shallow. In any case, she avoids relationships. The idea of being valid does not help her to act because, at that point, she paints herself as the *angry victim*, full of resentment, envy, and spitefulness toward others' moral flaws.

Her IRT revolves around worth. Before a meeting, she worries, when not avoiding, about the risk of being humiliated, while afterwards she ruminates about possible mistakes she has made and tries to reassure herself. Sara is also perfectionistic toward others (Hewitt et al., 2017): at work, she does not tolerate interruptions, phone calls, or being contradicted. This worsens interpersonal relationships and increases isolation.

Through therapy, Sara recalls memories in which she considered herself deserving and saw the others as welcoming. She begins to think of herself as up to it and capable of sharing with others and to understand how sometimes the idea that others exclude and criticize her is schema-driven and not necessarily true. Her perfectionism gets less and avoidance is reduced, and she is less isolated and angry. The exploratory system is activated, and Sara would like to do things she has always neglected.

They reformulate the contract; the new goal is to figure out what she likes and try to do it concretely. Since childhood, Sara has loved sailing; she used to go with her parents even though she feared their judgment. She has a sailing permit but has never used it. The first homework is to organize a tour in July to the Greek islands sailing with strangers. Sexuality drives her as well; she hopes to meet some interesting man. The first step is to go to a travel agency. The preliminary goal, as always in MIT, is to just try it and see what happens, not to succeed. It is enough for Sara to describe her internal states in the act of trying. Remember that even in advanced stages of therapy, any experiential work is, first and foremost, valuable as a new dynamic assessment. Success means to learn more about one's own internal world while undertaking new actions. Of course, the following goal is to try to change in reality. The session with Sara, however, does not work.

S: "Let's try it; let's hope for the best. I only pay a small advance in the worst case anyway, right?"
T: "We will find out together in the next meeting, won't we?"
S: "I just don't know. I'll meet new people, and maybe someone who doesn't like me will think I'm a klutz."
T: "And if that happens, then what? You fear that . . .?"
S: "That I'll be on the boat alone. Others will have fun, look at me and giggle behind my back."
T: "That's it, the schema's back in town, correct?"
S: "Oh shit. I know . . . but how can I be sure it won't end that way?"
T: "Look, let's not think about it now; just try. Let's see how you feel; you know you're not obliged to succeed anyway."
S: "Okay."

The therapist ends the session thinking that Sara will do the behavioral homework. But she is wrong because she does not pay attention to non-verbal markers indicating that Sara was leaving the session driven by her schema and by avoidance. She was already planning not to engage in the task! We are in the presence of a withdrawal fracture: the proposed behavioral experiment activates the schemas, and Sara protects herself by avoiding.

The therapist tries to support agency by pushing her to act but does not monitor non-verbal feedback. If she did, she would notice that Sara is ashamed and agrees to the task only to please her.

Sara starts the next session talking about something else, but therapy involves focusing on the results of homework.

T: "Let's take a moment to see how the attempt to go to the agency and book the vacation went."
S: [*Embarrassed*]: "I couldn't, I put it off. I was late, hoping to find it closed, and it was. I got anxious about asking for information and signing up: it was going to get real and once I got the brochure and signed up, I was caught!"

The rupture generated by the homework falls into pattern 2: during the proposal of the technique and even more so while carrying it out, Sara experienced negative affects that blocked her. The problem was not generated by the task alone. Sara gave clear signs that the mere idea of trying to fulfill her wish reactivated the schemas with which she tried to cope with avoidance. The correct intervention would have been to give up pushing toward task completion and to point out to her that the schema was back in control. However, the therapist overlooked this step, and Sara returned home ready to avoid.

But now, the therapist is aware of the rupture and faces it.

T: ". . . fear and shame have taken over; evidently, the idea of being excluded and unfit to be with others has come back powerfully: the usual empty and worthless Sara. I understand that. Perhaps a preliminary step is necessary, but first of all, do you feel up to trying again, or do you somehow prefer to give up for now?"

S: "No, holy shit, I want to try. If I keep hanging on to my fears, I won't live."

T: "To be sure, are you completely calm, and are you doing it because you want to and not to please me? Are you afraid that I would be disappointed if you don't?"

S: "No, doctor, really, I don't feel judged. I mean . . . during the week, I felt ashamed; I was sure I would disappoint you, but now it's okay."

T: "Very good. So, you certainly have the desire to experience positive things, but the task is challenging. Shall we practice together? Shall we do an exercise to prepare for the next trip to the agency?"

S: "Actually . . . yes."

Now, the therapist pays attention to the relationship, repairs it, and creates the basis for renewed agreement on the tasks needed to reach the goal. The therapist proposes a guided imagery exercise.

T: "Close your eyes, see yourself on a boat, in the Greek islands. Visualize the details."

S: [*Sara remembers pleasant feelings from other journeys*]: "I'm on the bow of the boat with a book. I have sunscreen on, I can smell it. I watch the sea, hear the rocking, the sound of the wind. I hear the hubbub of fellow passengers."

T: "What is it like?"

S: "Pleasant; they are pleasant, calm voices."

T: "Focus on these physical sensations."

S: "I feel calm, my heart beats slowly, and my breath is quiet."

T: "How do you describe Sara in the boat right now?"

S: "I'm full of energy, I'm doing well, I'm capable, I feel equal to others . . ."

T: "Do you remember what we called this Sara?"

S: [*Smiles*]: "The full and valid Sara."

T: "There, that's exactly what we need! Keep this full and valid Sara in mind, as well as the associated feelings, savor them, and take them with you; we will need them for the next steps."

S: [*Finished imagery*]: "Okay, if I keep in touch with the things I like, I feel solid, and maybe I can make it. Look, doctor, in the bad times, if I get anxious, I'll just shut up and get in the bow to calm down."

T: "Very good. So what do you say? Do you feel up in the next few days to trying again to go to the agency?"

S: "Yes."

T: [*Jokingly*]: "Sara . . . is that a 'yes yes' or yes like last time?"

S: "Yes, really! I mean, I'm already scared. Though I have two options. Option one: I try. Option two: I try as I'm fed up living like this!"

Even in these advanced procedural steps, it is important to monitor the therapeutic relationship, which the therapist now does.

T: "How did you experience my presence during all these transitions, the guided imagery, the request to return to the agency?"

S: "It's good for me that you do these things with me. Although stressful, I feel helped."

We see that the technique-relationship interaction pattern 2 has occurred. Sara accepts the task but within a withdrawal rupture. Once the rupture is repaired, the therapist proposes the task again, and this time, they move to pattern 4: the active work proposal strengthens the relationship, and the patient confidently agrees to engage in the task.

Coping with avoided or feared relational situations

What happens when patients prepare to act in everyday life by facing what they have always avoided? Coping with feared relational situations consists of exploring what happens if patients try to give up the coping strategies they use to regulate, maladaptively, their negative emotions. For example, avoidance to protect oneself from criticism, perfectionism, pleasing others, binge eating or self-injury to downregulate unbearable emotions, alcohol and substance use, and so on. Patients may anchor themselves to their healthy self-parts and decide not to sacrifice themselves, work less, expose their ideas during a work meeting, and so on. The aim is to train them in new ways of acting, enhancing their ability to master their inner states.

As in the previous step, here we work to de-automatize patterns embedded in the mind and body. The focus at this stage is behavioral experiments, but in-session exercises that prepare for behavioral change are also important.

Patients then act in the real world, but this path is not without obstacles and relapses that must themselves be discussed. Experiential techniques, again, are central. The risk of ruptures at this stage is low but still exists.

Carmine, 38 years old, is a freelance engineer suffering from obsessive-compulsive PD and usually copes with work situations by swinging between submission and angry protest. He asks for therapy because of anxiety and addiction to his cell phone, which leads him to spend hours and hours on social media "hypnotizing" himself, watching videos of all kinds, losing track of time, and neglecting commitments. At the beginning of therapy, Carmine abuses alcohol in the evening. He is also a perfectionist, which further worsens his functioning by leading him to miss deadlines due to his excessive attention to detail.

Carmine's wish underlying his schemas is social rank: he hopes to be appreciated for his professional and human qualities but thinks the other is critical. The core negative self-image is *incapable and inferior*, associated with shame and anxiety at the idea of being laughed at for his mistakes. Simultaneously, he has a *worthy and efficient* self-image, supported by memories in which he was valued. The therapist points out that this positive idea tends to fade quickly and be replaced by the dominant negative one.

Carmine learns to recognize that his ideas about himself and others originate in family history: he was the black sheep; his every action was wrong. Now he recognizes that these are learned ideas, not necessarily true, but at work, he still tends to consider them true: he describes his bosses as dismissive, goes along with them, and submits even when he has the possibility to express his own views. He cannot take it anymore and is very motivated to break these mechanisms.

C: "Doctor, I realize that when I remember my worth, I feel like saying what I think, refusing to accept the umpteenth assignment! Only in the end, I think again that if I speak, I will say bullshit, and they will kick my ass, so I shut up. Or I get pissed off because they look like bullies, but I shut up, and it gnaws me up inside. When I talk . . . I blurt out, and it's no good! I want to retort quietly, but I don't know how to do it."

The first agreed goal is to try and express disagreement and say 'no' instead of pleasing others. They begin with a role-play, which will activate negative arousal but is less risky than actual exposure. Three days from now, there will be a meeting to discuss a project, and Carmine will try to express his disagreement to his boss, *Rock*, and explain why. In the role-play, Carmine tries to make his case by embodying the healthy self instead of submitting. The fear of the reaction immediately emerges.

C: "Just the idea makes me anxious . . . in front of him I can't do it."

Despite the fact that Carmine knows that in his schema it is he who sees himself as *nothing,* he has learned to see himself as *solid*; the mere idea of facing the boss makes the negative image true and dominant again. It is, therefore, necessary to reinforce the solid self to make the role-play possible. The therapist asks him to visualize the two *Carmines* in the room and to mark their positions on the floor with two pieces of paper: one indicates the *solid Carmine* and the other the *nothing*

Carmine. She then asks him to stand on the *nothing Carmine* paper, close his eyes, and embody it:

T: "In this position, you are the last wheel of the wagon. Try to feel it in your body, and pay attention to the sensations. What do you feel by standing here? Thoughts about yourself, feelings."
C: [*Embodies this position, notices his shoulders drooping*]: "Yes, I feel the usual nothingness and shame . . . on my cheeks. I'm a jerk."

The therapist asks him to observe the flow of thoughts, emotions, and feelings. Moving his legs, Carmine feels restless at the idea of facing *Rock*. After a few moments, the therapist asks him to look at *solid Carmine*'s paper and walk toward it, breathing deeply and regularly.

T: "Recover the feeling of solidity . . . what's happening? What do you notice in your body? Any feelings rising? What thoughts do you have about yourself and the situation by being here?"
C: "My legs are stronger, straight . . . I feel it in my pelvis and navel area . . . a sense of energy. I feel good., I can do things."
T: "Looking at it from here, what do you think of the jerk-Carmine?"
C: "I see one who always toils and submits."
T: "What do you think of him?"
C: "He thinks he's a wimp and that others are always better than him. Even when he is right, he thinks he is wrong . . . especially if he faces *Rock*. It pisses me off, he doesn't speak out of fear of being wrong! Rock is tough. But if one doesn't speak his mind, others prevail! Besides, I could help Rock if I spoke. The problem is difficult, and if he listens to me he would find a solution!"

Carmine has gained access to the healthy self and looks with different eyes at the *nothing* self. He has regained differentiation, albeit it is volatile. This is the moment we previously described: the therapist voluntarily embodying the negative other, the villain, so to speak, to reactivate the schema and its automatic tendency to surrender. Then the therapist tries to let Carmine react differently, supporting his own wish, but under the pressure of the role-played negative other.

T: "Now let's make it more difficult, okay? I'm impersonating Rock, and you will be the solid Carmine and will answer me. Let's sit around the desk, we're in a meeting, there are other colleagues besides us. Suggest a couple of realistic, technical expressions that I will try to repeat in Rock's style, I know him by now anyway! Do you agree?"
[*Carmine nods*]
T: [*As Rock, speaking in the contemptuous tone of one who does not accept an answer*]: "So, up, up! This hassle of redoing the façade with steel inserts must

be solved within a week! [*Then, returning to herself*]: What did you feel while
I was Rock?"

C: "Angry! He's overbearing, it's not fair to treat me like this!"

T: "Did you feel anything else?"

C: "As usual . . . legs trembling . . . red cheeks . . . shame: I would like to have
my say, but nothingness is back. Anxiety."

T: "Okay, good that you see it clearly. Let's try not to fall into it . . . Remember the earlier exercise? Let's go with our mind to the solid Carmine paper.
Breathe deeply . . . and then respond to Rock."

C: [*After a few seconds and struggling*]: "In my opinion, it cannot be done as you
say, there is a legal issue . . ." [*He stops.*]

T: "What's going on?"'

C: [*In a feeble voice, folding in on himself*]: "I'm afraid I was wrong. Now he will
surely bullshit me because there must be a way to overcome the obstacle, and
I'm the only one who doesn't know it."

T: "So, Carmine, let's breathe deeply. I'd like you to observe what's going on.
Your body has changed posture and lost tone; do you notice that?"

C: "Yeah."

T: "Let's try to recover the solid Carmine. Regulate your posture and breath, and
straighten your back . . ."

C: [*Carmine straightens his arms and back, breathing deeply until his face
relaxes*]: "Okay, got it."

T: "Try answering again, this time louder."

C: [*More convinced*]: "There is a legal constraint, and I honestly don't know how
to get around it. There are no solutions, and you know it."

T: "How are you doing now?"

C: "Anxiety, but less than before."

The therapist invites him to repeat it a third time, and Carmine succeeds, more
calmly and steadily. He is satisfied, relaxed, and smiling. It seems that the conditions are now in place for the behavioral experiment: facing the real *Rock* in a
meeting. Carmine turns serious again.

C: "Doctor, here is ok, but outside, I have the real Rock Scoglio facing me, not
you! I'll get anxious. I'll feel like a moron. Besides, I will sign the documents,
so there might be legal consequences. I'm a little skeptical . . . Do you see
that, doctor? Will I really be able to get out of this? Look, we'd better drop the
homework; maybe I'm not ready."

We are in the presence of a withdrawal rupture that needs to be addressed.

T: "Carmine, compared to the two papers that are still on the floor, where are you
now? On which one?"

C: [*more relaxed*]: "On the first one. I'm a loser, and I'm going to disappoint you too."

T: "I guess the loser is really back! Can we try to move? Physically go back to the lame Carmine sheet. Then, from there, try moving to the solid Carmine sheet."

Carmine follows the path, and when he gets to the *solid Carmine* paper, he straightens his back and says, "Okay, being here, I feel I can try."

T: "Do you see that? Carmine lost ground, but found that he could regain it!"

C: "Boy, it's really automatic. I guess I'll take the papers home! I'll walk around the room from one to the other . . . [*Laughs*]. They'll think I'm crazy, but who cares!"

What happens in this exchange? Proposing a behavioral experiment generates negative emotions and thoughts, and the patient constructs the therapist as judgmental. At first, it is technique-relationship interaction pattern 2: the patient giving up on the exercise. The therapist's metacommunication repairs the rupture and restores Carmine's confidence in her and in the exercise. Now, pattern 3 takes place: despite transient negative states, the patient carries on with the exercise, and the relationship is good. Now, it is possible to schedule the behavioral experiment, and Carmine will be able to cope with Rock for real! Carmine knows that he will tend to relapse, and so they continue for months with the homework until the healthy part is consolidated.

Promoting wishes and interrupting coping

Al, 40-year-old blacksmith, suffers from obsessive-compulsive PD and presents work-related anxiety and anger. He argues with customers who do not appreciate his meticulousness and precision: "They want everything right away, and they don't pay for my efforts." The problem is that too much attention to detail causes delays in delivery, and this, together with his tendency to argue, leads him to lose customers. He is anxious at the idea that customers will criticize him instead of the appreciation he longs for. In therapy, he finally realizes that he has structured his life to prevent mistakes through perfectionistic control. He is driven by fear of being caught making mistakes and considered morally reprehensible in the eyes of a stern and punitive internal and external judge. He is physically tense and invents strategies to avoid this happening so as not to have to compare himself with this self-image and then experience guilt and shame. Thanks to therapy, he has also seen a *valid and appreciable* self-image. However, it is a shaky image that does not guide him in daily life.

This is the moment to help him think something that sounds like "I'm valid, and I feel like it, so now I'm going to try to face my fears, to create the conditions in real life to reach my goals instead of staying stuck in frustration." This operation cannot be just an intention. After a reformulation of the contract, Al is asked to make it concrete.

T: "Let's try to think about taking concrete action. Are you up to it? What do you think you can do at work? Can you attempt that quantum leap, opening a bigger business, which you always secretly wanted but thought you were unable to?"

The therapist 1) uses in-session techniques to coach Al to pursue his goals and deal with problematic exchanges anchoring himself to the healthy self; 2) based on the results of in-session experiments, she plans behavioral homework with Al, to be revised in the next session.

Al decides to follow his dream: opening a larger place by investing a small amount of money in machinery and personnel. The first step is to visualize the desired scene. The therapist uses guided imagery focused on future scenarios. She asks Al to contact his healthy self, whom he names *Mode Arthur* (his beloved grandfather), adopt a posture that embodies him, say what he thinks, and feel the related emotions. Al stands up, dwells on the sensations of his feet anchored to the floor, straightens his back, and breathes deeply. The therapist asks him to physically imagine the new location, the employees, and his works of craftsmanship. During each step, she asks him what he is thinking and feeling. Al visualizes the place, likes it, and thinks he is up to it; he feels strong, his posture is erect and energetic, and his face is relaxed.

T: "From this perspective, what do you feel you want to do?"
Al: "I feel good vibes. I will go tomorrow to the bank to make a business plan."

The exercise ends, and they plan the behavioral experiment: going to the bank to inquire about financing. The perfectionistic coping is still powerful; however, without interrupting it, it will be difficult to fulfill the wish for real.

The therapist asks him to give up perfectionism, and Al agrees to counter it: he has a delivery in two weeks, a wrought-iron gate. From his point of view, some of the work is imperfect, but he knows that only an expert eye will notice. The customer is in a hurry and apparently not particularly "obsessional like me." The *adequate and valid* self-moves in, and Al senses perfectionism as egodystonic: "I know very well that nothing would happen if it wasn't perfect. I would just struggle less and live better."

Al decides to deliver the gate by leaving it as it is, and he succeeds.

Patterns resurface after improvements

The next step in the procedures involves a series of operations designed to master the natural tendency of patients to return to being driven by maladaptive patterns after successful experiments. Remember that treating PD or PTSD requires changing structures embedded in both mind and body. If therapists imagine that momentary therapeutic success corresponds to stable long-term change, they are likely to be surprised, displeased, worried, and disappointed by the inevitable steps backward. This is why we have updated the decision-making procedures by showing how to deal with a return to schema-driven readings and behaviors after patients have begun to function healthily in real life. In this way, therapists who have just observed improvement will expect relapse and act promptly. Relapse can occur even within seconds! The shift between the attainment of schema-free mental states and behaviors and the return of schema-driven mental images, usually aggravated by repetitive thinking, is instantaneous: a patient seamlessly returns to question the progress made and almost forgets it!

Relapse can also occur with a wider interval. The therapist and patient say goodbye at the end of a session in which they have discussed the success of behavioral exposures, and the patient has more benign ideas about herself accompanied by pleasant emotions. But then she comes back to the next session suffering as if change never happened. Usually, the trigger is a specific event, and therapists need to be prepared to analyze the new episode in accordance with the procedures and assess to what level of functioning patients have slipped back.

In simple terms, at the end of a session, patients have accessed healthy parts and differentiated, but they do not in the next session. Therapists must therefore deal with patients who do not differentiate, no matter how well they did the previous week.

Often, therapists forget the inevitability of these swings, and this memory lapse causes ruptures in the relationship. These are problems in which the main contribution is the therapist's. It originates, on the one hand, from an illusion about the therapeutic process; on the other hand, from therapists' own patterns related to ideas of failing, disappointing others, being able to care as expected, and then experiencing shame, guilt, or sadness. The first step in preventing ruptures, or repairing them once generated, is to consider relapse normal, first and foremost in therapists' eyes.

When relapse happens in the next session after a good, successful one, therapists can think, "Okay, there must be a reason; it's not my fault." It is more difficult when, on the other hand, it happens in the same session, when patients abruptly change mental state: they were functioning better but immediately go back to IRT and schema-laden ideas.

Therapists must first say to themselves: "I am worrying, and there is nothing wrong with that. But what I observe is normal; fluctuations are part of the therapeutic process. I just need to get back to work on something I thought was solved." Once alarm, urgency, guilt, or shame have subsided, therapists can return to focusing on patients and anchoring their interventions in the case formulation.

In these passages, patients are generally sufficiently aware of their functioning, and that in emotionally intense situations, schemas can take over control and, transiently, sound true again. But when patients return to think in a schema-driven way, under the influence of repetitive thinking, awareness vanishes, and therapists have to point it out to them: "Look, you're reading the situation again through the lens of your schemas; you're just ruminating!"

We now offer the example of a sudden shift from a positive to a negative state, the type of swing that most often puzzles therapists.

At the beginning of therapy, Sara has a partner with whom she does not get along and with whom a cycle of mutual recriminations has crystallized. Sara wants to end the relationship but, believing she is unworthy, fears that she will never find another partner. Through the recovery of a sense of personal worth, Sara makes space for her wish to break up.

After a few months, she begins a relationship with a man with whom she is very much in love. She says that, for the first time, she has found a kindred spirit, one who is emotionally available and by whom she feels appreciated and loved. She does not fear abandonment and does not spend time worrying about it. She feels free to express herself without fear of judgment and is convinced he likes her.

Sara is now more in touch with her own wishes. She understands that she would like to live together with him; it seems reasonable and feasible, and she yearns for it. Nevertheless, when revealing this intention to the therapist, she appears anxious, her face tense, she rubs her hands together, and huddles on her shoulders. The therapist explores these non-verbal markers, and Sara admits that she is afraid to think about her plan for fear of rejection and being disappointed. The therapist tries to figure out what happened during the week that acted as a trigger for the relapse. Sara replies, "Absolutely nothing; in fact, we had happy moments."

In the absence of triggers, the hypothesis is that in session, at the idea of abandoning protective mechanisms and relying on a partner, schema-dependent fears are reactivated as if to protect herself from residual risks. The negative self-image at that moment has taken over: Sara again sees herself as *empty and worthless*, and, as a result, she predicts her boyfriend can only say no. She starts worrying.

S: "I'm sure he's not convinced. He doesn't really love me, or else he would have asked me to live together. I better leave him first. But if I leave him then I will miss him and not find anyone who wants me. I will be alone; it's my fate."

As she worries, her anxiety grows, and she no longer has the capacity to differentiate and understand that she is back to seeing herself through the lens of her schemas. The therapist, therefore, proposes a regulatory practice. Sara knows that anxiety must be regulated, so she agrees to lie down and focus her attention on the points of contact of her body with the couch. She breathes slowly, bringing one hand to her chest and one to her diaphragm. After a few minutes, she calms down. The therapist asks her what has happened. Sara seems to differentiate anew.

S: "I finished in my old place, the same old feelings."
T: "Shall we take a moment to understand what happened before? How come you were so bad when you were talking to me about living together? At first, you seemed happy, but then something happened, and you face changed."
S: "I felt like I used to feel: empty, useless. As soon as I thought about clinching living together . . . like when I was a girl, always rejected and shunned by my

classmates. I'm glad I found a way to calm down right away with the exercise. It helped me."

T: "How did you perceive me when I suggested that you do something to calm yourself down? What about during the exercise? Did you have my presence in mind?"

S: "Well, as always, I knew it would calm me down. We've done it before, and I know it helps."

Sara regained good self-regulation, calmed down, and quickly returned to having better metacognitive capacities. At this stage of therapy, her trust in the therapeutic process is quite solid, so she immediately agrees to practice the regulatory exercise and feels immediate benefits. This is, therefore, pattern 4 in our taxonomy: the proposal of the technique right away rekindles the patient's trust in both the exercise and the therapist.

The next step is passing to behavioral exposure. As an experiment, the therapist proposes trying and actually asking her partner to live together. Sara accepts but returns unhappy to the next session. After she started talking with her boyfriend, she froze, changed the subject, and gave up: "I can't do it, I'm too afraid of rejection."

The therapist asks her to retell the scene and zoom in on the moment when the shift to schema-related functioning happened. She suggests role-playing the moment when Sara and her partner are in the living room listening to music. Sara agrees, and the therapist asks her to arrange the room so that it mimics reality. Sara sits on the sofa and imagines her partner to her right. Before beginning, the therapist asks her to contact the desire to live together, imagine things to do together, and describe how she feels. Sara seems relaxed; she is sitting comfortably.

T: "How do you feel right now?"

S: "I feel good, peaceful. I feel good with him; I see he loves me."

T: "Then start talking, repeat what you said the other session."

S: [*Tense, bites her lips, gesturing, frowning, barely speaking*]: "Honey . . . I wanted to tell you something. But . . . I don't know . . . I wanted to tell you that . . . [*blushes*]"

T: "What's going on? I see you tense, what are you feeling?"

S: "Agitated, my heart pounds . . . angry too . . . I would like to beat him! It will be the same old story; he's gonna say no, sure as hell. Holy Mother, he pisses me off."

It is necessary to regulate Sara's emotions to continue the role-play, and the therapist invites her to breathe deeply and feel her feet resting on the ground, resuming a grounding exercise that Sara now knows well. Sara suddenly bursts into tears, not wanting to continue.

S: "I'm too sick . . . Everything you and I did, I lost. It didn't help. Either I'm not made for therapy, or this is the wrong therapy."

Sara has collapsed, and the rupture is evident: she angrily protests. It is true that, on the one hand, she sees herself as incapable, stupid, and disappointing the therapist, but at this moment, she makes the shift from passive to active, a frequent form of coping in patients. In practice, the only way patients have learned to cope with pain is to reverse roles: to assume, for example, the dominant one by placing the other in a submissive position (Gazzillo et al., 2022). In Sara's case, challenging the therapist allows her to reverse roles, transforming a sense of inferiority into contemptuous superiority in the face of the other seen as inferior.

It is crucial that the therapist responds in a well-regulated manner, avoiding entering into a power struggle. In fact, if the therapist does not react by either submitting to or berating the patient, she serves as a healthy role model. That is, she shows through her own behavior how one can remain whole in the face of devaluation.

In a well-regulated state, the therapist points out to Sara that she has probably stumbled into her schema. On the one hand, she has self-doubts; on the other, she questions the therapy. She points out to her that criticizing her is most healthy and indeed valuable.

T: "It means you feel free to disagree safely, just what you fail to do in your everyday life!"

Sara is very relieved by this observation and feels ready to try to work on self-regulation. The therapist reminds her that she has already learned to have power over her own mind. She again invites her to breathe slowly, and Sara calms down: she looks at the therapist with renewed confidence.

T: "That's better now. So bring to mind again situations in which you felt you were valid, solid, confident, and focus on the bodily sensations, describe them and contact the related emotions and thoughts."
S: "Okay, got them."
T: "Good. Now, keep in mind the bodily sensations and emotions associated with the thought of being fine the way you are, being valid. Do you feel up now, from this state, to going back to your boyfriend and talking to him?"
S: [*Nods, puts her hand on her belly*]: "How nice if we lived together, I would love it. How about you? [*Now turns to the therapist*] Okay, that can be fine."
T: "Great. How are you?"
S: "Hm . . . a little bit tired, kinda after a university test . . . but I said it."
T: "Would you like to try again to get some more exposure and learn how to regulate anxiety? Kind of like in the gym, when you need some more training."
S: [*breathes in and tries again. The next few times, she appears more and more relaxed*]: "At the end of the day, it's just a simple request, I can do it!"

Contact with healthy self-aspects gets consolidated with repetitions: Sara begins to understand that under stress she loses contact with her positive self and learns to recover it even when the negative parts have taken control.

Acting repeatedly in real life is essential to make change concrete and break the procedural aspects of schemas. The therapist, therefore, again proposes behavioral experiments involving talking to her boyfriend. Sara knows that she might freeze or he might refuse, but neither thought hinders her from trying.

The situation could be classified as technique-relationship interaction pattern 2: while performing an exercise, the patient experiences negative affects that generate a relational rupture. Sara, in fact, fears that she has failed in therapy as well, and soon afterward, moves on to devaluing the therapist. As per procedure, the therapist interrupts the exercise and works through the rupture first and then on Sara's emotion regulation. Once the relationship is repaired, the therapist continues to follow the procedures aimed at change. We will tell more about Sara in the next chapter.

In general, when patients begin to display these swings, it will take many repetitions, as in the steps described, both in session and in real life, to break schemas and adopt new behaviors while achieving higher levels of metacognitive mastery.

In this chapter, we have seen how to support healthy wishes while interrupting avoidance and other maladaptive coping. We have described how techniques can foster the process and how to handle possible alliance ruptures. If we have achieved these goals with sufficient certainty, it is time to bring attention from the internal world to another aspect of concrete reality: the actual relationships patients describe as problematic and the interpersonal cycles in which they are entangled. The next goals will be enhancing their capacities to read interpersonal exchanges from different perspectives, to form a more mature theory of the others' mind so as to achieve more freedom, spontaneity, and flexibility when acting in the real world. In the next chapter, we will see how to implement these goals in accordance with the decision-making procedures.

Chapter 12

Forming a more mature theory of others' minds

Recognizing one's own contribution to relational dysfunction and building an integrated model of self and others

Promoting relational effectiveness

We have brought patients to understand their inner world, so that they are, for example, aware that their tendencies to expect rejection when they ask for care and protection have origins in repeated episodes where they were sick, and their parents were distant, cold, and unavailable. They recognize that the idea of being unlovable that plagues them was formed back then. Through these reconstructions, along with other therapeutic operations, they realize that what was true in the past is not necessarily true today. Yes, these ideas still surface, laden with painful emotions, but they recognize them as ideas and know how to keep them at bay, prevent them from taking control of their stream of consciousness, and make room for alternative, more benign self-images.

Patients now enter sessions already accustomed to trying to achieve their wishes and being guided by their own preferences and aspirations, driven as they are by the exploratory system. They expose themselves to previously feared situations and counteract their coping. Sometimes they swing between reading the world from a lucid and flexible perspective and falling prey to patterns again, but they recognize when the shift happens and try not to let the schema take over control. So far, operations have aimed at changing internalized patterns. Concrete actions in everyday life have started, and this time patients follow an updated map of reality.

Time is finally ripe to aim for relational efficacy. If a patient wants to live with her partner, we expect not necessarily that it will happen, but that she will feel that it is a realistic scenario and make attempts. If she is looking for new friends, she will try to expose herself to groups that she feels have common interests. If she desires esteem and appreciation from colleagues, she will expose her plans and her own point of view without needing to please, submit, or avoid. In summary, this patient now visualizes the hope that her wishes, frustrated in the past, might be fulfilled concretely.

When facing impending negative reactions, the new and positive self-images that emerged should lead patients to read the behaviors of others not as signs that their core negative self-images are true, but as the opinions of others: "He criticizes me because he does it out of bad temper or because he fears me and he wants to

DOI: 10.4324/9781003570967-12

belittle me." In sum, the theory of mind has improved but very often needs further honing.

Tendencies to think: "My boss makes me feel . . ." and "If only my partner . . ." should be replaced by thoughts such as: "My boss is hypercritical, but he doesn't question my worth"; "I make mistakes, but overall I'm competent"; "I'm waiting for him to make up his mind to tell me if we're still together, and I feel bad about it. But he's not the type to search for long-term commitments, I clearly see now. So, even if he breaks up with me, it doesn't mean my life is over."

What steps should be taken when patients reach this awareness? Clinicians now focus on making the map of the world more detailed and realistic and increasing the effectiveness of actions in the real world. Patients recognizing that they have been guided by maladaptive patterns and adopting new perspectives is okay, but often insufficient for change. They must actually open the updated and detail-rich map of the world and, most importantly, actually follow its new paths to travel more safely, quickly, and in line with their own wishes, also guided by a more mature and realistic understanding of how real others react to their initiatives (Figure 12.1, Box 7).

A reminder: MIT is not a therapy in phases. We are not talking about initial and advanced moments of treatment. MIT steps are organized according to hierarchies. We, therefore, work on the steps we are going to expound when the steps described in the previous chapters are achieved in that session or series of sessions. If patients return to previous modes of functioning, clinicians have only to, as in the game of the goose, go back. Are patients returning to intellectualizing or worrying? The therapist asks, "Can you give me an example of a situation when . . .?"

That said, how do we get patients to take action for behavioral change? We start with how we help them understand others' minds in a more articulate way, build more flexible hypotheses, and move away from schema-dependent readings where they only read others as critical, disinterested, tyrannical, and so on.

We also lead them to decenter, to understand that others' acts are guided by their typical mental states, by their personality, and that patients, for the most part, are not the protagonists in others' streams of consciousness (Figure 12.1, Box 7). But even when the others' reactions are actually directed at the patient, they learn to see them as contextual so that they do not undermine their identity: "I bought my

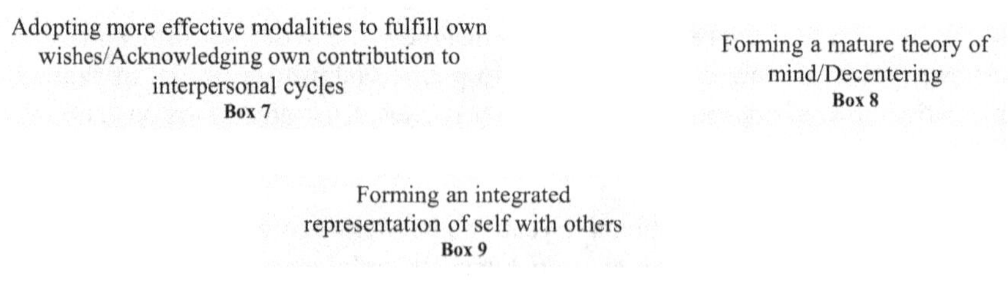

Adopting more effective modalities to fulfill own wishes/Acknowledging own contribution to interpersonal cycles **Box 7**	Forming a mature theory of mind/Decentering **Box 8**

Forming an integrated
representation of self with others
Box 9

Figure 12.1 Promoting relational effectiveness and building integration

partner the train ticket for the wrong day. She called me a jerk, but she was right! But then she's aware I'm overwhelmed these days. Well, by dinner time the air was cleared."

Understanding others' minds is one of the elements needed to dismantle dysfunctional interpersonal cycles. A parallel task is for patients to understand how they contribute to generating and maintaining relationship problems in the family, in romantic relationships, among friends, and at work (Figure 12.1, Box 8). Deactivating one's own contribution requires that patients: (a) recognize they are acting under the pressure of the schema; (b) realize that others can generate suffering, but up to a point, and that the rest of their pain depends on the prediction that their own wishes will remain unfulfilled and their core negative self-image confirmed; (c) recognize how they are acting out maladaptive copings that not only prevent them from fulfilling their goals but also harm a relationship; (d) want to interrupt these copings for the sake of the relationship itself; and (e) reach an attitude of curiosity and desire to explore: "What can I do differently and more functionally?"

Here's how the process works:

The other day, I made a mistake at my office, and it was pointed out to me. At other times, I would have resented it and reacted by shutting down, being offended. But I know now this is the very reason why my colleagues do not get along with me. This time, I felt a tinge of anger, sure, but I acknowledged what we said in therapy: I was feeling stupid, and I'm the one who believes it! My colleagues had nothing to do with it. At that point, instead of being offended and showing clear signs that I was, I joked: "Boys, I fucked up, what should I do? Do a walk of shame?" They jokingly answered: "Sure please do, wait a minute, we'll get some rotten tomatoes." We laughed and end of story.

Sara is the 27-year-old mathematician that we saw asking her partner to live together (Chapter 11). Her partner replies he would rather wait some more. Sara is sorry and sad, but does not feel *empty and worthless* as usual. She is satisfied with how she handled the conversation; she knows that expressing her wish was legitimate, and she feels solid. She did not get angry with her partner or attack him, risking triggering endless conflicts as in her past stories. She was disappointed but remained calm, thanks to her capacity to better understand her partner:

Larry is afraid to take this step. It's not about me, I mean, I'm still annoyed, but truth is he can't separate himself from his mother. I'm worried, I don't know how it's going to end . . . Look . . . this time, at least, I don't think he doesn't love me enough because I'm not worth a dime. I mean, the problem is in his head!

This change generates a first indirect contribution toward deactivating interpersonal cycles (Safran & Muran, 2000). Sara, in fact, experienced frustration but did not read it in light of the pattern: she sensed that her partner was driven by his own fears and not by a lack of love, so she did not enact any dysfunctional behaviors.

As a result, the relationship did not enter the usual spirals of tension, and her mood remained good.

Most often, however, patients, although changed, still report interpersonal difficulties, and active work in therapy is needed to reduce them. In these transitions, we expect difficulties mostly in close relationships, with for example, partners, children, parents, siblings, or colleagues, where interpersonal cycles have probably crystallized. It is not enough for patients to change the way they see themselves; they must deliberately want to change their behavior, this time to affect the actual relationship. It is crucial that they set aside their tendency to externalize responsibility and hold themselves accountable for changing: "If there is a path that leads to the improvement of the relationship, I must be the first one to walk it."

Patients may not realize that, although eager to be appreciated and now feeling valuable, they still enter relationships following old habits. Modalities of which they are unaware, and which make it difficult for relationships to succeed. They may, for example, still not be quite free from their dysfunctional coping behaviors and/or transiently fall prey to schema-related mental states. Think of the paranoid PD tendency to distrust (Lee, 2017), which leads patients to control others. They tend to behave like this even if they have begun to be inhabited by healthy self-images. Their tendencies are procedural, automatic, to the point of enacting them without awareness.

Integrating the various self-images (Figure 12.1, Box 9) or parts of the self (Bell et al., 2021) is also difficult. It involves making patients aware that different representations, some benevolent and some negative, lie inside them and may still surface. The latter will look more like areas of vulnerability, no longer pervasive and all-encompassing ideas as in the past. They are no more than characters among other characters in their internal theatre. We aim to make patients aware of how their self consists of a multiplicity of parts and characters and how, consequently, they see others in various ways. To discover how distinct and sometimes opposing wishes guide them at different moments, sometimes at the same moment. We try to lead them to weave a coherent, organized self-narrative (Singer, 2013; Lind et al., 2020), that includes positive aspects of self and others that were previously hidden and under-nurtured.

Patients, moreover, know what elicits their problematic self-parts and see them come on stage as events flow. They name them and take the leading actor role away from them. They also see the good in what used to make them suffer: perfectionistic aspects, for example, turn into normal prodding and conscientiousness. Self-sacrificial tendencies give way to a wonderful ability to help loved ones. These are ambitious goals, and techniques help us, as we will see later.

A patient with a pattern rooted in social rank complains of problems with his son:

> I know that when my son does things I don't approve of, I think I've done everything wrong for a moment. I used to impose my will to make him the way I wanted him to be, because only then would I feel like a good father. I recognize that demanding part of me. I still see it and feel it a little in my body.

Memories surface; my mother made me feel so wrong. Now I look at them, breathe and let them go. I have recovered a sense of dignity, and can talk to my son differently; I joke with him. I also know that I may still fluctuate between worry, stiffness and playfulness, but that's life.

Each of these described steps requires reformulating the contract (Radcliffe & Yeomans, 2019) and assessing whether or not patients wish to continue. Not everyone decides to go further. For example, a patient with dependent PD told one of us that, all things considered, pleasing others a little and submitting is not something she hates; she sees the benefits and knows that if she just modulates this tendency, the life she lives is fine with her.

Conversely, engaging in this last stretch of therapy necessarily comes through an additional commitment that patients must, as always, decide to make. Otherwise, the risk is that unknowingly, it is therapists generating ruptures, pushing patients where they do not intend to go.

Techniques are central to these operations as well, and we will see examples; however, the purposes and, thus, consequently, some of the steps change. In a role-play, a patient takes on the role of the other person and can expand his theory of mind to notice aspects he did not notice before. Sometimes the discovery is surprising: "My boss was rubbing his hands while he was talking to me . . . He seemed afraid; I hadn't noticed before"; "When playing with? my boyfriend I had my eyes downcast before saying goodbye . . . I think it was sadness and not boredom, he was sad probably, and I never realized that was possible."

When working on a dysfunctional interpersonal cycle, interventions such as role-play or two-chair play in which therapist and patients make a series of role reversals are useful. Patients can observe themselves from the outside and then, returning to their own shoes, train new skills, such as assertiveness or more effective communication. Exercises are repeated several times until patients feel they can enact new behaviors.

Alliance ruptures are rare in this step but not impossible. In fact, therapists are now saying to patients that their styles are really dysfunctional, and thus run the risk of inducing schema-related reactions, such as "You are criticizing me."

The repair operations are the same as those already covered throughout the volume and allow us to capture residual, still active aspects of the schemas and overcome them again.

Promoting understanding of others' minds and the difference in their perspective

Schemas generate bias in the attribution of thoughts, emotions, and intentions to others: it is a basic projective mechanism (Ames, 2004; Andermann et al., 2022; Bertsch et al., 2022). Immersed in the feeling of being alone, patients see the other as distant, focus attention on signs of rejection, and neglect schema-discrepant information (Dimaggio et al., 2020).

Inhabiting the healthy self often helps to modify these attributional styles. The process starts almost automatically as soon as patients deprive negative self-images of power: if I see myself as vulnerable, I will expect others to be threatening. If I see myself as strong, I will read a variety of intentions in others. This is one reason why we prescribe decision-making procedures to promote first differentiation and only later theory of mind. Once patients understand they were schema-driven, the ability to read others in a varied, flexible, realistic way blossoms almost automatically.

At other times, this process requires active work in session after a reformulation of the contract. Developing a more mature and articulate theory of the other's mind and decentering often go in parallel with work on interpersonal cycles.

Techniques are, as always, very helpful. The first type of intervention concerns past memories and prototypical episodes. We can go back again to some of the scenes and relive them, for example, with guided imagery.

This time, however, the focus is different: we explore patients' inner world to look at the other with curiosity. It is necessary for patients to try and look at the other with the eyes of the healthy self-parts. A young man now glimpses that his father seems critical but is afraid, that he accuses him but is actually ashamed, and that he displays anger but is sad inside.

We aim here for a two-level change. On the one hand, we try to build a nuanced picture of others, that is, to think that others have a wide range of reactions, not just those predicted by schemas. On the other hand, we try to help patients discover who "real" others are, guided by curiosity and exploration. We can, for example, help them read a partner's absence in light of factors that make it understandable: he is grieving, has lost his job, is ill, tired, and so on. Patients understand others in a more complex, articulate way and contemplate the idea that they display different and even contradictory aspects because it is in their nature. This skill needs, ça va sans dire, training.

Ruptures in the therapeutic relationship, while rare, do not disappear entirely in this step. Guided imagery, role-play, or body interventions can reactivate patterns and trigger ruptures.

His therapist attempts to improve the theory of mind of Gary, a 50-year-old, ophthalmologist with narcissistic PD and generalized anxiety. He sought help because of conflicts with his wife. When Gary saw himself as lonely, he sought treatment, but his wife did not respond, and he became very sad. His busy parents neglected him in terms of care while praising him for his school performance. It was, however, an appreciation that alternated with the classic "You only did your duty," and so Gary also developed the idea of worthlessness with associated shame. He thus shifted from needing care to rank: "If I am flawless, maybe they will appreciate me," and this ignited perfectionistic behaviors. In therapy, he learned to see himself as lovable and worthwhile, images he already had in the outskirts of his mind when therapy started but were blurred, fuzzy, and pale.

Therapy is advanced, and anxiety at the idea of making mistakes and IRT has been reduced. Gary now feels lovable, and his self-esteem is more stable. Since he feels more lovable, he pays less attention to his wife's neglect of him, so arguments are less frequent. However, he cannot resolve conflicts with his boss. He describes him as genuinely critical and manipulative: "He carries out the *divide-and-conquer* policy." He has now learned not to feel challenged but continues to suffer: "He is my boss, he has ties . . . understand? If I mess up, he will ruin my career." He still mulls over the possible causes of his boss's attitude but is beginning to realize that this is who the boss is: he treats everyone this way. There is, therefore, the basis for expanding Gary's theory of mind. The therapist, therefore, elicits a recent episode in which Gary again felt anxious about possible criticism from the boss.

Meeting time, the goal is to open a nursing unit in the hospital. The boss makes his point, as usual:

> Are you sure you can do it? You haven't put much effort in lately, have you? I've been chasing you for weeks to have this meeting and you always have something else to do, just Lawrenson did something, thank you Tony. If it goes like this, things are going to go south . . . By the way, Dr. Bettancourt [Gary], you were on vacation, am I right?

Gary feels hurt but no longer blushes nor sees red. He feels inadequate and manipulated, but less than in the past. He has learned to remain calm and firm. However, he remains angry at these constant jibes which, he is clear, are typical of his boss. "It's who he is, doctor, a mobster," he says with a laugh. The therapist suggests that he view the episode in guided imagination to help him better decode what the boss has in mind, given the risk that Gary will still read him in light of his own attributional biases, a legacy of the schemas.

Gary repeats the boss's words to himself and falters but feels strong; his self-esteem does not collapse. He feels embodied aspects of stability and self-confidence, and anchors himself to the theme. The therapist asks him for details about the boss's tone, manner, and words and suggests that he metaphorically press the button "hold" on his face without losing touch with his sense of steadfastness.

G: "He's fiddling with his pen, his face is sweaty . . . the face of a stern father. Like my father. But . . . No, fuck . . . he's worried."

T: "About what?"

G: "Like being reprimanded, but yes, basically by the general manager, his boss. Who is terrible! He would like our support . . . he feels left in the lurch. I mean, it's so clear! With the manager, he's all bowing and scraping . . . strong with the weak and weak with the strong . . . Whatever . . . like me! I guess he's been under a lot of pressure since this whole organization change thing started."

During imagery, we leave no room for reflection or association (Chapter 10). The therapist immediately brings Gary back into the scene.

T: "Do you see him under pressure now?"

G: "Yes. Sweat. I can almost see it in his face."

T: "What thoughts do you read seeing that face?"

G: " 'If it goes wrong, it will blow up in my face'. The problem is he's never very open with us."

T: "Observe it again, what do you see?"

G: ". . . Shame?"

T: "Because he fears that . . .?"

G: "That we see how weak he is."

> Having finished the imagery, Gary is surprised: he has never seen his boss in this light and says that he now has a different way to deal with him. Gary's face, however, also displays mild anger toward the therapist.

T: "Gary, is everything alright? Am I mistaken, or did you look at me askance? Or am I getting paranoid myself [*smiles*]?"

G: "I feel a little irritated as if you were blaming me. You showed me that I've been misreading the situation over the years, like I didn't understand anything."

Gary, on the one hand, thinks he is wrong, and on the other hand, imagines that the therapist is criticizing him unfairly. He has fallen into the pattern trap. The therapist begins to metacommunicate, which comes smoothly given she knows the bond is very good overall. Gary then realizes he is back to swinging between seeing himself as incapable and reacting angrily to the unfair humiliation: "To cut a long story short: same old me," he smilingly says. The session ends after they agree to work on breaking the interpersonal cycle with his boss.

The technique was not the factor triggering the alliance rupture. The problem was subsequent to the imagery and was not attributable to the technique per se but to the attempt to show Gary his contribution to the cycle. It happens easily, and this is why this is one of the later change operations in the decision-making procedures.

Learning how to satisfy wishes and break interpersonal cycles

PD sufferers enter real relationships representing themselves and others in dysfunctional ways. Guided by these ideas, their actions elicit negative responses (Dimaggio et al., 2007; Safran & Muran, 2000). In addition to schemas, both coping and poor metacognition contribute to triggering and maintaining interpersonal cycles (Messman-Moore & Coates, 2007).

If a person always feels disappointed in his need for care, representing himself as lonely and unaided and having no awareness of the healthy parts, he will not enter into relationships with *real* others. He will only read others through the lens of his schemas, thus expecting that they will respond frustratingly to his needs. When he needs care, therefore, his attention will be biased towards words and non-verbal cues that indicate potential abandonment. As a result of these schema-dependent readings, he does not ask for help or show he is suffering. Instead, he adopts coping such as forcing himself to fend for himself or retreating, offended and resentful, silently.

These behaviors influence the other and help maintain a negative interaction pattern in reality, which feeds the pattern and confirms its assumptions: a dysfunctional interpersonal cycle is established. If a patient shows himself as self-sufficient, the others think he does not need care and do not provide it; if a patient displays signs he has been offended, the others will become worried or angry. In no case will they respond to his very attachment need, and at the end of the story, he will see himself as more abandoned than at the beginning. And he will very likely persist with communicative behaviors that have already failed or resort to different but dysfunctional ones. He is unaware of the role of his actions in making his desire founder.

MIT prescribes working on interpersonal cycles only during advanced steps of the decision-making procedures, which is useful when patients have understood their inner world, achieved a good critical distance from schemas, and made room for healthy self-images. After they manage to differentiate and can understand with more flexibility and realism social interactions and understand the others' minds in a more articulate way, therapists can work on curbing their own contribution to interpersonal cycles for the sake of the therapeutic relationships.

In fact, as with theory of mind, work on interpersonal cycles begins to some extent automatically when patients differentiate and access their healthy parts. A patient with dependent and avoidant traits, accustomed to pleasing others for fear of being criticized and left alone, realizes that he is "being nice" to others as a coping strategy. The disadvantage is that others respond to this strategy by teasing him. At times he considered this okay: "They joke with me, which means they include me in the group," but underneath remains the fear that others will not take him seriously and consider him a loser. This reinforces the idea of unworthiness and, as a result, leads him to accentuate his "jester" behaviors.

Stopping submissiveness and pleasing others and inhabiting the healthy self already help to elicit different responses. For example, during a dinner party, this patient no longer frets about trying to please but speaks only if the topic interests him and he has something to say. He refrains from telling out-of-place jokes and smiling constantly. Others are likely to treat him differently now.

More often than not, however, it is necessary to devote time to building adaptive ways of relating. Techniques are valuable in helping patients see themselves while trying new behaviors and notice all those procedural and automated aspects with which they have positioned themselves in social interactions. In helping them discover how they evoke those very reactions that will cause them pain and frustrate their goals.

We work on two levels: the first, in-session, is about paving the way for training in everyday life. Therapists monitor patients' behavior in session and offer genuine feedback:

I noticed that in the role-play, when you were telling your colleague that this time the vacation plan should be agreed between you first, you had your jaw clenched and your gaze tense. I myself felt a bit tense, like you were angry at me, and if this happens in your interactions, it will probably spread further tension in the air [*the patient agrees*]. Would you like to figure out what was going on and try again with a different voice and facial expression?;

Earlier, during the guided imagery, in which you were telling your boyfriend that you are fed up with his jealousy and that you did not cheat on him as he fears, your voice trembled, and you blushed. You were almost about to apologize for telling him this.

Relational rupture fractures are possible, although less frequent or deep. Patients may find the exercises distressing, falling back into the meshes of their schemas. Therapists offer feedback on a plane of reality, pointing out, as in the previous examples, that patients have been too aggressive or submissive. Patients may feel criticized or invalidated.

In the example here, the patient agrees to dismantle the interpersonal cycle, but the role-play activates a problem that breaks the alliance. We will be in pattern 2 of our classification.

Felicia, a 50-year-old prison social worker, suffers from paranoid PD. At the beginning of therapy, she had hypochondria and generalized anxiety and frequently quarreled with colleagues. After two years, she has realized that when she asks for closeness and care, she thinks she is inadequate, unlovable, and an underdog compared with others she portrays as liars and manipulative. She knows, thanks to therapy, that these readings originate from her cold and distant mother who always criticized her and from an absent, drug-addicted father who lied all his life and squandered the family's fortune. She has discovered her lovable and valid self; however, she still reports relationship difficulties on several levels. She has conflicting relationships at work with two younger colleagues on her team. Felicia describes them as conceited and narcissistic, and in the past, she used to get angry, ruminating for days about humiliation, feeling sad and lonely, and without anyone who loved her in the end analysis. Felicia has now overcome her "the other makes me feel . . ." reasoning and senses that she can elicit hostile reactions from others. She has realized that she always expects they will offend her. She arrives at meetings laden with angry rumination. It is not clear to her, however, how she triggers treating her with hostility in others.

F: "I don't see? myself from the outside, I don't understand what I'm doing. I try to be calmer, but I feel like I don't understand what's going on. My colleagues always attack me even when I stay put."

She tells of a meeting in which a convict she takes care of is the topic. Her female colleagues object that Felicia has not agreed on her decisions with the team, creating a problem. Felicia is now less sensitive to criticism, anchors herself to the good self-esteem she has regained, and defends her actions: "You never agree things with me . . . You are just good at pointing fingers!" Her colleagues reply that she is always aggressive and cannot be reasoned with and that she always thinks she knows everything. Felicia is fully unaware of this aspect of herself and is surprised now that she discovers that others can see her as arrogant and conceited, like she always thought others were.

The therapist suggests that she observe herself in action through a role-play: when she sees herself through her colleagues' eyes, she may perhaps better understand the self-aspects she is unaware of. At first, the therapist impersonates the colleague who has spoken the most, while Felicia plays herself.

T: [*Playing the colleague*]: "In my opinion, you should learn to communicate with us about your decisions before you go off on your own."

F: "Yes, okay. But you girls never do that, you're always pointing at my faults, never seeing yours!"

T: [*Coming out of role-play*]: "How do you feel now?"

F: "Angry. They are like two little girls, and are bossy. I'm twice as experienced as they are, and they believe they can give me orders."

T: "How does your colleague seem to you?"

F: "A witch."

Felicia feels humiliated but recognizes that, for a few moments, she "fell into the pattern," then mastered her mental state and regained a sense of personal worth, which then triggered anger at the injustice suffered. The following steps aim at two purposes. The first is to bring Felicia to look at herself through the other's eyes since perspective-taking is a pillar of adaptive social action. The second is to develop relational mastery: Felicia will try to observe her own behavior, evaluate its effectiveness and its impact on the other, and try to visualize more functional behaviors and experiment with them.

The roles are reversed: Felicia plays the colleague, and the therapist plays her, trying to repeat her words and adopt her posture and tone.

F: [*On the colleague's side*]: "Felicia, you need to communicate your decisions with us."

T: [*In Felicia's part*]: "Yes, okay. You guys never do that! [*Back in the role of therapist.*] What did you feel when, as Felicia, I was responding to you like that?"

F: "How strange. As if I saw myself in a movie. I see a totally unlikable, aggressive person, with a tense face, arms crossed and not smiling, on their guard, and aggressive."

T: "And how do you feel in the shoes of the colleague who finds Felicia in front of her?"

F: "That I have to defend myself. What does this person want? [*She steps out of her colleague's shoes and reflects.*] They can't stand me anymore; we've fought so many times."

T: "Does that help you see the situation differently? I mean, it makes us think about how we could act differently."

F: "Sure, so it doesn't work!"

T: "And, in fact, you see it now, don't you? I have to say that even when I was your colleague, I felt the impact of your aggression. I wanted to defend myself. It's okay if I say this, isn't it?"

F: "Yes, yes, doctor, it is."

T: "How do you feel?"

F: "A little down."

T: "Sad? Like you're thinking: 'I have to fix something'?"

M: "A lot of things!"

T: "No, no, not a lot! Yes, we have stuff to work on, sure, but you have already made the most important step, that is to understand that some changes need to be made. It's natural that you're a little bit down, of course! It's just a matter of figuring out how you can do it, but it shouldn't be difficult, you have the right attitude now. We can start trying now if you want to."

The therapist validates Felicia's difficulties and, at the same time, realistically appraises the problematic aspects of her behaviors. Decision-making procedures suggest that we have solid ground to undertake this agreed-upon behavioral change step. Now the therapist is ready to continue the role-play to experiment with new attitudes in the protected environment of the session. The goal is to build advanced social mastery skills. Relational ruptures at such moments are possible, albeit minor. Continuing the role-plays, Felicia remains head-bowed, gloomy, and pensive. The therapist notices these non-verbal markers.

T: "Is everything all right? You still look down."

F: "It's difficult. Am I really that unbearable?"

T: "Listen, how do you see me now? What am I thinking about you?"

F: "That you can't stand me . . . no, wait!"

T: "Tell me."

F: "I got it!"

T: [*smiles*]: "Same old story?"

F: "Exactly. No one loves me because I'm a pain in the ass."

T: "And imagine your therapist is feeling a huge pain in her ass now!"

F: [*Laughs*]: "She most of all!"

Exploration of the relationship reveals that this part of the role-play has a transiently negative impact on the relationship: we are in pattern 2. It is necessary to stop the technical work and repair the relationship. The rupture is mended, the climate becomes playful and cooperative, and role-play can continue.

The therapist invites Felicia to act differently. She cannot imagine how to act and asks the therapist to try first to put on her shoes. Now, it makes sense for the therapist to use modeling. For much of therapy, therapists should not display their virtuous behaviors and their problem-solving skills (which they often do not use when they need them in their everyday life) as examples of virtue and social effectiveness. They would put themselves on a pedestal, motivated by their wish for social rank.

In these more advanced therapy steps, modeling is instead necessary. Therapists are constructing something new, and patients are asking to learn new modes of social behavior. The former are now fully empowered to adopt the role of the teacher, the coach: they illustrate a new gesture and invite patients to try it, repeat it, practice it, and change it until they feel it is their own and, through continued practice, harmonious.

The therapist and Felicia repeat the sequence. Felicia plays her colleague, and the therapist responds as Felicia:

F: [*In the colleague role*]: "Felicia, you need to communicate your decisions!"
T: [*As Felicia*] "Yes, you are right! We are always rushing, and sometimes we forget. I mean, it's right that we pass information to each other; it's just that I act on impulse. I'm convinced I'm doing the right thing, and I go straight. I just forget that we have to communicate in advance. Look, shall we put this issue on the agenda? Then we can think together about how to solve the problem. [*Returning to the therapist role*] How is it for you to feel this way?"
F: "Yikes. Thank you. I just don't know how to do this."
T: "Try it! Shall we switch roles?"
    Another round of role-play begins: the therapist repeats her colleague's comment. Felicia assumes a more relaxed posture and smiles.
F: "Okay, girls, I was in a rush and didn't brief you, you are right. However, I think the problem of not sharing information is generalized. It happens to all of us a little bit. Maybe we need to find a way to pass information to each other, what do you say?"
T: [*Explaining how she felt in her colleague's shoes*]: "Do you know that this time I heard your words and they sounded ok to me? You were gentler, and I didn't feel attacked. I even felt a bit guilty; I realized it was somewhat my fault. And, look, how was it for you speaking like this?"
F: "Certain attitudes are so automatic, fuck! I'm not used to being more cooperative."
T: "Which you were this time! How did you feel?"
F: "I was feeling envious! I mean, the urge to eat them was there! But also . . . calmer, you live better this way . . . it's just so difficult."
T: "Sure it's hard, believe me, I know. But you can do it, I've seen it, and I've felt in myself your communicating was ok; I didn't feel hurt this time . . . . It's just a skill you need to practice."
F: "You know what I'm going to do? I'm going to enroll in a theater class . . . workshop . . . whatever."

While waiting for the theater course, they agree on a behavioral experiment: during the week, Felicia will try changing attitudes with her colleagues, as in the role-play. There will be a team meeting, which can be an opportunity to practice.

F: "Let's see, doctor . . . I' will sure give it a shot."

In the next session, the patient recounts that during the meeting her colleagues raised a new issue: they disagreed with a technical decision made by Felicia about a convict. For a moment, she is about to respond aggressively. She feels herself flaring up; her instinct tells her to attack. However, she has the previous session in mind and restrains herself; she knows it will make things worse. She then seeks contact with the healthy self, breathes deeply, anchors herself in the chair, and remembers she is competent. And she says, "Ladies, so . . . I've known this inmate for years. What you say makes sense, but with him, believe me, it doesn't work. That's why we decided to overlook it and go the route that I later took. You are missing this bit of the story and, in fact, I should have told you . . . let me tell the whole story . . ."

Felicia is satisfied with her behavior and has seen its effectiveness: her colleagues understand her course of action and approve it.

F: [*laughing*]: "Hey, doc, just between us . . . they're still spoiled brats, right?"
T: [*laughing in turn*]: "I Never asked you to marry them. We don't want you to be made a saint by therapy, at least that was not my goal!"

At this stage, therapeutic change depends primarily on repeated exercise. Acquiring new modes of action requires training, as in any form of learning. The in-session work described now is only the initial step. Once functional modes of action are illustrated, it is up to the patient to apply himself, to enter a process of trial and error and refinement of skills. Health depends on the repetition of an effective gesture until it becomes an internalized habit, a new automatism.

What is missing before treatment is complete? Here, we describe how to get to higher metacognitive functioning: forming an integrated, accepting view of self and others, taking into account the many facets, the characters that inhabit our internal theatre, recognizing them as our own, and understanding others are also populated by internal multitudes, of aspects we like and dislike, sometimes coherent, sometimes contradictory. Then, in the next chapter, we will explain how to deal with residual dysfunctional symptoms and behaviors.

Forming an integrated representation of self and others

Achieving an awareness that there are different ideas within us about who we are and who others are, some benign and some negative, and holding them together in a unified sense of self is not easy (Fuchs, 2007; Hermans et al., 1992). It involves recognizing that we and others are often driven by goals and experiences that vary and may seem inconsistent. Nevertheless, we feel we are a whole person, and so are others. At the same time, it is difficult to recognize who we were, who we have become, and what generated the change, if any, all elements shaping a coherent narrative identity (McAdams, 1996), which is something hard to achieve for many with PD (Lind et al., 2020; Lind, 2021). This is the metacognitive function of integration (Carcione et al., 2021). Achieving it requires a rich and lucid awareness of the different aspects that lurk within people, starting with ourselves.

Integration manifests itself in the clinic in different declinations. At low overall metacognitive monitoring, it involves the difficulty of recognizing a mental state that suddenly appears in the stream of consciousness as one's own: "How come I was calm before and now I have a terrible fear that he's cheating on me, or that I'll get sick?"; "I get tense, feel restless, just like that, out of the blue"; "I felt threatened when my colleague came into the room. But he didn't cause it, I'm sure. Some stuff hovering in the air, but I can't say."

The impact of the emergence of these non-integrated mental states leads to fright, confusion, loss of emotional control, and at times dysregulation. We discussed in chapter 8 how to deal with these symptoms and problems when patients lack these basic aspects of integration.

In this section, we focus on the difficulty of integrating at higher metacognitive levels. Even when patients differentiate, it may happen that, at times, they do not recognize aspects of themselves as their own or cannot understand what makes them switch from one state of mind, from one character or part of the self taking control, to another. They see themselves, therefore, as incoherent or feel parts of themselves are foreign, alien (Bateman & Fonagy, 2004): "I did something that disgusts me: I brought home a boy I met just before in a bar. Am I immoral, am I a whore?"

In other cases, patients do not differentiate under stress, which also indicates a transient loss of integration: "My manager told me that the document was badly written. I'm an idiot." At this moment, patients believe their negative ideas about themselves to be true and forget that, until the previous session, they thought they were valid and competent.

Clinicians must help patients progressively build an integrated view of themselves that holds together the different aspects of personality, strengths and weaknesses, and differences in behaviors and feelings in various situations. The goal is for them to recognize themselves in the different aspects, feel them as "self," and inhabit different psychological positions with flexibility and security (Gonçalves et al., 2011). For example, they may root their self-esteem in being a good spouse even if they doubt their work qualities at a problematic moment.

A coherent self-image stabilizes identity. It is a process well described by narrative identity (Lind, 2021; McAdams, 1996). Moreover, dialogical self-theory (Hermans et al., 1992; Hermans & Dimaggio, 2004) shows how we are inhabited by a cast of characters, voices, and positions of the self that enter into conversation with each other until we reach a sense of greater unity or balance among the various self-aspects: "I can be serious, focused, and stern, but at the same time leave more room for my light side, which likes to go to the pizzeria with friends to joke and tease each other."

This level of integration requires that therapists and patients draw a shared map of recurrent mental states, the interpersonal patterns that guide patients' social action. On this map, they observe how transitions between mental states are guided by the patient's position within a schema or by the transition from one motivational system to another.

Clare, a 37-year-old lawyer, is feeling confused and judging herself because her long-time friends are planning a night out in her hometown, but she would rather go to a business dinner. She is torn between two desires that are both healthy and adaptive: group belonging and a mixture of curiosity and ambition. She gets stuck, though, because she thinks she is an insincere friend if she chooses the business dinner. The activation of schemas is not powerful: yes, she judges herself and feels excluded. But she realizes that exclusion for the most part is just real, not her sensation: she would not be there with her cherished friends, and it depends on her, so she does not feel rejected. In a way, Clare has to realize that she now feels less like belonging to a group with which she once identified. The therapist validates both desires and helps her recognize herself in both aspects. Then he points out to her that she is just making a difficult choice that has an emotional cost, that involves suffering and that he himself experienced something similar at various moments in his growing up.

Experiential techniques help a lot: in imagery, the therapist brings Clare to relive moments when she is with her friends and points out her influencing feelings, which fluctuate between affectionate, critical, and distant. He echoes Clare's words when she talks about her friends: "I don't like what Helene says" "I love Laura," "I see them as still living in the past; I have changed." Clare recognizes these aspects of herself and begins to make peace with herself.

After this, the therapist brings Clare, again in imagery, to a moment where she works with motivation and energy and lets the inner world emerge. The therapist continually validates what surfaces and emphasizes Clare's sense of *ownership* of the experience. At the end, Clare says: "I want to pursue this project at work. I believe in my ideas. The working dinner is important. I will definitely go there, I'll miss my friends, but that's ok." Clare anchors her decision to something she feels as her own without judging herself. She is just left with the human sorrow of discovering herself distant from past friends.

In such situations, there is usually minimal impact on the therapeutic relationship. A transient type 3 pattern may surface: during the exercise, the patient feels pressured for a moment by the therapist, who puts her in touch with a painful loss. But this does not hinder the exercise, and soon after, when they talk about it, Clare knows that she has to say out loud what she thinks and feels about her friends' meeting, and she is grateful to the therapist for helping her.

A second aspect of integration to be promoted concerns awareness of one's evolution throughout life history. This serves to have a sense of consistency and continuity of identity, allowing us to understand that we are still the same despite the changes that have occurred. Or, if we discover ourselves to be different, we make sense of the change and accept who we have become. (McAdams, 1996; Semerari et al., 2003). It is a type of integration already recognizable in the previous example: the patient needs to integrate two different aspects of herself but also to discover herself as different from the past.

The realization of this process of integrating different parts of the self over time involves a capacity close to what Janet (1928) called *personification* and *presentification*: "That lonely, neglected child was me, but it is a me of the past, now I am different." Patients, therefore, are aware of their history and accept the multiplicity of their inner world. They realize that apparent inconsistencies often simply mean that they are driven by various goals at different times. They can describe their own mental states and have a more mature and accurate theory of the other's mind. They are aware of their positive self-images and have agency and good mastery over their own minds when things become a bit trickier. They have integrated new patterns of action at the "somatic" level (Ogden et al., 2006) and have rewritten endings of painful scenes, experiencing more benevolent and effective feelings, emotions, and thoughts about themselves.

We aim for this specific type of integration at the end of therapy through the reconstruction of the therapeutic process: "Who was I at the beginning? How have I changed? Who am I now? What do I accept about myself, and what areas do I want to continue working on when therapy is over?"

Often, however, specific interventions are needed. It is very helpful to engage the patient in joint reframing, to have the patient say

> Yesterday I still felt lousy to my wife when she criticized me, but I know that I am not the way she describes me; I am not selfish or overbearing. On the contrary, I care a lot about others. It was really hard for me to let myself act without always having to think that I might hurt someone. Obviously, when my wife calls me selfish, I still believe her for a while. I think I am! But then I anchor myself in what I am doing and like doing and it's really important to me.

Even more specifically, we can make this shared formulation clearer and richer using drawings or letters that summarize what has been achieved so far. This is most useful if it is patients who ask how the work is going. Therapists do not make the effort alone; instead, they involve patients in a shared reflection that they often put together with them in writing or in a chart. If we are at the end of therapy, one naturally summarizes the whole process in preparation for the upcoming separation (Ryle & Kerr, 2002).

Patients are asked to describe, including in writing as homework, how they saw themselves at the beginning of therapy and how they see themselves now, pointing out progress, any areas they think they still need to work on, and aspects of themselves that used to be problems and they now consider mere attitudes. Sometimes, patients show uncertainty; they are gripped by fear about residual areas of vulnerability that might make them feel bad again. We then invite them to describe themselves based on the elements in the shared formulation: "What schema moved me? What wish was driving me? What negative idea of myself was making me suffer?" Then, "What didn't work and what allowed me to feel better?" Above all, "What healthy, benevolent, effective aspects of myself did I discover? In what ways was I able to give them space?"

These reconstructions serve to anticipate problems that will arise normally, equip patients to deal with difficulties, and prevent relapses: "How much and when are negative ideas still taking control? How do I deal with problems and old fears when they resurface? How do I stop when I tend to adopt the old mechanisms?"

End-of-treatment integration includes an awareness that therapy, by definition, leaves a share of *unfinished business* (Greenberg, 2002): patients know how they function, know how to cultivate well-being, but are aware of the vulnerabilities that will accompany them and are equipped to deal with them.

What role do experiential techniques play in achieving such advanced aspects of metacognitive functioning and identity integration? They offer the possibility of sequentially embodying various aspects of self and others. We can, for example, use bodily techniques. We ask patients to imagine themselves in a positive situation and embody it, adopting a posture that allows them to feel it clearly. Then, we invite them to embody another part of themselves and adopt a congruent posture. We ask them to make several transitions from one posture to the other until they feel both parts as their own. Above all, they do not have to reject the negative images; they recognize they are part of them and can sometimes emerge.

Angelina, 35 years old, is an accountant, and at the beginning of therapy suffered from dependent PD with obsessive-compulsive traits and depression. After three years, she has almost fully recovered; she has just separated from her partner, ending a troubled relationship that lasted for years. She is relieved because she has overcome lifetime emotional dependence. During the first summer after her separation, she travels alone to the Greek islands and, to her surprise, has sexual relations with two men she meets on different islands. She returns to therapy after the vacation and is happy; she feels alive again, has surfed for the first time in her life, and talked to locals, sometimes expressing herself almost only in gestures. At the turn of autumn, her depression is coming on again. Instead of locking herself in her home, she signs up on a dating app, again for the first time, and sleeps with a man with whom she found a match that same day. In the weeks that follow, she has more encounters. She describes them at times with pleasure and playfulness, but at some point, moral self-criticism emerges.

A: "I don't like to see myself like that."
T: "How?"
A: "Come on doctor . . . I don't like myself."
T: [*smiling*]: "I see you don't like yourself! In what way? What do you think . . . I am . . .?"
A: "That stuff . . ."
T: [*Smiling, the therapeutic relationship is very good, and humor often characterizes it*]: "Yes, the famous that stuff. Come on, say it!"
A: "Phew . . . I mean . . . I feel like a whore."
T: "Wow! We said it!"

In fact, there are many positive aspects to this part of herself: feeling physically attractive again after her sexuality with her partner has died down; discovering her body capable of feeling pleasure after some physical problems that plagued her;

rekindling her taste for exploration and knowledge; and keeping herself alive and not falling into depression.

The therapist leads her to select a series of moments experienced during the years of therapy. Some are depressive, dull, and lifeless. Others have been laden with anger and frustration. Yet others describe moments of competence at work. After these, they pick out moments together in which she flirts with the first man she met in Greece. The therapist asks her to imagine the scene and embody it in a posture. Then move on to the next scene and adopt the congruent posture. And then repeat it for each of the reenacted episodes.

In this way, Angelina re-inhabits characters from her own internal scenario and, each time, she realizes that the character belongs to her, including the *Angelina who flirts and sleeps with men she has just met*. This is not what she wants for the future, she is aware, but now she knows that even this aspect of herself has a role, a utility, and fully deserves to exist.

Therapy may close here with most patients. At these levels, however, it is common for some symptoms and coping mechanisms to reappear. Patients still have a clear and integrated view of self, but health anxiety, problematic eating behaviors, loss of anger control, perfectionism, and so on reappear at times again. We devote the next chapter to this last step of the decision-making procedures. It is no longer the time for understanding, meaning-making, and returning to explore the past. It is only necessary to devote focused work on symptoms, maladaptive behaviors, and residual coping.

Chapter 13

Dealing with relationship problems, coping, and residual symptoms

We are in the most advanced stages of therapy. Patients are fully aware of the internal structures that guide their functioning and are going in the direction of fulfilling healthy, adaptive wishes. Metacognition is improved: they grasp the various aspects of mental states that run through their mind and recognize their schema-dependent ideas as old thinking habits, which they usually no longer take as true. At the same time, they anchor themselves to more benevolent images of themselves and others and let them be the guide when navigating through social relationships. They have developed a sense of agency over mental states and, when suffering returns, they recognize the mechanisms underlying its re-insurgence and counteract them promptly.

They have also formed an integrated view of themselves in relationships; they see the various aspects of themselves as parts of a more complex play and can adopt different roles as events unfold. They recognize themselves as competitive at times and affectionate at others. There are moments when they return to walking in the shoes of a losing, inferior, unlovable, passive character, but they can see it happening and switch to a different self.

What if symptoms or problem behaviors persist at the end of therapy?

Even in advanced therapy, residual relational problems, symptoms, and dysfunctional behaviors often remain. If therapy works, patients, in the cold winds of reality, sometimes fall back on schema-dependent thinking but come out of it, at least if events do not fit their negative forecasts too closely. In other words, they can counteract an abandonment-centered schema if, for example, their partner does not respond to messages or forgets an appointment. But if a partner leaves them, it is easy for the old schema to seem pretty darn true once again.

In the final stages, however, they maintain differentiation even in the face of major frustrating events: serious problems at work, the end of a romantic relationship, lack of real support from family in times of need, and so on. They think,

> The responses I've received do not make me happy. I feel bad about it, but I keep a good idea of myself. I have limitations, difficulties, flaws, and vulnerabilities, and it's normal, but if I look in the mirror, I like the image I see.

DOI: 10.4324/9781003570967-13

Treating residual symptoms,
behaviural coping and
interpersonal repetitive
thinking using fully-fledged
metacognitive capacities

Forming more sophisticated
and effective mastery
strategies for dealing with
interpersonal situations
according to a richer
understanding of self and
others

Box 10

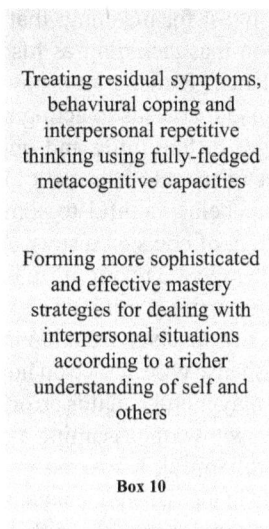

Figure 13.1 Advanced treatment of symptoms and coping and promotion of relational mastery

Additionally, when faced with problems, patients use effective mastery strategies instead of falling into the usual coping.

Despite these skills, relapses occur at the end of successful therapies; schemas regain control even though patients recognize them as such, and tendencies to resort to coping resurface, sometimes tenaciously. At the same time, patients are faced with situations that require social intelligence. Promoting problem-solving strategies through a more articulate knowledge of self and others to deal with residual psychopathology and relational problems is the final therapy step (Figure 13.1., Box 10).

How do we proceed before we get to the moment for shaking hands and waving goodbye to patients, to make sure that they are able to master any return of suffering independently?

Handle the problem in line with the metacognitive levels achieved

First, it is important to know what not to do! Digging into the past again is useless; therapists have to carefully avoid it. Schemas are now known, the history is known, so if patients bring recent narrative episodes we do not go back to asking for remote associations. If they tell episodes from the past, unless they include new, surprising elements that lead us to a substantial revision of the formulation, we do not spend time working on them.

Whatever narrative patients bring to us, therapists should, in essence, ask both themselves and the patients: "Well, what you just told me, in what way does it invite us to act now in session and during the coming week?" We must resist the temptation to go back to the quest for meaning: that would only be pandering to intellectualizations, rumination masquerading as historical and existential reflections, or, even worse, avoidance. Patients steer towards reflections on the past instead of driving down the road that leads to acting better tomorrow.

Therapists sometimes linger in this futile and unproductive search for meaning. Sometimes, they err out of naiveté because old stories sound relevant, and it seems to them that they are being faithful to some kind of higher mission of psychotherapy: making meaning of one's own story. At other times, they err out of fear of creating tension in a therapeutic relationship they find comfortable. Calling patients to therapeutic actions carries a minimal risk of ruptures, minor ones for sure, and yet therapists protect themselves from having to face them.

Another temptation is to dispense wise advice on how to deal with everyday problematic situations. Therapists may indulge in this error, moved by excessive caretaking or the need to assert their own worth: assuming a charismatic role is rewarding; it boosts our self-esteem. And harmful. Nurturing or pretending we are wise only contributes to keeping patients in a passive, dependent, subservient position.

Instead, when patients report minor or major difficulties, therapists are, now that treatment has advanced, expected even more than before to step back and invite patients to cooperate. They should not offer solutions but ask patients to actively seek them: "I understand; the situation you described is challenging. How do you want to work on it now in session with me? How can we deal with this problem during the week?"

Patients talk about residual relationship difficulties, relapses, and resistant symptoms. Therapists listen and validate, but the minimum necessary for patients to feel welcomed. And immediately after, they ask: "How is it that the problem persists, despite us having explored, understood, and even successfully dealt with it over and over again? What behavioral coping mechanisms or forms of repetitive thinking are in place?"

Almost in real time, they turn the question over to patients. The solution to this dilemma is not the responsibility of the therapist alone; it must become a shared quest. We repeat: allowing limited time for the recounting of episodes, particularly historical ones, does not mean approaching patients' suffering superficially. We know that pain originates from life experiences; we understand that patients want to tell us about them again. This is human. We make ourselves, once again, for a few moments, witnesses to the sources of pain. We listen, we validate, we empathize. Now, however, as soon as possible, we point out that the episode just recounted speaks of the schemas that we have already identified, shared, and dealt with many times. There is no need to work on this further unless episodes surface that speak of unexplored areas of the self. In this case, we need to treat them as if it were session 1. The decision-making procedures, by definition, ask us to go back to the initial steps. New problems: ask for episodes. But now we are in the advanced stages of therapy; metacognition is high, and problems have been dissected and treated. Patients just need to actively address their symptoms, coping, and residual relational problems. Dwelling in past pains does not lead to more fertile lands.

Instead, therapists identify with the patients what pattern they have let possess them and what coping strategies they are enacting. We invite patients to summarize their own functioning: "In your opinion, what makes you behave that way or ruminate again? Are there any new elements, or is it something we already know?" We should devote much attention to any type of IRT and dysfunctional protective behaviors, especially avoidance.

Patients believe they can allow themselves to go back to ruminating or implementing behaviors such as self-sacrifice, perfectionism, and so on instead of healthy actions. Almost like saying to themselves: "After all, I just thought about it a little more," or "I know, I just didn't feel that going by my parents was that much of a cost." Patients need to learn and call it self-indulgence, being aware these mechanisms are very likely to snowball and fuel relapse.

Therapists rephrase the contract:

Okay, I see, that pain we know has reoccurred. When the other does X, you feel Y, and at that moment, even if you? do not realize it, you? assume that Y is your? real defect. As a result, you ruminate about it or avoid exposure (or, of course, whatever other residual coping the patient is doing). We know that this will worsen your problems, but we also know that it gives? you power over your reactions. Can we agree that, in this final stage of therapy, we aim to counter repetitive thinking and avoidance (or any other coping) as much as we can?

As can be seen, therapists probe whether patients want their residual pathology treated. In terms of history and functioning, they are only interested in what is useful for planning activities. They stimulate problem-solving instead by involving patients in designing plans to deal with current difficulties. It is necessary to be pragmatic and concrete. If a patient, for example, agrees to counter behavioral coping, we immediately ask: "Well, when are you going to try?"

It may seem like an overly directive, hierarchical attitude, but it is not. If we have come this far, it means that therapy has worked and the alliance is solid. Yes, there is a rank component present, but it is the one inherent in the cooperative system. The two agree on roles, with therapists as a kind of coach suggesting the form, frequency, and pace of exercises and spurring patients on when, as in everything that requires exercise, they tend to give up.

Patients visualize their wish and reenact healthy parts. Therapists ask them to act in the desired direction without allowing themselves to be blocked by repetitive thinking of any kind or enacting their usual coping behaviors. Therapy now takes place mostly in-between sessions. The lion's share of the time goes to exposure procedures. In sessions, we use experiential techniques but only to anticipate *in vitro* the work that the patient will do *in vivo* in the form of homework.

Once patients entrust themselves, the therapeutic relationship becomes just a background that allows patients to turn the exploratory system on and to experience new and beneficial ways of being until they make them their own. The therapist's presence is at the same time diminishing and becoming internalized and stronger. Patients can work in a safe space, take care of themselves, and feel how this reduces symptoms and increases well-being.

Treating residual symptoms and dysfunctional behaviors: an agenda

We now describe the principles that guide therapists in working on symptoms when metacognition is high, and the relationship is solid. In Chapter 8, we described how to work when metacognition is low and the therapeutic relationship unstable, on three areas: dysfunctional symptoms and behaviors, emotional dysregulation, and IRT. We made the case for behavioral intervention procedures, such as a food diary for eating disorders, behavioral activation for depression, experiential techniques for reducing emotional dysregulation in session, and lastly, an eight-step pathway for managing IRT.

Now that metacognitive skills are high, and the relationship is solid, how do these procedures change? At this point, emotional dysregulation is usually no longer a problem. If it occurs, it is short-lived and less intense; patients manage it with strategies they already know: they bring their attention to their body, adjusting their breathing and muscle tension; they accept the temporary increase in emotionality and remember that, as it came, so it will fade away.

Behavioral problems such as binge eating, substance use, behavioral addictions, or emotional dependency may lead patients to return to enacting avoidance. Similarly, it is common to start adopting IRT, which in turn generates relapses into anxiety, depression, or obsessions and compulsions.

Find a renewed agreement on abstaining from any coping

The first step is always setting agreed goals. Therapists ask patients if they are going to actively address the problems:

> At this time, your symptom (or behavior or IRT) is resurfacing. By now, you know where it stems from, what the underlying schemas are and the stimuli triggering it. Yet, when you tend to feel X or behave Y or ruminate, you seem to find it difficult to counteract the pain without resorting to the mechanisms that, we know, make things worse. Now I think, having come to this point, we have to decide how much you want to get rid of your symptoms and problems. We have to be crystal-clear: if you don't actively counteract them, they will come back; it's almost inevitable. If we let you adopt what were your habitual repetitive thinking styles or problem behaviors, symptoms or problems will stay; I have to be frank about on that. If you want to tell me about your symptoms and problems and worries, I need to know that you will be willing to counteract them and not just tell about them. If not, I need to know why you repeat things that you and I know very well. We know that dealing with these symptoms and curbing these tendencies will come at a cost. It will require dealing with pain quotas

and committing to regulating them in a functional way, as we have learned. It is a matter of choosing to reduce or eliminate the pain or, at any rate, knowing that, whenever it recurs, you can counteract it; you will no longer feed it. The alternative, we must be explicit, is to accept that a share of suffering will remain. Clearly, I am on the side of trying, but what do you think?

Introducing, at the end of therapy, an ongoing commitment in the contract to refrain from coping and dysfunctional behaviors is most important. It is a choice between health, understood as significant symptom reduction, relapse prevention, or full recovery on the one hand, and chronicity on the other. Therapists portray possible future scenarios and ask patients which ones they would like to inhabit. Patients know that they can get better, prevent relapses, or manage them quickly, and achieve full recovery. But they must make a commitment. And indeed, pay a price.

Refraining from avoidance, binge eating, and angry outbursts, persisting in autonomy, knowing that loved ones will be hurt, and stopping ruminating generate guilt, shame, and vulnerability – feelings that patients would like to keep at bay, confining them to the distant outskirts of their mind. Therapists, therefore, ask them "Which direction do you choose?" They then perform a simple operation. Just one; that is all that is needed.

Therapists wait for the answer.

Only when they have received an answer do they move forward in the direction of health or chronicity. They have to be ready to accept both scenarios, as in the face of an explicit, clear, insistent question, patients have chosen one of them.

From here onward, sessions almost always follow the principles of exposure-based therapies. Goals need to be operationally defined: for example, deciding to stop tendencies to react with contempt when partners criticize them, or tendencies to drink or binge when shame, loneliness, and vulnerability resurface. Exposure steps are then planned. We can use imagery exposures followed by homework or homework directly. The next session immediately focuses not so much on recounting the problem again but on the patients' actions to deal with it. If they have made efforts, it will already be a success; if they have not tried, we will nonjudgmentally ask: "What happened that prevented you from becoming a therapist of yourself?" Once the obstacles in taking action against the problem have been identified, therapists agree with patients on how to deal with them and schedule new homework.

Therapists now function much like a sport coach or a music teacher; they must continually motivate patients to act therapeutically throughout the week, encourage them to persevere, and maintain commitment, effort, and perseverance in the face of difficulties. Failures are part of the journey; the only problem now is *not trying*. In the face of commitment, therapists visibly display satisfaction. If patients improve, the therapist can celebrate with a light heart: "How nice! Do you realize how easily you were able to be the maker of your well-being and to get rid of that problem that was still bothering you?"

Interrupting behavioral coping and perseverative thinking

In the advanced stages of decision-making procedures or at the end of therapy, coping may resurface, or now that relational problems are resolved, its presence is more easily detected. One patient continues to use cocaine from time to time, another occasionally indulges in alcohol consumption, and another has sporadic binges followed by restriction and compensation with exercise. Others maintain high levels of perfectionism or workaholism. Many return to ruminating about their mistakes or wrongs suffered or worrying about how others will react if they continue to be independent. Above all, however, a great many continue to practice the quintessential behavioral coping: avoidance.

As always, the pivotal operation is to update the contract. The therapist must get a crystal-clear answer to this question: do patients intend to abstain from a behavior or not? Some answers indicate that the intention is "no." Therapists should not let themselves be fooled by answers like: "Okay, I hope I can avoid giving in binge eating when I'm alone at home in the evening" or "Alright, I'll see if I can stop avoiding and will call my colleagues to go out to a restaurant." Therapists should become as alert as an animal in the savannah to these responses, listening for a suspicious rustling. They immediately intervene because "I hope to . . ." or "I'll see if I can, maybe I . . ." almost always indicate that patients are already deciding to avoid at that very moment in session.

Therapists are satisfied only when they have, with patients, identified the precise time of the week, sometimes the exact time of the day, when patients will engage in counteracting a dysfunctional behavior. For example, in the case of binge eating, they may tell a patient:

T: "Okay, so you have decided that you will try to deal with late evening loneliness by resisting the temptation to binge. Very good, and so, when do we start? Tomorrow night? No, maybe better tonight. What do you say? It's not worth waiting, is it?"

It helps if a therapist can combine firmness and inflexibility with irony and playfulness. She can then, with the patient, go over potential adaptive mastery strategies to implement instead of bingeing.

T: "We know that tonight, when you get on the couch, you will feel lonely, right? At that point what is there to help you?"

Imagery rescripting is useful: patients picturing the scene in their mind try to react differently, practicing adaptive behaviors.

T: "Close your eyes and try to visualize the scene you will be in. How would you like to respond to that sense of emptiness and loneliness? Can you imagine doing something healthy or otherwise different than going to the fridge? Do you like that part of yourself that can do something good for you? What qualities does it have?"

When patients recall a healthy self-aspect, the final step is simple:

T: "Good, now try and do it."

After updating the contract and, if necessary, coaching adaptive behaviors with imagery rescripting or role-playing, the rest of the work takes place in-between sessions: behavioral exercises, followed by behavioral exercises, reinforced by behavioral exercises until patients recover or are satisfied with their coping skills, knowing that problems can resurface, yes, but will not overwhelm them.

Use articulated metacognitive skills to move through relationships

As we have seen, many patients have limited strategies for acting in social relationships, solving problems and conflicts, negotiating their goals with others, modifying behaviors flexibly as contexts change, or adapting to the rules of the environment. If they realize that a social situation does not suit them, they see walls and barriers, but not a way out, which instead exists. They therefore lack mastery strategies (Carcione et al., 2011). In chapter 8, we describe how to promote them when metacognition is low.

We now show how to develop the highest levels of mastery, that is, the ability to devise strategies for adaptively realizing one's goals and solving social problems based on a rich, articulate, and mature knowledge of one's own mind and that of others.

It is a step partly already initiated in the procedures described in chapter 11, in the points where we illustrate how patients can interrupt dysfunctional interpersonal cycles and use a richer and more mature theory of the others' minds and attempt to realize their own nuclear wishes in reality.

Remember that, without awareness of one's role in causing problems, it is not possible to solve them: if an individual realizes that it is his or her own submissive attitude that causes others to underestimate him or her, he or she can attempt to communicate more openly and directly, increasing the chances of being appreciated.

Realizing how we cannot give up certain goals, that if we let them go we would pay too high a cost in terms of psychological health, joy, and personal fulfillment, is the driver to keep striving for them. We also need to become skilled at understanding what others are thinking and why, so as to devise strategies for cooperating and paths for overcoming conflicts. To express our desires in a way that maximizes the likelihood that our requests will be accepted. Good theory of mind also allows us to recognize when it is futile to insist, when the others are inflexible, and none of our efforts have the power to make them change their mind. A refined understanding of others, a decentered knowledge of how they function, also allows us to decide what are the best times to enter their attentional span and call them to interact with us. Finally, it is beneficial to know who we are as our self-facets change, to know the multiplicity of purposes and goals that drive us, so that we can define hierarchies among them and implement appropriate, goal- and context-specific strategies (Semerari et al., 2003).

In short, when therapy is at advanced stages or nearing completion, patients need to use psychological knowledge pragmatically: "How can I behave at work to carry out my project, avoiding incidents?"; "How do I deal with my teenage daughter who rebels against rules, doesn't study, and stays stubbornly in silence at dinner?"

We now help patients plan and implement behaviors based on full awareness of their goals: "What do I want?" means-ends relationship: "What do I have to do to get what I want?" or cost-benefit: "What will I have to spend, what will I have to give up? What will be the gain in well-being, health and satisfaction if I achieve the purpose?," and of the social context: "How can I lead others to support me?"

Therapists actively help patients build strategies, and experiential techniques are valuable. For example, they simulate interaction with role-play or chairwork. We suggest following precise steps to promote advanced mastery, although in a non-mandatory sequence.

1. Summarize what is understood about schema structure and remember that one is moving to achieve a core wish or to cope with the consequences of its frustration. It is then a matter of trying to ask others in adaptive ways, enriching strategies and making them more flexible, or regulating one's emotions and behaviors in case of negative responses.
2. Make patients anchor themselves to their core wishes and feel them emotionally. They must act by feeling that the purpose is relevant. Simultaneously, they must be invited to form an articulate representation of how others would think, feel, and behave, considering different possibilities and remembering that they do not have to take for granted that these will be the actual reactions.
3. Lead patients to move in new ways, entering an atmosphere of discovery without certainty of what will happen. One must make sure that patients act guided by the exploratory motive, knowing that searching for something new involves emotional risks and deciding to take them.
4. Assess if setting new therapeutic tasks, the most important component of the alliance (Bordin, 1979) at stake here, activates schemas in the therapeutic relationship. It is possible, in fact, for schemas to be activated, even at this late stage in therapy, for two reasons. The first is that we assume that patients' behaviors are indeed dysfunctional or that their repertoire of action is really limited. We are therefore pointing at some, so to speak, real flow. It is possible that patients blame themselves for this or read the therapists' invitations as criticism. If this happens, it is good that it emerges immediately so that the schema activation or

micro-rupture can usually be overcome quickly. Secondly, it is easy for patients to feel disoriented, and this elicits helplessness, inability, and fear of loneliness, that often best anyone treading a new path. These are normal reactions to accompany the process of discovery, but again, it is good to bring them out and regulate them.

5. Plan the new action, designing adaptive strategies based on knowledge of one's own wishes, aptitudes, and limits, as well as knowledge of others. And remember, as we noted earlier, that we will likely discover something new about ourselves and others.

6. Simulate the action in session. One excellent exercise is role-play, in which therapists and patients repeatedly switch roles. Patients attempt to express themselves in various ways while therapists offer feedback, and together they assess whether the style adopted worked or what problems it generated. In the role exchange, therapists can mimic patients' behavior so that the latter, in the others' shoes, evaluate its impact. Or, therapists can try modelling different styles so that patients learn alternative possibilities. Next, patients wear their own shoes again and try to make the innovations proposed by the therapist their own, modifying them as desired. Alternatively, future-focused imagery exercises can be used in which patients evaluate the impact of their own actions with as realistic a knowledge of the other as possible. They evaluate how the imagined others react and what impact the actions generate. At the end of the imagery, they have a viable action plan.

7. Agree on behavioral experiments. This is the decisive step: trying to act differently in the real world. The previous steps are about getting there free of schemas, ready for discovery, and with a flexible repertoire already partly trained.

8. Reflect on the behavioral experiments in the next session. Were they successful, or were there problems? Most importantly, what did we discover about the patient and the people around them? How can the findings be used during subsequent experiments?

9. Monitor the therapeutic relationship. While performing an exercise, did a patient see the therapist as benevolent and supportive, or critical and disappointed? Or pushy and constricting? Or demanding but, like a good coach, able to encourage one to overcome difficulties under pressure with confidence and tenacity?

We repeat that none of the preceding steps is mandatory, and it is not always necessary to use role-play and guided imagery before behavioral experiments: very often, just discussing alternative strategies and then inviting patients to implement them does the job. The impact on the therapeutic relationship is often marginal, and investigating it can be a scholastic exercise if the atmosphere appears positive and patients, even with the inevitable difficulties, carry out the experiments and remain curious about the emerging self.

It is a moment of discovery; schemas can reappear, but what is important is to find new, more effective ways of expressing oneself and communicating based on a more open and realistic view of the world and an accurate knowledge of others.

The examples are many and various: entering the world of work after prolonged social withdrawal, coping with independent living after having always depended on parents, and opening up to relationships after years consumed by behavioral and substance addictions. In all these cases, an obstacle to overcome manifests itself: a lack of knowledge of others' minds.

Daniel is 23 years old and suffers from avoidant PD. He has never had a girl-friend. He knows that his tendencies toward shame, passivity, and giving up any goals are schema-driven, and he is overcoming them. But romantic relationships are unknown to him. He agrees with the therapist to use Instagram. He starts following comic book authors and music groups he loves. He starts posting comments and responding to some girls' comments. Then he follows their profiles and posts what a female friend explains to him as "tactical likes." That is, likes added to old posts on that girl's profile, indicating attention. At this stage, the idea of being and looking like "a moron" emerges, but he quickly overcomes it. Except that he does not know how to carry forward the conversation. The therapist and Daniel use role-play and imagery on future scenarios: they write messages and responses. They also design preliminary behavioral experiments: consulting with friends again and asking them how they would react to Daniel's approaches. The friends willingly lend themselves to the game: Daniel tells of several "female support sessions," cheerful evenings from which he comes out with new ideas on how to court a girl. He now has tools, albeit certainly imperfect ones, but it is a starting point.

He soon finds a good icebreaker and starts a conversation with a girl who shares his musical tastes. He invites her for an aperitif, and she accepts. When he talks about the rendezvous to the therapist, they both sense that Daniel really likes her. He engages with the therapist, amid much laughter, in a series of role-plays with various role switches to communicate to the girl that he likes her: "How might you express yourself? How might the girl react?" After a couple of weeks, Daniel has his first sexual intercourse and begins a romantic relationship.

These steps are a prelude to the conclusion of therapy. Patients now move through the world with more confidence, free of the influence of schemas. When these bite, they do not sink their teeth; they stay for only a limited time. Patients recognize them and can shake them off. When negative self-images surface, they know they are part of the cast of characters in their internal theater but no longer protagonists. They are inhabited by small insecurities; they have limits and flaws, but they accept them, and these no longer prevent them from moving forward, playing, and exploring the world with hope.

Chapter 14

Conclusions

Technically active yet relationship-conscious

Our goal has been to explain how to treat patients with personality disorders and post-traumatic disorders, which co-occur with all sorts of symptom disorders. Letting such patients discover more benevolent, future-oriented images of themselves and others, in which self-directedness, curiosity, and hope are present, requires commitment. Reducing symptoms requires commitment. Disrupting many and various coping strategies, such as avoidance, perfectionism, submissive addiction, aggression, binge eating and compensatory mechanisms, alcohol and substance use, and all forms of repetitive thinking, requires commitment.

Our key aim was to show how it is unthinkable to treat these patients only through attention to the therapeutic relationship. Just as it is unrealistic to use the repertoire of experiential and behavioral techniques without paying enormous attention to the therapeutic relationship.

We started with an attempt to classify patterns of interaction between techniques and therapeutic relationships. We summarize them:

1. The very proposal of a technique causes a major disruption that requires immediate attention instead of continuing with the technique itself.
2. The technique generates negative effects that cause a minor rupture. It needs to be repaired, but immediately afterward, therapists can go back to using the technique.
3. The technique generates negative, often not visible effects. Patients are able either with minimal work or spontaneously to overcome them without discontinuing it. An initial micro-rupture is followed by consolidation.
4. The technique strengthens the relationship: patients become curious, experience a sense of activity, and see the therapists as competent and able to help.
5. The positive results that the technique produces create a sense of confidence and security.

It should be clear after having read this volume how radically far our approach is from the scared attitude of many therapists who do not use the techniques or delay their application for fear of breaking the alliance and causing dysregulation.

DOI: 10.4324/9781003570967-14

One of the most frequent mistakes seems to be not intervening actively. Our work, throughout this volume, has been to design specific, detailed procedures for being active, for using experiential techniques and behavioral experiments full steam, while paying continuous attention to the vicissitudes of the therapeutic relationship.

We hope to have taken a step forward from our previous work, and this volume will guide therapists in effectively dealing with the widest possible range of clinical situations. It will help them quickly recognize when they are acting too cautiously or too hastily. Or when they are being driven by their haste and not by case formulation. The procedures designed here may help them step back and ask themselves: "What is the necessary action with this patient right now, based on the formulation?"

We note that young colleagues, during their first years of clinical practice, often make mistakes from too much caution or too much momentum. Here, we offer procedures that will enable them to correct errors, refine formulation, reformulate the therapeutic contract – which is one of the most effective and most neglected ingredients of psychotherapy – and move toward treating interpersonal problems and symptoms. The hope is that treatments guided by these principles will be effective and, as long as it is reasonably possible with a particular pathology and in light of a particular functioning, rapid.

Is it about proposing short-term treatments? No. It is about aiming for the fastest possible speed in alleviating suffering and relational dysfunction. With some patients, a few months will be enough; with others, it will still take years. What matters is that, throughout the time of working with a person, therapists remain firm, alert in their formulation, attentive to the relationship, and active, stopping only when the patient asks. At that point, they revisit the contract and redefine goals and tasks.

Being therapists of patients with personality disorders and their comorbid conditions requires attention to the barriers they unintentionally put up to treatment. We must be unyielding with ourselves, not stopping at these barriers unless patients ask us aloud. It requires us to tolerate helplessness and frustration while sustaining an ongoing sense of confidence and orientation to the future, of inner peace when therapy stagnates, while we wonder how to get out of the swamp together with the patients. Every step achieved, no matter how tiny, brings a little joy to us.

As this book comes out, studies are continuing on the effectiveness of MIT in its various formats and for various problems. Our deep-seated personal wish is to gather growing empirical evidence to support our efforts and to keep on improving our model as data comes in and points to what to change and what is working.

References

Alexander, F., & French, F. (1946). *Psychoanalytic therapy: Principles and application.* Ronald Press.

American Psychiatric Association. (2022). *Diagnostic and statistical manual of mental disorders* (5th ed., text revision). https://doi.org/10.1176/appi.books.9780890425787

Ames, D. R. (2004). Inside the mind-reader's toolkit: Projection and stereotyping in mental state inference. *Journal of Personality and Social Psychology, 87,* 340–353. https://psycnet.apa.org/doi/10.1037/0022-3514.87.3.340

Andermann, M., Izurieta Hidalgo, N. A., Rupp, A., Schmahl, C., Herpertz, S. C., & Bertsch, K. (2022). Behavioral and neurophysiological correlates of emotional face processing in borderline personality disorder: Are there differences between men and women? *European Archives of Psychiatry and Clinical Neuroscience, 272*(8), 1583–1594. https://doi.org/10.1007/s00406-022-01434-4

Arntz, A. (2012). Imagery rescripting as a therapeutic technique: Review of clinical trials, basic studies, and research agenda. *Journal of Experimental Psychopathology, 3*(2), 189–208. https://psycnet.apa.org/doi/10.5127/jep.024211

Austin, T. M. (2011). *A task analysis of metacommunication in time-limited dynamic psychotherapy* [Doctoral dissertation, Antioch University, OhioLINK Electronic Theses and Dissertations Center].

Bamelis, L. L., Evers, S. M., Spinhoven, P., & Arntz, A. (2014). Results of a multicenter randomized controlled trial of the clinical effectiveness of schema therapy for personality disorders. *American Journal of Psychiatry, 171*(3), 305–322. Https://doi.org/10.1176/appi.ajp.2013.12040518

Bateman, A. W., & Fonagy, P. (2004). Mentalization-based treatment of BPD. *Journal of Personality Disorders, 18*(1), 36–51. https://psycnet.apa.org/doi/10.1521/pedi.18.1.36.32772

Beck, A. T., Baruch, E., Balter, J. M., Steer, R. A., & Warman, D. M. (2004). A new instrument for measuring insight: The Beck Cognitive Insight Scale. *Schizophrenia Research, 68*(2–3), 319–329. https://doi.org/10.1016/s0920-9964(03)00189-0

Beck, E., Bo, S., Jørgensen, M. S., Gondan, M., Poulsen, S., Storebø, O. J., Fjelldad Andersen, C., Folmo, E., Sharp, C., Pedersen, J., & Simonsen, E. (2020). Mentalization-based treatment in groups for adolescents with borderline personality disorder: A randomized controlled trial. *Journal of Child Psychology and Psychiatry, 61,* 594–604. https://doi.org/10.1111/jcpp.13152

Bell, T., Montague, J., Elander, J., & Gilbert, P. (2021). Suddenly you are King Solomon: Multiplicity, transformation and integration in compassion focused therapy chairwork. *Journal of Psychotherapy Integration, 31*(3), 223–237. https://psycnet.apa.org/doi/10.1037/int0000240

Bennett-Levy, J. (2019). Why therapists should walk the talk: The theoretical and empirical case for personal practice in therapist training and professional development. *Journal of*

Behavior Therapy and Experimental Psychiatry, *62*, 133–145. https://doi.org/10.1016/j. jbtep.2018.08.004

Bertsch, K., Buades-Rotger, M., Krauch, M., Ueltzhöffer, K., Kleindienst, N., Herpertz, S. C., & Krämer, U. M. (2022). Abnormal processing of interpersonal cues during an aggressive encounter in women with borderline personality disorder: Neural and behavioral findings. *Journal of Psychopathology and Clinical Science*, *131*(5), 493–506. https://doi.org/10.1037/abn0000756

Bohus, M., Kleindienst, N., Hahn, C., Müller-Engelmann, M., Ludäscher, P., Steil, R., Fydrich, T., Kuehner, C., Resick, P. A., Stiglmayr, C., Schmahl, C., & Priebe, K. (2020). Dialectical behavior therapy for posttraumatic stress disorder (DBTPTSD) compared with cognitive processing therapy (CPT) in complex presentations of PTSD in women survivors of childhood abuse: A randomized clinical trial. *JAMA Psychiatry*, *77*(12), 1235–1245. https://doi.org/10.1001/jamapsychiatry.2020.2148

Bordin, E. S. (1979). The generalizability of the psychoanalytic concept of the working alliance. *Psychotherapy: Theory, Research & Practice*, *16*(3), 252. https://psycnet.apa.org/doi/10.1037/h0085885

Boterhoven de Haan, K., Lee, C., Fassbinder, E., Van Es, S., Menninga, S., Meewisse, M., & Arntz, A. (2020). Imagery rescripting and eye movement desensitisation and reprocessing as treatment for adults with posttraumatic stress disorder from childhood trauma: Randomised clinical trial. *The British Journal of Psychiatry*, *217*(5), 609–615. https://doi.org/10.1192/bjp.2020.158

Bowlby, J. (1988). *Clinical applications of attachment: A secure base*. Routledge.

Brand, R. M., Bendall, S., Hardy, A., Rossell, S. L., & Thomas, N. (2021). Trauma-focused imaginal exposure for auditory hallucinations: A case series. *Psychology and Psychotherapy: Theory, Research & Practice*, *94*, 408–425. https://doi.org/10.1111/papt.12284

Broomhall, A. G., Phillips, W. J., Hine, D. W., & Loi, N. M. (2017). Upward counterfactual thinking and depression: A meta-analysis. *Clinical Psychology Review*, *55*, 56–73. https://psycnet.apa.org/doi/10.1016/j.cpr.2017.04.010

Browning, C. (1999). Floatback and float forward: Techniques for linking past, present and future. *EMDRIA Newsletter*, *4*(3), 12.

Caligor, E., Clarkin, J. F., & Yeomans, F. E. (2019). Transference-focused psychotherapy for narcissistic and borderline personality disorders. In D. Kealy & J. S. Ogrodniczuk (Eds.), *Contemporary psychodynamic psychotherapy: Evolving clinical practice*. Elsevier.

Carcione, A., Dimaggio, G., Conti, L., Fiore, D., Nicolò, G., & Semerari, A. (2010). *Metacognition assessment scale-R, scoring manual V.4.0*. Unpublished manuscript.

Carcione, A., Nicolò, G., & Semerari, A. (2021). *Complex cases of personality disorders*. Springer.

Carcione, A., Semerari, A., Nicolò, G., Pedone, R., Popolo, R., Conti, L., Fiore, D., Procacci, M., & Dimaggio, G. (2011). Metacognitive mastery dysfunctions in personality disorder psychotherapy. *Psychiatry Research*, *190*, 60–71. https://doi.org/10.1016/j.psychres.2010.12.032

Carver, C. S., Scheier, M. F., & Weintraub, J. K. (1989). Assessing coping strategies: A theoretically based approach. *Journal of Personality & Social Psychology*, *56*(2), 267–283. https://psycnet.apa.org/doi/10.1037/0022-3514.56.2.267

Caselli, G., & Spada, M. M. (2015). Desire thinking: What is it and what drives it? *Addictive Behaviors*, *44*, 71–79. https://doi.org/10.1016/j.addbeh.2014.07.021

Centonze, A., Popolo, R., MacBeth, A., & Dimaggio, G. (2021). Building the alliance and using experiential techniques in the early phases of psychotherapy for Avoidant Personality Disorder. *Journal of Clinical Psychology: In Session*, *77*, 1219–1232. https://doi.org/10.1002/jclp.23143

Chanen, A. M., Jackson, H. J., McCutcheon, L. K., Jovev, M., Dudgeon, P., Yuen, H. P., & McGorry, P. D. (2008). Early intervention for adolescents with borderline personality disorder using cognitive analytic therapy: Randomised controlled trial. *The British Journal of Psychiatry, 193*(6), 477–484. https://doi.org/10.1192/bjp.bp.107.048934

Cheli, S., Lysaker, P. H., & Dimaggio, G. (2019). Metacognitively oriented psychotherapy for Schizotypal Personality Disorder: A two cases series. *Personality and Mental Health, 13*, 155–167. https://doi.org/10.1002/pmh.1447

Choi-Kain, L. W., Masland, S. R., & Finch, E. F. (2023). Corrective experiences to enhance trust: Clinical wisdom from good (enough) psychiatric management. *Journal of Personality Disorders, 37*(5), 559–579. https://psycnet.apa.org/doi/10.1521/pedi.2023.37.5.559

Chow, D. L., Miller, S. D., Seidel, J. A., Kane, R. T., Thornton, J. A., & Andrews, W. P. (2015). The role of deliberate practice in the development of highly effective psychotherapists. *Psychotherapy, 52*(3), 337–345. https://psycnet.apa.org/doi/10.1037/pst0000015

Cosmides, L., & Tooby, J. (2013). Evolutionary psychology: New perspectives on cognition and motivation. *Annual Review of Psychology, 64*(1), 201–229. https://doi.org/10.1146/annurev.psych.121208.131628

Critchfield, K. L., Gazzillo, F., & Kramer, U. (2022). Case formulation of interpersonal patterns and its impact on the therapeutic process: Introduction to the issue. *Journal of Clinical Psychology, 78*, 379–385. https://psycnet.apa.org/doi/10.1002/jclp.23322

Del Giudice, M. (2014). An evolutionary life history framework for psychopathology. *Psychological Inquiry, 25*(3–4), 261–300. https://doi.org/10.1080/1047840X.2014.884918

Deng, W., Hu, D., Xu, S., Liu, X., Zhao, J., Chen, Q., & Li, X. (2019). The efficacy of virtual reality exposure therapy for PTSD symptoms: A systematic review and meta-analysis. *Journal of Affective Disorders, 257*, 698–709. https://doi.org/10.1016/j.jad.2019.07.086

Dimaggio, G. (2022). Treatment principles for pathological narcissism and narcissistic personality disorder. *Journal of Psychotherapy Integration, 32*, 408–425. https://doi.org/10.1037/int0000263

Dimaggio, G., MacBeth, A., Popolo, R., Salvatore, G., Perrini, F., Raouna, A., Osam, C. S., Buonocore, L., Bandiera, A., & Montano, A. (2018). The problem of overcontrol: Perfectionism and emotional inhibition as predictors of personality disorder. *Comprehensive Psychiatry, 83*, 71–78. https://doi.org/10.1016/j.comppsych.2018.03.005

Dimaggio, G., Montano, A., Popolo, R., & Salvatore, G. (2015). *Metacognitive interpersonal therapy for personality disorders: A treatment manual*. Routledge.

Dimaggio, G., Ottavi, P., Popolo, R., & Salvatore, G. (2020). *Metacognitive interpersonal therapy body, imagery and change*. Routledge.

Dimaggio, G., Salvatore, G., MacBeth, A., Ottavi, P., Buonocore, L., & Popolo, R. (2017). Metacognitive interpersonal therapy for personality disorders: A case study series. *Journal of Contemporary Psychotherapy, 47*, 11–21. https://psycnet.apa.org/doi/10.1007/s10879-016-9342-7

Dimaggio, G., Semerari, A., Carcione, A., Nicolò, G., & Procacci, M. (2007). *Psychotherapy of personality disorders: Metacognition, states of mind and interpersonal cycles*. Routledge.

Dimaggio, G., & Shahar, G. (2017). Behavioural activation as a key principle of change in the psychotherapy of adult mental disorders. *Psychotherapy, 54*(3), 221–224. http://dx.doi.org/10.1037/pst0000117

Dimaggio, G., & Valentino, V. (2024). The ongoing rewriting of the therapeutic contract in Metacognitive Interpersonal Therapy for narcissistic personality disorder: The case of Mark. *Journal of Clinical Psychology: In Session, 80*(4), 776–794. https://doi.org/10.1002/jclp.23621

Dimaggio, G., Vanheule, S., Lysaker, P. H., Carcione, A., & Nicolò, G. (2009). Impaired self-reflection in psychiatric disorders among adults: A proposal for the existence of a network of semi independent functions. *Consciousness and Cognition, 18*, 653–664. https://psycnet.apa.org/doi/10.1016/j.concog.2009.06.003

Duffy, K. E. M., Simmonds-Buckley, M., Haake, R., Delgadillo, J. M., & Barkham, M. (2023). The efficacy of individual humanistic-experiential therapies for the treatment of depression: A systematic review and meta-analysis of randomized controlled trials. *Psychotherapy Research*, *34*, 323–338. https://doi.org/10.1080/10503307.2023.2227757

Dufresne, L., Bussières, E. L., Bédard, A., Gingras, N., Blanchette-Sarrasin, A., & Bégin, C. (2020). Personality traits in adolescents with eating disorder: A meta-analytic review. *Journal of Eating Disorders*, *53*(2), 157–173. https://doi.org/10.1002/eat.23183

Dugué, R., Renner, F., Austermann, M., Tuschen-Caffier, B., & Jacob, G. A. (2019). Imagery rescripting in individuals with binge-eating behavior: An experimental proof-of-concept study. *International Journal Eating Disorders*, *52*, 183–188. https://doi.org/10.1002/eat.22995

Ehret, A. M., Joormann, J., & Berking, M. (2015). Examining risk and resilience factors for depression: The role of self-criticism and self-compassion. *Cognition and Emotion*, *29*(8), 1496–1504. https://doi.org/10.1080/02699931.2014.992394

Ehring, T., & Watkins, E. R. (2008). Repetitive negative thinking as a transdiagnostic process. *International Journal of Cognitive Therapy*, *1*(3), 192–205. https://doi.org/10.1521/ijct.2008.1.3.192

Elliott, R., Bohart, A., Larson, D., Muntigl, P., & Smoliak, O. (2023). Empathic reflections by themselves are not effective: Meta-analysis and qualitative synthesis. *Psychotherapy Research*, *33*(7), 957–973. https://doi.org/10.1080/10503307.2023.2218981

Ellis, A. (2010). *Overcoming destructive beliefs, feelings, and behaviors: New directions for rational emotive behavior therapy*. Prometheus Books.

Fairburn, C. G., Cooper, Z., & Shafran, R. (2003). Cognitive behaviour therapy for eating disorders: A transdiagnostic theory and treatment. *Behaviour Researach and Therapy*, *41*(5), 509–528. https://doi.org/10.1016/s0005-7967(02)00088-8

Farina, B., Liotti, M., Imperatori, C., Tombolini, L., Gasperini, E., Mallozzi, P., Russo, M., Simoncini Malucelli, G., & Monticelli, F. (2023). Cooperation within the therapeutic relationship improves metacognitive functioning: Preliminary findings. *Research in Psychotherapy: Psychopathology, Process and Outcome*, *26*(3). https://psycnet.apa.org/doi/10.4081/ripppo.2023.712

Fioravanti, G., Dimaggio, G., MacBeth, A., Nicolis, M., & Popolo, R. (2023). Metacognitive interpersonal therapy-eating disorders versus cognitive behavioral therapy for eating disorders for non-underweight adults with eating disorders: Study protocol for a pilot pre-registered randomized controlled trial. *Research in Psychotherapy: Psychopathology, Process and Outcome*, *26*(2), 690. https://doi.org/10.4081/ripppo.2023.690

Fioravanti, G., MacBeth, A., Cheli, S., Popolo, R., Nicolosi, V., & Dimaggio, G. (2024). Metacognitive Interpersonal Therapy for Eating Disorders (MIT-ED) including underweight participants. Study protocol for a single arm feasibility study.

Fioravanti, G., MacBeth, A., Popolo, R., Travagnin, F., Nicolis, M., & Dimaggio, G. (2025). Metacognitive interpersonal therapy-eating disorders (MIT-ED) versus CBT-E for adults: A proof-of-concept randomized controlled trial. *International Journal of Eating Disorders*, *58*(5), 993–998. https://doi.org/10.1002/eat.24408

Fioravanti, G., Popolo, R., MacBeth, A., & Dimaggio, G. (in press). Metacognitive interpersonal therapy eating disorders (MIT-ED) in the case of an 18-year-old girl with avoidant and obsessive-compulsive personality disorders, binge eating disorder and obesity. *Journal of Clinical Psychology: In Session*.

Flückiger, C., Del Re, A. C., Wampold, B. E., & Horvath, A. O. (2018). The alliance in adult psychotherapy: A meta-analytic synthesis. *Psychotherapy*, *55*(4), 316–340. https://doi.org/10.1037/pst0000172

Fonagy, P., Gergely, G., & Jurist, E. L. (2018). *Affect regulation, mentalization and the development of the self*. Routledge.

Fuchs, T. (2007). Fragmented selves: Temporality and identity in borderline personality disorder. *Psychopathology*, *40*(6), 379–387. https://doi.org/10.1159/000106468

Gazzillo, F. (2023). Toward a more comprehensive understanding of pathogenic beliefs: Theory and clinical implications. *Journal of Contemporary Psychotherapy: On the Cutting Edge of Modern Developments in Psychotherapy, 53*(3), 227–234. https://doi.org/10.1007/s10879-022-09564-5

Gazzillo, F., Curtis, J., & Silberschatz, G. (2022). The plan formulation method: An empirically validated and clinically useful procedure applied to a clinical case of a patient with a severe personality disorder. *Journal of Clinical Psychology, 78*(3), 409–421. https://doi.org/10.1002/jclp.23299

Goldman, R. N., & Goldstein, Z. (2023). Guiding task work in the context of an emotion-focused relationship. *Journal of Clinical Psychology, 79*, 1627–1640. https://doi.org/10.1002/jclp.23472

Goldman, R. N., Vaz, A., & Rousmaniere, T. (2021). *Deliberate practice in emotion-focused therapy*. American Psychological Association. https://doi.org/10.1037/0000227-000

Gonçalves, M. M., Ribeiro, A. P., Stiles, W. B., Conde, T., Matos, M., Martins, C., & Santos, A. (2011). The role of mutual in-feeding in maintaining problematic self-narratives: Exploring one path to therapeutic failure. *Psychotherapy Research, 21*(1), 27–40. https://doi.org/10.1080/10503307.2010.507789

Gordon-King, K., Schweitzer, R. D., & Dimaggio, G. (2018). Metacognitive interpersonal therapy for personality disorders featuring emotional inhibition: A multiple baseline case series. *Journal of Nervous and Mental Disease, 206*(4), 263–269. https://doi.org/10.1097/nmd.0000000000000789

Greenberg, L. S. (2002). *Emotion-focused therapy: Coaching clients to work with their feelings*. American Psychological Association.

Harned, M. S., Schmidt, S. C., Korslund, K. E., & Gallop, R. J. (2021). Does adding the dialectical behavior therapy prolonged exposure (DBT PE) protocol for PTSD to DBT improve outcomes in public mental health settings? A pilot nonrandomized effectiveness trial with benchmarking. *Behavior Therapy, 52*, 639–655. https://doi.org/10.1016/j.beth.2020.08.003

Harrington, S., Pascual-Leone, A., Paivio, S., Edmondstone, C., & Baher, T. (2021). Depth of experiencing and therapeutic alliance: What predicts outcome for whom in emotion-focused therapy for trauma? *Psychology and Psychotherapy: Theory, Research & Practice, 94*, 895–914. https://doi.org/10.1111/papt.12342

Hermans, H. J. M., & Dimaggio, G. (Eds.). (2004). *The dialogical self in psychotherapy: An introduction.* Brunner-Routledge.

Hermans, H. J. M., Kempen, H. J. G., & van Loon, R. J. P. (1992). The dialogical self: Beyond individualism and rationalism. *American Psychologist, 47*(1), 23–33.

Hewitt, P. L., Flett, G. L., & Mikail, S. F. (2017). *Perfectionism: Conceptualization, assessment, and treatment*. Guilford Press.

Hill, C. E., Kivlighan, D. M. III, Rousmaniere, T., Kivlighan, D. M., Jr., Gerstenblith, J. A., & Hillman, J. W. (2020). Deliberate practice for the skill of immediacy: A multiple case study of doctoral student therapists and clients. *Psychotherapy, 57*(4), 587–597. https://doi.org/10.1037/pst0000247

Hoppen, T. H., Lindemann, A. S., & Morina, N. (2022). Safety of psychological interventions for adult post-traumatic stress disorder: Meta-analysis on the incidence and relative risk of deterioration, adverse events and serious adverse events. *The British Journal of Psychiatry, 221*(5), 658–667. https://doi.org/10.1192/bjp.2022.111

Horowitz, M. J. (1979). *States of mind: Analysis of change in psychotherapy.* Springer.

Inchausti, F., Garcia-Mieres, H., Garcia-Poveda, N. V., Fonseca-Pedrero, E., MacBeth, A., Popolo, R., & Dimaggio, G. (2023). Recovery-focused metacognitive interpersonal therapy (MIT) for adolescents with first-episode psychosis. *Journal of Contemporary Psychotherapy, 53*, 9–17. https://doi.org/10.1007/s10879-022-09569-0

Inchausti, F., García-Poveda, N. V., Ballesteros-Prados, A., Fonseca-Pedrero, E., MacBeth, A., Popolo, R., & Dimaggio, G. (2024). Metacognitive interpersonal group therapy for adolescents (MIT-GA) with personality disorders: A randomized controlled trial. *Submitted.*

Inchausti, F., Moreno-Campos, L., Prado-Abril, J., Sánchez-Reales, S., Fonseca-Pedrero, E., MacBeth, A., Popolo, R., & Dimaggio, G. (2020). Metacognitive interpersonal therapy in group (MIT-G) for personality disorders: Preliminary results from a pilot study in a public mental health setting. *Journal of Contemporary Psychotherapy, 50*(3), 97–203. https://doi.org/10.1007/s10879-020-09453-9

Janet, P. (1928). *L'évolution de la mémoire et de la notion du temps* (Vol. 1). A. Chahine.

Kadriu, F., Claes, L., Witteman, C., & Krans, J. (2022). Imagery rescripting of autobiographical memories versus intrusive images in individuals with disordered eating. *Cognitive Therapy and Research, 46*(4), 764–775. https://doi.org/10.1007/s10608-021-10258-w

Kaplan, D. M., Palitsky, R., Carey, A. L., Crane, T. E., Havens, C. M., Medrano, M. R., & O'Connor, M. F. (2018). Maladaptive repetitive thought as a transdiagnostic phenomenon and treatment target: An integrative review. *Journal of Clinical Psychology, 74*(7), 1126–1136. https://doi.org/10.1002/jclp.22585

Kelley, K., Miller, J. A. M., Mason, C. K., & DeShong, H. L. (2024). Investigating the transdiagnostic potential of rumination in relation to Cluster B personality disorder symptoms. *Personality Disorders: Theory, Research, and Treatment, 15*(6), 469–478. https://doi.org/10.1037/per0000690

Kelly-Weeder, S., Kells, M., Jennings, K., Dunne, J., & Wolfe, B. (2018). Procedures and protocols for weight assessment during acute illness in individuals with anorexia nervosa: A national survey. *Journal of American Psychiatry and Nurses Association, 24*(3), 241–246. https://doi.org/10.1177/1078390317717790

Kiesler, D. J. (1996). *Contemporary interpersonal theory and research: Personality, psychopathology, and psychotherapy.* Wiley.

Kip, A., Schoppe, L., Arntz, A., & Morina, N. (2023). Efficacy of imagery rescripting in treating mental disorders associated with aversive memories-An updated meta-analysis. *Journal of Anxiety Disorders, 102772.* https://doi.org/10.1016/j.janxdis.2023.102772

Kramer, U. (Ed.). (2019). *Case formulation for personality disorders. Tailoring psychotherapy to the individual client.* Academic Press.

Lazarus, R. S., & Folkman, S. (1984). *Stress, appraisal, and coping.* Springer.

Leahy, R. L. (2008). The therapeutic relationship in cognitive-behavioral therapy. *Behavioural and Cognitive Psychotherapy, 36*(6), 769–777. https://doi.org/10.1017/S1352465808004852

Leahy, R. L. (2019). Introduction: Emotional schemas and emotional schema therapy. *International Journal of Cognitive Therapy, 12*(1), 1–4. https://doi.org/10.1007/s41811-018-0038-5

Leboeuf, I., & Antoine, P. (2023). Exploring the processes of connection and disconnection in imagery work in a patient with depression and dependent personality disorder. *Journal of Clinical Psychology, 79,* 1641–1655. https://doi.org/10.1002/jclp.23464

Lee, R. J. (2017). Mistrustful and misunderstood: A review of paranoid personality disorder. *Current Behavioral Neuroscience Reports, 4,* 151–165. https://doi.org/10.1007/s40473-017-0116-7

Leiman, M., & Stiles, W. B. (2001). Dialogical sequence analysis and the zone of proximal development as conceptual enhancements to the assimilation model: The case of Jan revisited. *Psychotherapy Research, 11*(3), 311–330. https://psycnet.apa.org/doi/10.1093/ptr/11.3.311

Lewinsohn, P. M. (1974). A behavioral approach to depression. In R. J. Friedman & M. M. Katz (Eds.), *The psychology of depression: Contemporary theory and research* (pp. 157–185). Winston-Wiley.

Lind, M. (2021). ICD-11 Personality disorder: The indispensable turn to narrative identity. *Frontiers in Psychiatry, 12*, 642696. https://doi.org/10.3389/fpsyt.2021.642696

Lind, M., Adler, J. M., & Clark, L. A. (2020). Narrative identity and personality disorder: An empirical and conceptual review. *Current Psychiatry Reports, 22*, 1–11. https://doi.org/10.1007/s11920-020-01187-8

Linehan, M. (1993). *Cognitive-behavioral treatment of borderline personality disorder.* Guilford Press.

Links, P. S., Mercer, D., & Novick, J. (2015). Establishing a treatment framework and therapeutic alliance. In W. J. Livesley, G. Dimaggio, & J. F. Clarkin (Eds.), *Integrated treatment for personality disorders: A modular approach.* Guilford Press.

Liotti, G. (2006). A model of dissociation based on attachment theory and research. *Journal of Trauma & Dissociation, 7*(4), 55–73. https://doi.org/10.1300/J229v07n04_04

Liotti, G., & Gilbert, P. (2011). Mentalizing, motivation, and social mentalities: Theoretical considerations and implications for psychotherapy. *Psychology and Psychotherapy: Theory, Research and Practice, 84*, 9–25. https://doi.org/10.1348/147608310X520094

Luborsky, L., & Crits-Christoph, P. (1990). *Understanding transference: The core conflictual relationship theme method.* Basic Books.

Magistrale, G., Hasson-Ohayon, I., Lysaker, P. H., & Dimaggio, G. (2024). Is time ripe for introducing behavioral homework in relational psychoanalysis? *Journal of Clinical Psychology: In Session, 80*, 871–883 https://doi.org/10.1002/jclp.23600

Mahon, D. (2023). A scoping review of deliberate practice in the acquisition of therapeutic skills and practices. *Counselling and Psychotherapy Research, 23*(4), 965–981. https://doi.org/10.1002/capr.12601

Marconi, E., Monti, L., Fredda, G., Kotzalidis, G. D., Janiri, D., Zani, V., Vitaletti, D. Simone, M. V., Piciollo, S., Moriconi, F., Di Pietro, E., Popolo, R., Dimaggio, G., Veredice, C., Sani, G., & Chieffo, D. P. R. (2023). Outpatient care for adolescents and young adults (AYA) mental health: Promoting self- and others understanding through a Metacognitive Interpersonal Therapy-informed psychological intervention. *Frontiers in Psychiatry, 14*, 1221158. https://doi.org/10.3389/fpsyt.2023.1221158

Markowitz, J. C., Petkova, E., Neria, Y., Van Meter, P. E., Zhao, Y., Hembree, E., Lovell, K., Biyanova, T., & Marshall, R. D. (2015). Is exposure necessary? A randomized clinical trial of Interpersonal psychotherapy for PTSD. *American Journal of Psychiatry, 172*, 430–440. https://doi.org/10.1176/appi.ajp.2014.14070908

Martell, C. R., Dimidjian, S., & Herman-Dunn, R. (2022). *Behavioral activation for depression. A clinician's guide.* Guilford Press.

Martinussen, M., Friborg, O., Schmierer, P., Kaiser, S., Øvergård, K. T., Neunhoeffer, A. L., Martinsen, E.W, & Rosenvinge, J. H. (2017). The comorbidity of personality disorders in eating disorders: A meta-analysis. *Eating and Weight Disorders, 22*, 201–209. https://doi.org/10.1007/s40519-016-0345-x

Matos, M., & Dimaggio, G. (2023). The interplay between therapeutic relationship and therapeutic technique: It takes two to tango. *Journal of Clinical Psychology, 79*, 1609–1614. https://doi.org/10.1002/jclp.23500

Matos, M., Petrocchi, N., Irons, C., & Steindl, S. R. (2023). Never underestimate fears, blocks, and resistances: The interplay between experiential practices, self-conscious emotions, and the therapeutic relationship in compassion focused therapy. *Journal of Clinical Psychology, 79*, 1670–1685. https://doi.org/10.1002/jclp.23474

McAdams, D. P. (1996). Personality, modernity, and the storied self: A contemporary framework for studying persons. *Psychological Inquiry, 7*(4), 295–321. https://doi.org/10.1207/s15327965pli0704_1

McCarthy, P. R., & Betz, N. E. (1978). Differential effects of self-disclosing versus self involving counselor statements. *Journal of Counseling Psychology, 25*, 251–256. https://psycnet.apa.org/doi/10.1037/0022-0167.25.4.251

Messman-Moore, T. L., & Coates, A. A. (2007). The impact of childhood psychological abuse on adult interpersonal conflict: The role of early maladaptive schemas and patterns of interpersonal behavior. *Journal of Emotional Abuse, 7*(2), 75–92. https://psycnet.apa.org/doi/10.1300/J135v07n02_05

Miller, W. R., & Rollnick, S. (2012). *Motivational interviewing: Helping people change.* Guilford Press.

Misso, D., Velotti, P., Pasetto, A., & Dimaggio, G. (2022). Treating intimate partner violence with metacognitive interpersonal therapy: The case of Aaron. *Journal of Clinical Psychology, 78*(1), 50–66. https://doi.org/10.1002/jclp.23294

Moos, R. H. (2002). Life stressors, social resources, and coping skills in youth: Applications to adolescents with chronic disorders. *Journal of Adolescent Health, 30*(4), 22–29. https://doi.org/10.1016/s1054-139x(02)00337-3

Morina, N., Lancee, J., & Arntz, A. (2017). Imagery rescripting as a clinical intervention for aversive memories: A meta-analysis. *Journal of Behavior Therapy and Experimental Psychiatry, 55*, 6–15. https://doi.org/10.1016/j.jbtep.2016.11.003

Muran, J. C., & Eubanks, C. F. (2020). *Therapist performance under pressure: Negotiating emotion, difference, and rupture.* American Psychological Association.

Nader, K., & Einarsson, E. Ö. (2010). Memory reconsolidation: An update. *Annals of the New York Academy of Sciences, 1191*, 27–41. https://doi.org/10.1111/j.1749-6632.2010.05443.x

Nolen-Hoeksema, S. (2000). The role of rumination in depressive disorders and mixed anxiety/depressive symptoms. *Journal of Abnormal Psychology, 109*, 504–511.

Nordahl, H., Vollset, T., & Hjemdal, O. (2022). An empirical test of the metacognitive model of generalized anxiety disorder. *Scandinavian Journal of Psychology, 64*(3), 263–267. https://doi.org/10.1111/sjop.12884

Ogden, P., & Fisher, J. (2015). *Sensorimotor psychotherapy: Interventions for trauma and attachment.* Norton.

Ogden, P., Pain, C., & Fisher, J. (2006). A sensorimotor approach to the treatment of trauma and dissociation. *Psychiatric Clinics of North America, 29*(1), 263–279. https://doi.org/10.1016/j.psc.2005.10.012

Osoro, A., Villalobos, D., & Tamayo, J. A. (2021). Efficacy of emotion-focused therapy in the treatment of eating disorders: A systematic review. *Clinical Psychology & Psychotherapy, 29*, 815–836. https://doi.org/10.1002/cpp.2690

Ottavi, P., Passarella, T., Pasinetti, M., MacBeth, A., Velotti, P., Buonocore, L., Popolo, R., Salvatore, G., Velotti, A., & Dimaggio, G. (2019). Metacognitive interpersonal mindfulness-based training for worry about interpersonal events: A pilot feasibility and acceptability study. *Journal of Nervous and Mental Disease, 207*, 944–950. https://doi.org/10.1097/nmd.0000000000001054

Ozier, A. D., & Henry, B. W. (2011). American Dietetic Association. Position of the American Dietetic Association: Nutrition intervention in the treatment of eating disorders. *Journal of the American Dietetic Association, 111*, 1236–1241. https://doi.org/10.1016/j.jada.2011.06.016.

Paivio, S. C., Jarry, J. L., Chagigiorgis, H., Hall, I., & Ralston, M. (2010). Efficacy of two versions of emotion-focused therapy for resolving child abuse trauma. *Psychotherapy Research, 20*(3), 353–366. https://psycnet.apa.org/doi/10.1080/10503300903505274

Pascual-Leone, A., & Yeryomenko, N. (2017). The client experiencing scale as a predictor of treatment outcomes: A meta-analysis on psychotherapy process. *Psychotherapy Research, 27*(6), 653–665. https://doi.org/10.1080/10503307.2016.1152409

Pasetto, A., Misso, D., Velotti, P., & Dimaggio, G. (2021). Metacognitive interpersonal therapy for intimate partner violence: A single case study. *Partner Abuse, 12*, 64–79. https://psycnet.apa.org/doi/10.1891/PA-2020-0016

Pasetto, A., Misso, D., Velotti, P., & Dimaggio, G. (2024). Metacognitive interpersonal therapy for domestic offenders with personality disorders: A case series. *Submitted for Publication.*

Pincus, A. L., Cain, N. M., & Halberstadt, A. L. (2020). Importance of self and other in defining personality pathology. *Psychopathology*, *53*(3–4), 133–140. https://doi.org/10.1159/000506313

Popolo, R., MacBeth, A., Brunello, S., Canfora, F., Ozdemir, E., Rebecchi, D., Toselli, C., Venturelli, G., Salvatore, G., & Dimaggio, G. (2018). Metacognitive Interpersonal Therapy in Group (MIT-G): A pilot noncontrolled effectiveness study. *Research in Psychotherapy: Psychopathology, Process and Outcome*, *21*, 155–163. https://doi.org/10.4081/ripppo.2018.338

Popolo, R., MacBeth, A., Canfora, F., Rebecchi, D., Toselli, C., Salvatore, G., & Dimaggio, G. (2019). Metacognitive interpersonal therapy in group (MIT-G) for young adults personality disorders. A pilot randomized controlled trial. *Psychology and Psychotherapy: Theory, Research & Practice*, *92*, 342–358. https://doi.org/10.1111/papt.12182

Popolo, R., MacBeth, A., Lazzerini, L., Brunello, S., Venturelli, G., Rebecchi, D., Morales, M. F., & Dimaggio, G. (2022). Metacognitive interpersonal therapy in group versus TAU + waiting list for young adults with personality disorders: Randomized clinical trial. *Personality Disorders: Theory, Research, and Treatment*, *13*(6), 619–628. https://doi.org/10.1037/per0000497

Pugh, M., Dixon, A., & Bell, T. (2023). Chairwork and the therapeutic relationship: Can the cart join the horse? *Journal of Clinical Psychology*, *79*, 1615–1626. https://doi.org/10.1002/jclp.23473

Radcliffe, J., & Yeomans, F. (2019). Transference-focused psychotherapy for patients with personality disorders: Overview and case example with a focus on the use of contracting. *British Journal of Psychotherapy*, *35*(1), 4–23. https://psycnet.apa.org/doi/10.1111/bjp.12421

Rafaeli, E., Maurer, O., & Thoma, N. C. (2014). Working with modes in schema therapy. In N. C. Thoma & D. McKay (Eds.), *Working with emotion in cognitive-behavioral therapy: Techniques for clinical practice* (pp. 263–287). Guilford Press.

Rizzo, A. A., Reger, G. M., Gahm, G. A., Difede, J., & Rothbaum, B. O. (2009). Virtual reality exposure therapy for combat related PTSD. In P. Shiromani, T. Keane, & J. LeDoux (Eds.), *Post-traumatic stress disorder: Basic science and clinical practice* (pp. 375–399). Humana.

Romano, M., Moscovitch, D. A., Huppert, J. D., Reimer, S. G., & Moscovitch, M. (2020). The effects of imagery rescripting on memory outcomes in social anxiety disorder. *Journal of Anxiety Disorders*, *69*, 102–169. https://doi.org/10.1016/j.janxdis.2019.102169

Rossi, R., Corbo, D., Magni, L. R., Pievani, M., Nicolò, G., Semerari, A., Carcione, A., & CLIMAMITHE Study Group (2023). Metacognitive interpersonal therapy in borderline personality disorder: Clinical and neuroimaging outcomes from the CLIMAMITHE study – A randomized clinical trial. *Personality Disorders: Theory, Research, and Treatment*, *14*(4), 452–466. https://doi.org/10.1037/per0000621

Rousmaniere, T. (2019). *Mastering the Inner skills of psychotherapy: A deliberate practice manual*. Gold Lantern Books.

Rousmaniere, T., Goodyear, R. K., Miller, S. D., & Wampold, B. E. (Eds.). (2017). *The cycle of excellence: Using deliberate practice to improve supervision and training*. Wiley Blackwell

Ryle, A., & Kerr, I. B. (2002). *Introducing to cognitive analytic therapy: Principles and practice*. Wiley.

Sacks, D., & Vaz, A. (2023). The use of deliberate practice in cognitive behavioral therapy supervision: From declarative to procedural knowledge. In M. D. Terjesen & T. Del Vecchio (Eds.), *Handbook of training and supervision in cognitive behavioral therapy*. Springer.

Safran, J. D., & Muran, J. C. (2000). Negotiating the therapeutic alliance: A relational treatment guide. Guilford Press.

Safran, J. D., & Segal, Z. V. (1990). *Interpersonal process in cognitive therapy*. Jason Aronson.

Sagui-Henson, S. J. (2017). Cognitive avoidance. In V. Zeigler-Hill & T. Shackelford (Eds.), *Encyclopedia of personality and individual differences*. Springer.

Schmeck, K., Weise, S., Schlüter-Müller, S., Birkhölzer, M., Fürer, L., Koenig, J., Krause, M., Lerch, S., Schenk, N., Valdes, N., Zimmermann, R., & Kaess, M. (2023). Effectiveness of adolescent identity treatment (AIT) versus DBT-a for the treatment of adolescent borderline personality disorder. *Personality Disorders: Theory, Research, and Treatment, 14*(2), 148–160. https://doi.org/10.1037/per0000572

Seitz, K. I., Leitenstorfer, J., Krauch, M., Hillmann, K., Boll, S., Ueltzhoeffer, K., & Bertsch, K. (2021). An eye-tracking study of interpersonal threat sensitivity and adverse childhood experiences in borderline personality disorder. *Borderline Personality Disorder and Emotion Dysregulation, 8*(1), 1–12. https://doi.org/10.1186/s40479-020-00141-7

Semerari, A., Carcione, A., Dimaggio, G., Falcone, M., Nicolò, G., Procacci, M., & Alleva, G. (2003). How to evaluate metacognitive functioning in psychotherapy? The Metacognition Assessment Scale and its applications. *Clinical Psychology and Psychotherapy, 10*, 238–261. https://doi.org/10.1002/cpp.362

Sibrava, N. J., & Borkovec, T. D. (2006). The cognitive avoidance theory of worry. In G. C. L. Davey & A. Wells (Eds.), *Worry and its psychological disorders: Theory, assessment and treatment* (pp. 239–256). Wiley.

Simonsen, S., Popolo, R., Juul, S., Frandsen, F. W., & Dimaggio, G. (2022). Treating avoidant personality disorder with combined individual metacognitive interpersonal therapy and group mentalization based treatment: A pilot study. *Journal of Nervous and Mental Disease, 210*, 163–171. https://doi.org/10.1097/nmd.0000000000001432

Singer, J. A. (2013). Lost in translation? Finding the person in the emerging paradigm of clinical science: Introduction to a special issue on personality psychology and psychotherapy. *Journal of Personality, 81*(6), 511–514. https://psycnet.apa.org/doi/10.1111/jopy.12017

Skinner, E. A., Edge, K., Altman, J., & Sherwood, H. (2003). Searching for the structure of coping: A review and critique of category systems for classifying ways of coping. *Psychological Bulletin, 129*, 216–269. https://doi.org/10.1037/0033-2909.129.2.216

Solms, M. (2021). *The hidden spring: A journey to the source of consciousness*. Profile Books.

Steindl, S. R., Matos, M., & Dimaggio, G. (2023). The interplay between therapeutic relationship and therapeutic technique: The whole is more than the sum of its parts. *Journal of Clinical Psychology, 79*, 1686–1692. https://doi.org/10.1002/jclp.23519

Stiegler, J. R., Molde, H., & Schanche, E. (2018). Does an emotion-focused two-chair dialogue add to the therapeutic effect of the empathic attunement to affect? *Clinical Psychology and Psychotherapy, 25*, 86–95. https://doi.org/10.1002/cpp.2144

Sukhodolsky, D. G., & Golub, A., & Cromwell, E. N. (2001). Development and validation of the anger rumination scale. *Personality and Individual Differences, 31*(5), 689–700. https://psycnet.apa.org/doi/10.1016/S0191-8869(00)00171-9

Trevarthen, C. (1979). Communication and cooperation in early infancy: A description of primary intersubjectivity. *Before Speech: The Beginning of Interpersonal Communication, 1*, 530–571.

Trevarthen, C. (1987). Sharing makes sense: Intersubjectivity and the making of an infant's meaning. In R. Steele & T. Threadgold (Eds.). *Language topics: Essays in honour of Michael Halliday* (pp. 177–199). John Benjamins.

Tripp, J. C., Haller, M., Trim, R. S., Straus, E., Bryan, C. J., Davis, B. C., Lyons, R., Hamblen, J. L., & Norman, S. B. (2020). Does exposure exacerbate symptoms in veterans with PTSD and alcohol use disorder? *Psychological Trauma: Theory, Research, Practice, and Policy, 3*(8), 920–928. https://doi.org/10.1037/tra0000634

Van Vliet, N., Huntjens, R., Van Dijk, M., Bachrach, N., Meewisse, M., & De Jongh, A. (2021). Phase-based treatment versus immediate trauma-focused treatment for post-traumatic stress disorder due to childhood abuse: Randomised clinical trial. *BJPsych Open, 7*(6), 211. https://doi.org/10.1192/bjo.2021.1057

von Below, C. (2020). We just did not get on: Young adults' experiences of unsuccessful psychodynamic psychotherapy – A lack of meta-communication and mentalization? *Frontiers in Psychology*, *11*, 1243. https://doi.org/10.3389/fpsyg.2020.01243

von Koch, L., Kathmann, N., & Reuter, B. (2023). Lack of speeded disengagement from facial expressions of disgust in remitted major depressive disorder: Evidence from an eye-movement study. *Behaviour Research and Therapy*, *160*, 104231. https://doi.org/10.1016/j.brat.2022.104231

Wahl, K., Ehring, T., Kley, H., Lieb, R., Meyer, A., Kordon, A., & Schönfeld, S. (2019). Is repetitive negative thinking a transdiagnostic process? A comparison of key processes of RNT in depression, generalized anxiety disorder, obsessive-compulsive disorder, and community controls. *Journal of Behavior Therapy and Experimental Psychiatry*, *64*, 45–53. https://doi.org/10.1016/j.jbtep.2019.02.006

Wakelin, K. E., Perman, G., & Simonds, L. M. (2022). Effectiveness of self-compassion-related interventions for reducing self-criticism: A systematic review and meta-analysis. *Clinical Psychology and Psychotherapy*, 1–25. https://doi.org/10.1002/cpp.2586

Waller, G., & Mountford, V. A. (2015). Weighing patients within cognitive-behavioural therapy for eating disorders: How, when and why. *Behaviour Research and Therapy*, *70*, 1–10. https://doi.org/10.1016/j.brat.2015.04.004

Watson, J. C., Gordon, L. B., Stermac, L., Kalogerakos, F., & Steckley, P. (2003). Comparing the effectiveness of process-experiential with cognitive-behavioral psychotherapy in the treatment of depression. *Journal of Consulting and Clinical Psychology*, *71*(4), 773–781. https://doi.org/10.1037/0022-006x.71.4.773

Wegner, D. M., & Erber, R. (1992). The hyperaccessibility of suppressed thoughts. *Journal of Personality and Social Psychology*, *63*, 903–912. https://psycnet.apa.org/doi/10.1037/0022-3514.63.6.903

Weiss, J. (1993). *How psychotherapy works: Process and technique*. Guilford Press.

Wells, A. (2008). *Metacognitive therapy for anxiety and depression*. Guilford Press.

Wells, A. (2009). *Metacognitive therapy for anxiety and depression*. Guilford Press.

Westen, D., Novotny, C. M., & Thompson-Brenner, H. (2004). The empirical status of empirically supported psychotherapies: Assumptions, findings, and reporting in controlled clinical trials. *Psychological Bulletin*, *130*(4), 631–663. https://doi.org/10.1037/0033-2909.130.4.631

Wilberg, T., Pedersen, G., Bremer, K., Johansen, M. S., & Kvarstein, E. H. (2023). Combined group and individual therapy for patients with avoidant personality disorder – A pilot study. *Frontiers in Psychiatry*, *14*, 118–168. https://doi.org/10.3389/fpsyt.2023.1181686

Wiltshire, T. J., Philipsen, J. S., Trasmundi, S. B., Jensen, T. W., & Steffensen, S. V. (2020). Interpersonal coordination dynamics in psychotherapy: A systematic review. *Cognitive Therapy and Research*, *44*, 752–773. https://psycnet.apa.org/doi/10.1007/s10608-020-10106-3

Wolpe, J. (1973). *The practice of behavior therapy* (2nd ed.). Pergamon.

Wright, A. G., Ringwald, W. R., Hopwood, C. J., & Pincus, A. L. (2022). It's time to replace the personality disorders with the interpersonal disorders. *American Psychologist*, *77*, 1085. https://psycnet.apa.org/doi/10.1037/amp0001087

Young, J. E., Klosko, J. S., & Weishaar, M. E. (2003). *Schema therapy: A practitioner's guide*. Guilford Press.

Zhou, Y., & Wade, T. D. (2021). Face-to-face imagery rescripting as a treatment adjunct for day patients with an eating disorder: A randomised controlled pilot study. *Journal of Behavioral and Cognitive Therapy*, *31*(1), 37–45. http://dx.doi.org/10.1016/j.jbct.2020.11.005

Zimmer-Gembeck, M. J., & Skinner, E. A. (2016). The development of coping: Implications for psychopathology and resilience (pp. 485–545). In D. Cicchetti (Ed.), *Developmental psychology: Risk, resilience, and intervention*. Wiley.

Index

For Product Safety Concerns and Information please contact our EU
representative GPSR@taylorandfrancis.com
Taylor & Francis Verlag GmbH, Kaufingerstraße 24, 80331 München, Germany

www.ingramcontent.com/pod-product-compliance
Lightning Source LLC
Chambersburg PA
CBHW071846270326
41929CB00013B/2115